Ann M. Voda, RN, PhD

Menopause, Me and You
The Sound of Women Pausing

Pre-publication
REVIEWS,
COMMENTARIES,
EVALUATIONS . . .

"**D**r. Voda's material is fascinating, combining a thorough scientific explanation of the female reproductive system with the voices of many women telling their experiences as they pass through menopause. In this unique book we hear the voice of a wise woman and experienced clinician and researcher.

Voda treats menopause as a natural event in women's lives, not an estrogen deficiency disease. She presents a thorough discussion of hormones and their effects on the entire body, including the cellular mechanisms through which they act. Her book is full of important suggestions for self-care, including a unique section on personal record keeping for women of all ages. Essential reading for the inquiring mind!"

Sadja Greenwood, MD
Author of Menopause Naturally;
Assistant Clinical Professor,
Department of Obstetrics
and Gynecology,
University of California,
San Francisco

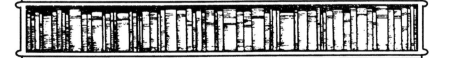

"**A**t last! A book that gives women the facts necessary to make an informed decision about whether to take hormone replacement therapy. Although women are routinely told 'it is up to them' to decide whether to take hormones, they are never informed about the facts necessary to choose wisely. Ann Voda's comprehensive book on menopause offers women the results of important medical research, written in a way that we can all understand. This book is a must for every woman eager to shed the myths about menopause and learn what medical research shows us about the best way to handle this significant period of life."

Myra Dinnerstein, PhD
Research Professor, Women's Studies
University of Arizona

"**T**his is a book with a feminist perspective, discussing the pros and cons of the management of menopause from a social, psychological, and physiological construct, not under the table or with only one voice. Ann takes herself as an example, tackling the menopause issue more humanistically and full of caring. Ann also demonstrates what 'women study' is and demonstrates that there is no value-free scientific research but rather a collection of way-of-life experiences involved in such study. She takes the research method both from qualitative and quantitative ways of exploration and tries to create new theories in menstruation, including the phenomenon of menopause. In her book, Ann provides many tools to help women and researchers communicate with their own bodies and understand the physiological and psychological changes in their bodies, which not only empower women but also provide a way to love their bodies, to learn the body messages. I read this book with great appreciation. Although the experiences are based on white, middle-class women of America, the confusions, the dilemma, and the needs of women facing menopause are all the same. Currently in Taiwan and Asia as a whole, physicians take the western concepts, strongly medicalize menopause, and even prescribe hormones without a second thought. This book will serve as a reference book for medical professionals; a conscious awareness guideline for women's health movement activists; a self-help book for middle-aged women; an introduction textbook for those students who are taking a 'women's study of health' course; and a handbook for those researchers who really care about women's menstruation health."

Chueh Chang, MPH, ScD
Associate Professor,
College of Public Health,
National Taiwan University;
Coordinator,
Women's Research Program,
Population Studies Center, NTU

More pre-publication
REVIEWS, COMMENTARIES, EVALUATIONS . . .

"This is a most comprehensive book on menopause. It is research-based and is written with the idea of empowerment of women. Menstrual events are presented as normal, with patterns of variability both within and between women.

Included are descriptions of Voda's own menstrual and menopausal experiences, also direct quotes from the many women who have been participants in her research. These include her work on the hot flash as well as her work as director of the Tremin Trust, following up the important longitudinal studies begun by Dr. Alan Treolar over sixty years ago.

Throughout, there is a strong focus on women as intelligent decision makers and monitors of their own bodies. Readers are given concrete tools for monitoring, such as temperature charts, monthly calendars, and scales for reporting bleeding patterns. I particularly appreciated the sections of the book labeled 'Ann's Advice,' which help women readers relate the more complex text to themselves and their own decisions.

This is not a self-care book, as Voda continues to refer women to their own providers. But she recommends that women seek providers who relate to them as informed persons, aware of their own bodies and participants in decision making.

This book is recommended for considered reading by these pro-fessional providers, as well as for the women in their care."

Effie I. Graham, PhD
Former Professor, College of Nursing,
University of Alaska, Anchorage;
A founder of the Society
for Menstrual Cycle Research

"*Menopause, Me and You: The Sound of Women Pausing,* by Ann M. Voda, is the book I and many women have been waiting for. For the past ten years I have conducted research, written, and lectured on the subject of menopause. I am always looking for better information, and this book definitely fills a void. Ann's solid academic background and professional experience make this book valuable for the lay reader who wants a clear understanding of the medical aspects of menopause. But the real strength of the book is the way Ann has used the voices of women, their questions, their concerns, and their ways of dealing with this time in their lives, to enlighten and inform. In the last section of the book, she encourages all women to become active in their own care by providing ways of gathering information about their own experiences. This is a resource every woman will want in her library."

Judy Mahle Lutter, MA
President, Melpomene Institute
St. Paul, MN

"This book provides something for women in all phases of life. Through a provocative combination of science, personal reflection, and the voices of many women, Ann Voda walks any woman through her menstrual life—from onset through menopause. The voices of real women, who have been part of a fifty-year study of their menstrual history, reflect the unique and diverse experiences of each through these transitions. I appreciated that a scholar was willing to actually give advice, not just the facts!

There is something for every woman in this book. Ann Voda finally gives women factual and personal knowledge about the role of hormones in our life phases. There is substantial information on how the body prepares and adapts to menopause so that any woman can find her own story within the pages and thus make decisions based on many pieces of the puzzle, not just the pharmaceutical pressures to replace hormones.

How sad that women entering menopause will read this book only to finally learn about the previous thirty years of their menstrual history. This book is not just about the last forty years of a woman's life, but also about the first forty. It should be required reading for all those clinicians, practitioners, and therapists who serve women.

Before any woman pops that first estrogen/progesterone pill or sticks on that first estrogen/progesterone patch, she should read Ann Voda's book about what this may mean. Voda's book finally explains the mystery of hormone replacement in terms of a woman's total menstrual history."

Patty Reagan, PhD, MPH
Associate Professor,
Health Education/Women's Studies,
University of Utah,
Salt Lake City, Utah

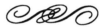

"*Menopause, Me and You* is a treasure trove of information. It is about scientific inquiry, about how women *do* science, *relate* to science, are *described by* science, and are currently *refining* what science says about the biology of women, and menopause in particular. It is theoretical *and* practical. Knowledge is power, and Ann Voda's book is a ready reference that will be consulted over and over again by readers who are eager to learn more about themselves and to reconcile their own experiences with what the experts say, as they try to make the best health care decisions they can during midlife and beyond."

Margaret L. Stubbs, PhD
Instructor, Department of Psychology,
Chatham College, Pittsburgh, PA;
Board Member, Society for
Menstrual Cycle Research

More pre-publication
REVIEWS, COMMENTARIES, EVALUATIONS . . .

"This is a most remarkable book, a personal memoir woven into a scholarly work providing the reader with considerable information about women's health, especially the menstrual cycle and menopause. The author has chosen to use not only her own voice, but the voices of women going through this life transition in our culture. It makes compelling reading, which is not frequent in books that provide us with medical data. Dr. Ann Voda is a distinguished scientist and nurse researcher who has chosen to summarize much of her years of work as director of the Tremin Trust Research Program on Women's Health, and combine it with current thinking and advice for women. This book differs from most of the writing in this field, where one reads either an entire book of personal views *or* a medical book. I would recommend it to health care providers as well as women and men who want more and accurate descriptions of menopause and women's reproductive health in general. It is a fine contribution to preventive health care of women."

Miriam B. Rosenthal, MD
*Associate Professor of Psychiatry
and Reproductive Biology,
Case Western Reserve University;
Chief of Behavioral Medicine,
Department of Obstetrics/Gynecology,
University MacDonald Women's
Hospital*

"Dr. Ann Voda's book honors the American woman's intelligence. She presents the physiological menstrual-life cycle in an understandable way, allowing the reader to make informed decisions on self-care.

Dr. Voda has been rallying the cry for information about menopause and menstruation for the past two decades. In an objective manner, she presents current research on menopause and outlines the strengths and limitations of the study to allow the reader to decide on the merits of the research being conducted today.

Voda's careful review of the history of hormone treatment over the past thirty years makes one wonder if science is listening to women's voices and concerns about menopause. Dr. Voda presents a thought-provoking review of the risks and benefits of hormone replacement therapy. Her chapter on selecting a health care provider gives support to a woman's ability to control and modify her own health care.

Dr. Voda has been a pioneer in women's health, and this book aptly demonstrates her conviction of informing women about their bodies. This book is thought provoking, stimulating, and is an affirmation of a woman's right to know."

Agatha A. Quinn, RN, PhD
*Assistant Professor,
University of Colorado
Health Sciences Center,
School of Nursing*

Menopause, Me and You

HAWORTH Innovations in Feminist Studies
Esther Rothblum, PhD and Ellen Cole, PhD
Senior Co-Editors

New, Recent, and Forthcoming Titles:

When Husbands Come Out of the Closet by Jean Schaar Gochros

Prisoners of Ritual: An Odyssey into Female Genital Circumcision in Africa by Hanny Lightfoot-Klein

Foundations for a Feminist Restructuring of the Academic Disciplines edited by Michele Paludi and Gertrude A. Steuernagel

Hippocrates' Handmaidens: Women Married to Physicians by Esther Nitzberg

Waiting: A Diary of Loss and Hope in Pregnancy by Ellen Judith Reich

God's Country: A Case Against Theocracy by Sandy Rapp

Women and Aging: Celebrating Ourselves by Ruth Raymond Thone

Women's Conflicts About Eating and Sexuality: The Relationship Between Food and Sex by Rosalyn M. Meadow and Lillie Weiss

A Woman's Odyssey into Africa: Tracks Across a Life by Hanny Lightfoot-Klein

Anorexia Nervosa and Recovery: A Hunger for Meaning by Karen Way

Women Murdered by the Men They Loved by Constance A. Bean

Reproductive Hazards in the Workplace: Mending Jobs, Managing Pregnancies by Regina Kenen

Our Choices: Women's Personal Decisions About Abortion by Sumi Hoshiko

Tending Inner Gardens: The Healing Art of Feminist Psychotherapy by Lesley Irene Shore

The Way of the Woman Writer by Janet Lynn Roseman

Racism in the Lives of Women: Testimony, Theory, and Guides to Anti-Racist Practice by Jeanne Adleman and Gloria Enguídanos

Advocating for Self: Women's Decisions Concerning Contraception by Peggy Matteson

Feminist Visions of Gender Similarities and Differences by Meredith M. Kimball

Experiencing Abortion: A Weaving of Women's Words by Eve Kushner

Menopause, Me and You: The Sound of Women Pausing by Ann M. Voda

Menopause, Me and You
The Sound of Women Pausing

Ann M. Voda, RN, PhD

Harrington Park Press
An Imprint of The Haworth Press, Inc.
New York • London

Published by

Harrington Park Press, an imprint of The Haworth Press, Inc., 10 Alice Street, Binghamton, NY 13904-1580.

Cover design by Becky J. Salsgiver.

Library of Congress Cataloging-in-Publication Data

Voda, Ann M. (Ann Mae), 1930-
  Menopause, me and you : the sound of women pausing / Ann M. Voda.
    p.   cm.
  Includes bibliographical references and index.
  ISBN 1-56023-911-5 (alk. paper)
  1. Menopause. I. Title.
RG186.V63   1997
618.1'75–dc21

96-52108
CIP

To the women of The Tremin Trust Research Program,
who have taught me so much.

To all my colleagues who work so very hard every day
to *demythify* and *demystify* the menstrual cycle and menopause.

And to C.A. — thanks for all your support and love.

ABOUT THE AUTHOR

Ann M. Voda, RN, PhD, is Professor of Adult Physiological Nursing and Director of The Tremin Trust Research Program on Women's Health at the University of Utah. The author of many articles and book chapters, Dr. Voda has researched and published extensively on topics such as the physiology and endocrinology of menopause, hormone use among middle-aged women, body composition changes in menopausal women, and sexual response changes in heterosexual mid-life women. The immediate past President of the North American Menopause Society and the former President of the Society for Menstrual Cycle Research, she continues to serve on the Board of Directors for both societies. She is the Chair of the North American Menopause Society Education Committee and is a member of the Editorial Advisory Boards of *Menopause Management* and *Menopause*. Dr. Voda is currently co-investigator on a study of mid-life women and has been supported by research grants from the National Institutes of Health. She frequently participates in research symposia, conferences, lectures, and demonstrations to present her work and expertise on the subject of menopause.

CONTENTS

Figures

Chapter 20

Chapter 21

Chapter 22

Tables

Preface

Within the pages of *Menopause, Me and You,* I have included the voices of many women, in various stages of menopause, who describe what they are feeling as well as what it means to be a midlife woman at the closure of reproductive life. This is not a book that presents menopausal women as sick, hysterical, or out of control, and it definitely is not a book devoted to clinical treatment, i.e., "how-to-treat" menopausal women. Instead, it is a book that describes the experiences of women who, with much ambivalence and some anxiety, both celebrate the end of menstruation and curse the changes they experience. In this book I have included several self-monitoring tools that I have found useful for observing and naming the changes that occur during the transition to menopause. The tools are designed to help women discover knowledge about themselves and to maximize the potential of the information they gather to understand the dynamics of the change process.

Like Gloria Steinem, who wrote personally to readers in *Revolutions from Within,* I, too, have written in a personal way as I describe my own professional and personal journey into women's health, the experiences I have had, and the research I have done. I am hopeful that my stories, the stories of Alan Treloar, and those of the women of The Tremin Trust who were in various stages of menopause, will strike a familiar chord with readers. I am convinced that as healthy women, we are the experts on menopause. If we just listen to each other, we will understand more about the experience from the perspective of women. In that way, we will come to understand menopause for what it really is: a normal growth and developmental event, not a disease to be treated. Until recently, the experts on menopause, albeit self-proclaimed, have been researchers who studied the effects of steroid hormones on tissues and organs, and clinicians who prescribed these hormones. My good colleague, Dr. Patricia Kaufert, at the third meeting of the

North American Menopause Society in 1992, asked conferees: "Who are the experts on menopause?" Kaufert argued that the women who experience the event are the real experts. She recommended that research first and foremost be grounded more holistically in the experience of women.

The experiences of the women included in this book are those of white, educated, mostly middle-class women. Consequently, some book content falls prey to a criticism leveled by Kaufert—that we have few descriptions of the menopause experience from the perspective of women in non-Westernized nations. A lack of cross-cultural research has supported a belief that the menopause experience of white women is a universal phenomenon. I make no such claim. Cross-cultural research conducted by Beyene, Lock, duToit, Davis, Wright, Flint, and others informs us that both the meaning and the experience of menopause are different for women in other cultures and races. I am grateful to these researchers for the pioneering work they have done.

I am most grateful to the thousands of women in The Tremin Trust Research Program on Women's Health, who willingly agreed to record menstrual histories, be interviewed, and fill out surveys over the course of many years. The data provided by these women suggest that even though they view menopause as a normal event, they are confused and made anxious by the rhetoric espoused in popular magazines, TV, radio, and newspapers that implicitly proclaims menopause as a medical condition that needs to be treated. I thank these women for their insights and their wisdom. They have taught me much! It is their need for anonymity, not lack of respect or space, that prohibits listing their names.

Ann M. Voda

Acknowledgments

This book had its beginnings years ago in a handbook created for workshops and conferences. It has been in the process of expansion and revision for more than five years. Special help and encouragement was provided by the following wonderful, talented, and computer-literate individuals: Sue Meeks, who has always been there for me; Lyn Pearse, who never complained when corrections and revisions seemed endless; Dori Fortune, who not only provided encouragement, but words of wisdom, as well as invaluable editing and typing; and finally, an angel named Miriam Romero, who provided support and invaluable technical computer wizardry—avoiding virus infestations and dealing calmly with crashes during the final stages of manuscript preparation.

I would also like to thank the following people for taking the time to do prepublication reviews of this book: Chueh Chang, PhD; Myra Dinnerstein, PhD; Effie I. Graham, PhD; Sadja Greenwood, MD; Judy Mahle Lutter; Agatha A. Quinn, RN, PhD; Patty Reagan, PhD; Miriam B. Rosenthal, MD; and Margaret Stubbs, PhD.

Introduction and Purpose

This is not your usual book on menopause. It has two purposes. The first is to present information on menopause, the changes women can expect to experience as they make the transition to and beyond menopause, risks associated with menopausal treatments, and sound advice based on facts and common sense. To fully understand what is happening at menopause requires an understanding of the hormonal and biochemical events associated with fertilization, conception, puberty, menarche, and the dynamic nature of the ensuing 30-plus years of the menstrual cycle. When these events are understood, menopausal changes such as atrophic vaginitis, urinary incontinence, hot flashes, mood swings, changes in menstrual bleeding pattern, changes in body weight and body composition, sexuality changes, heart disease, breast cancer, and osteoporosis are also understood.

A second purpose of the book is to provide women with several tools they can use to monitor themselves, in other words, tools to collect data on perimenopausal changes. These data-gathering methods are included because I have found through research and personal experience that keeping records is a way of staying in touch with one's self and one's body, a way of discovering knowledge about one's self. This is the kind of information that only women can provide about themselves. When it is considered, along with a care provider's assessment, a woman will have all the data needed to make an informed decision about health care.

Menopause, by definition, is that time in a woman's life when she experiences the last menstrual bleed. On October 7, 1981, I experienced my last bleed. I have been postmenopausal 15 years. For 12 of these 15 years, I have directed The Tremin Trust Research Program on Women's Health, a program begun in the 1930s at the University of Minnesota. For more than 20 years, I have been researching women's health issues related to menstruation and menopause. Since 1978, my research focus has been on menopause. I have conducted research on premenstrual tension, hormone fluctuations during the menstrual cycle, menopausal hot flash and mid-life body composition changes, bleeding changes, attitudes toward menopause, and common menopausal changes.

Now, in collaboration with Dr. Phyllis K. Mansfield of Pennsylvania State University, I continue to study common changes associated with menopause, resources women utilize to obtain information on menopause, sexuality changes at menopause, and how the bleeding pattern changes from premenopause to perimenopause.

All of this research experience, however, does not make me or any other menopause researcher *the* expert on menopause. The real experts, in my opinion, are the women who have experienced/are experiencing menopause. For example, the thousands of participants in The Tremin Trust Research Program (some of whom, since 1935, have unselfishly volunteered their time to complete research records, even donating money to support the research on women's health) are the real menopause experts. Only a very small portion of these women's voices, compiled over decades, are included in this book, expressed in the women's own words. Interestingly, the themes and concerns of contemporary women's voices resonate some of the same concerns that women had almost 60 years ago, e.g., if I had painful, miserable menstrual cycles, will my menopause be miserable, too? How long does a hot flash last? What causes it? Is heavy bleeding normal? Why am I so moody at this time?

Also included in the book are the voices of authors of both past and recent books, and lay or scientific articles, who, for better or worse, have shared with the world their understandings and misunderstandings of menstruation and menopause. Their influence and information is felt, considered, and evaluated throughout the book as it relates to understanding menopause. Unfortunately, many gaps in information still exist about the effects of estrogen on body systems and specific organs. As one article is published claiming that estrogen hormone is safe as related to breast cancer, close upon its heels is another article refuting the safety of hormones. One case in point involves two recently published articles (July 1995). One article in the *New England Journal of Medicine* concluded that hormone replacement therapy increases the risk of breast cancer in women, whereas the other article, in *The Journal of the American Medical Association*, refuted this conclusion. These kinds of contradictory statements will continue to emanate from sources we have learned to trust. So, what is a woman to do? Who is she to believe? Rather than doing a comprehensive review of the hormone/breast cancer literature, I will attempt to present information concerning the topics under discussion in as balanced an approach as possible, albeit realizing that I am only human and that I view the world through a woman-centered feminist lens. For this I make no apology. For far too long society has been denied the perspective of women about uniquely female experiences. Throughout history, scientific and philosophical thought as well as the creation of knowledge have primarily been the domain of male scientists. Consequently, the world has been denied women's perspective. This is especially true in the area of women's menstrual and reproductive processes.

WHY AM I WRITING THIS BOOK?

Over the past ten years, literally hundreds of menstrual and menopause books have been published–some based on traditional scientific research, others a result of consumer activism or journalistic hucksterism. Recently, the North American Menopause Society compiled a list of suggested readings for consumers on menopause/women's health, which included 42 titles. A market for these books, and more books to come, will endure if for no other reason than hundreds of thousands of women enter the menopause transition each year. When that first hot flash is experienced, or when the menstrual bleeding pattern changes, the search for information begins. This great interest in menopause is not because it is something new to women. Contrary to sociobiological and evolutionary theories (of which the latter claims that menopause is maladaptive–that women were never intended to live beyond reproductive years), women have lived past menopause for aeons, surviving into old age. According to anthropologist Margaret Lock (1993), a menopausal researcher, Homo sapiens have a life expectancy of 90 to 100 years. Whether or not one achieves the maximal longevity depends upon infant mortality; in other words, if an individual lives through infancy, there is a good chance of reaching old age. In all developed countries except for South Africa, infant mortality is less than 20 per 1,000 births, whereas in the least developed countries the mortality rate is estimated at 100 per 1,000 births, or higher (Diczfalusy, 1993).

By the end of the 1990s, based on projections from the United States Census Bureau, more than 50 million women will be over 50 years of age, and, most likely, postmenopausal. It is hoped that most of these women will experience menopause naturally, not artificially or precipitously. Current estimates indicate that the hysterectomy rate in the United States has decreased from around 650,000, to 550,000 a year (Graves, 1989). Still, this is a large number of U.S. women to have surgical removal of the uterus. These women, by definition, should be classified as menopausal; they will bleed no more. They do continue to cycle hormones if they have not had their ovaries surgically removed. Hysterectomy for women younger than age 50, who at the time of surgery were still experiencing menstrual bleeds, is problematic. These women now have no outward indicator, e.g., the natural stopping of menstrual bleeding, to know with certainty when they experience menopause, since cessation of menstruation was brought about through unnatural means: surgery. These women want information on how they can determine when they have stopped cycling and have become postmenopausal. Their only choice is to have an assay of FSH (follicle-stimulating hormone) performed, which requires a blood sample (an invasive procedure) and considerable cost.

Other women enter menopause quite precipitously and unnaturally when both ovaries are surgically removed along with the uterus. These women seek information about menopausal changes, such as hot flashes, mood swings, etc., which occur while still recovering from surgery in hospital. These women want to know why changes have occurred so suddenly and what other changes will occur, and they want to be reassured that the changes are normal. I question why some of these procedures are performed in the first place.

WHY SHOULD YOU READ THIS BOOK?

Unfortunately for women seeking information on menopause, some authors of published menopause books, even though not experts on menopause, have cashed in on a very lucrative market—50 million women around age 50, either pre- or postmenopausal, who want information. A major impetus to write nonmedical books occurred when author after author experienced that first hot flash, or heavy bleeding, and then set out to find information on the topic. Finding nothing, they wrote their books, some of which Dr. Patricia Kaufert (1992) labels as nothing more than "journalistic hucksterism." Other nonmedical books focus on menopause as a normal and natural event, celebrating it through poetry and song, advocating natural and/or nonmedical ways to intervene.

Books describing menopause as a medical event, written by medical and other health care experts, define women as estrogen-deficient at menopause, which, in effect, reduces women to the level of ovaries and uterus. These authors describe how women can best prevent the occurrence of postmenopausal disease. They may not explicitly describe all women as estrogen-deficient and in need of hormone replacement; they do, however, make a very powerful case for hormone replacement, if for no other reason than for women to obtain symptom relief and enhance quality of life.

So, into what category does *Menopause, Me and You: The Sound of Women Pausing* fall? The answer is that it falls into some of these categories, albeit packaged in a different way. Many of the published menopause books dogmatically insist that the most important thing a woman can do is to assume the responsibility for her health care, to take charge of this life transition, and to be in control. Several years ago, Art Ulene, on *The Today Show*, in the context of a discussion about whether or not to be a hormone user, said that it was not the physician or anyone else who should make that decision for a woman; that job, he said, was the woman's responsibility. Easy to say, Art; not so easy to do unless relevant information critical to making that decision is readily available.

Menopause, Me and You: The Sound of Women Pausing is divided into four sections. Section I includes content related to my own journey into women's health: my menopause. It also includes detailed information on conception and fertilization, reconceptualizing these events from a woman-centered, feminist perspective.

Section II discusses and reconceptualizes the menstrual cycle and menstruation, providing the knowledge base to understand menopause as the closure of menstrual life, not the end of life. Conceptualizing menopause as a natural process means it must be understood in terms of its relationship to the menstrual cycle. To understand the menstrual cycle implies understanding the physiological, endocrinological, and biochemical mechanisms that regulate the menstrual cycle and menstruation.

Section III defines and clarifies terms used to describe menopause. To understand the mechanisms that regulate the menstrual cycle, it takes readers on a journey into the center of the steroid hormone target cell. I explain hormone action at the cell-molecular level. Still another journey, into the nucleus of the cell, is necessary to understand that sex hormones function to initiate very powerful mechanisms that instruct body cells to divide or to make certain proteins—such as growth factors, which may be implicated in breast cancer. This journey provides the framework to appreciate at a scientific level that women were genetically programmed to end the production of reproductive hormones, and this message was written upon the union of egg and sperm.

Section III also discusses common menopausal changes and diseases attributed to being estrogen-deficient. To understand risks associated with hormone use and hysterectomy, it is necessary to understand the anatomy and normal function of the uterus and ovaries. Neither the ovaries nor uterus are excess anatomical or physiological baggage for a woman when she reaches menopause. Both organs play very important roles anatomically with respect to support for other internal organs. They are also very important for maintenance of hormone synthesis and the sexual response.

Section IV provides women with ways of gathering information, a way of "discovering knowledge" about themselves. In order to make informed decisions, whether about hormone use, for hot flashes, or how to manage bleeding changes associated with perimenopause (as one woman said, "Should I ride it out without anything? Do it 'hot turkey'?"), learning as much as one can about one's self is necessary. This means recording or writing down information about the experience and sharing that information with a health care provider. Certain information-gathering tools are provided in Section IV: a menstrual calendar card, hot flash body diagrams and diary, basal body temperature record, body composition record, menstrual bleeding scale, and factors to consider when choosing a care provider.

- The *menstrual calendar card* is especially valuable in understanding how the pattern of menstruation changes as the menopausal transition approaches as well as the benefit of having this information to share with a care provider.
- *Hot flash body diagrams* were developed when I began my hot flash research in the early 1980s. They are especially helpful in understanding what triggers a hot flash, how frequently it occurs, where it starts, and where it spreads.
- *The menstrual bleeding scale* was developed by Dr. Phyllis K. Mansfield in order to rate the quality of bleeding during perimenopause.
- *Other measures* developed by others, such as body composition and basal body temperature method of ovulation, provide ways of monitoring changes with aging. Such measures also provide noninvasive ways of determining whether menstrual cycles are ovulatory or not.
- Choosing a health care provider is perhaps the most difficult task confronting women. Drawing upon the work of an international colleague, Marie Londano, I have included a checklist of attributes associated with a humanistic versus a paternalistic care provider, and suggestions on how to interact with care providers in order to minimize the possibility of a paternalistic, e.g., "I know what is best for you. I am the doctor," approach.

Utilizing self-monitoring methods will become increasingly more important as health care delivery in the United States undergoes transformation and traditional roles of health care providers and patients change. People in general are already questioning the wisdom of clinicians in diagnosis and treatment, especially those that are high-cost or technologically advanced. Over the past two decades, all individuals are being urged to question whether they need to take drugs or hormones, or have surgeries to treat normal life events. People are beginning to realize that medical care is not necessarily health care, and that what may be normal for one person may not be normal for another. And, to a great extent, it is the myth of normalcy that has gotten us into trouble, creating many of the false impressions that riddle much of the thinking about women's health.

Keeping records takes time and work; it is not for those who want others to decide what is best for them. In the long run, I believe it is worth the effort. It is astonishing to imagine that a truly informed decision related to health care could result from a 10- or 15-minute visit to a care provider, based on information generated solely from a care provider's assessment.

The information, tools, and voices of women included in the book are intended to help both women and care providers understand the dynamic nature of the change process. The first voice "heard" in the book is mine. It will, by example, illustrate how at midlife, I was naive and blind to gender bias in research on women. I was so blind, in fact, that my first research study was designed to find out why menstruating women were out of control and a little crazy during the premenstruum.

SECTION I.
PREPARING FOR THE JOURNEY

No man has ever menstruated, ovulated, been pregnant and lactated, or experienced menopause. Yet until recently, it has been through the eyes of men that these experiences have been described and given meaning. Such meaning has in some cases banished women from daily activities during their menstruations, labeled them crazy during premenstrual days, and declared them useless to society once menopause arrived. Clearly, there is an undeniable need for development of different research paradigms which validate that women's experiences, sensations, and perceptions—as described by women—are the most reliable source of women's thinking. Call this process what you wish. Some of my feminist colleagues describe it as *woman-centered thought*, a concept that emerged as a result of the second wave of feminism and the women's movement in the 1970s. Sadly, however, despite more than 20 years of woman-centered thought, the world of science and women's health care research remains predominantly the domain of male scientists. Even in the mid-1990s, as the Women's Health Initiative becomes operationalized, the critical mass of researchers (those who direct the studies on women) are, for the most part, those individuals who created the knowledge and theories about women upon which the new research is based. In other words, these researchers will frame and study problems based on a preexisting, male-created knowledge base. They will interpret research findings based upon their attitudes and beliefs about women. Recommendations made as an outcome of this kind of research can only serve to perpetuate the status quo, reinforcing menopausal and menstrual disease ideologies.

Much ado has been made recently about the fact that women were deliberately excluded from participating in research studies on important diseases, such as heart disease. The reasons given were that hormone fluctuations during a menstrual cycle, or a pregnancy, during the course of research, would bias a study. The consequences of excluding women from research are that "standards" for "normalcy," with respect to what is "normal" biological function in diagnosing what is disease, were derived mostly from studies done on young, healthy, white males. Even in animal studies, a gender bias is evident—the rats used in research, except for reproductive studies, are white and male.

Inserting my views on issues does not mean that this will be a book that bashes physicians and scientists and makes women feel guilty about what has been done to them or what they could have done differently. Rather, I hope that the information in this book will empower women to take responsibility for their health, to question their care providers about treatment regimens, to raise questions within themselves about why women have been made out to be diseased simply because they are women (i.e., their reproductive function is different than that of males), and to help health care providers reconceptualize the meaning of menopausal and menstrual experiences.

As a woman, a nurse, and a scientist, I have lived through decades of discovery of invasive reproductive technologies, including the widespread use of oral contraceptives, and, more recently, injectable and implantable hormonal contraceptives. Also, from time to time, I have disagreed with feminist colleagues who claimed that these agents were the answer to the age-old question of how women, by gaining control of reproduction, gain control of their lives. My disagreement was based upon an analysis of risk/benefit criteria used to condone hormone use for women. For example, the pill was widely recommended for women to prevent pregnancy, a normal physiological process. Pregnancy, argued pill proponents, is very risky, as a woman could die during the pregnancy or during the birthing process. Therefore, it needs to be prevented, and the best, safest way to do this is to use oral contraceptives. In the early days of pill use, I argued that the pill was riskier for women than a pregnancy, since the hormones in the pill were drugs, and little information was available on either short- or long-term side effects.

More recently, however, I have modified my view of risk versus benefit associated with the use of hormones. When I removed the lens of a white, middle-class, educated nurse/feminist and viewed the situation from the perspective of women living in developing countries (developing implies using Westernized cultures as the standard for being "developed"), I realized that my feminist colleagues were right—the risks to health from pregnancy for women in developing countries was indeed very great. These women needed ways to gain control of their fertility and reproduction. In 1993, Diczfalusy reported that the lifetime risk of dying from pregnancy-related causes is 1:38 in South Asia and 1:24 in Africa (p. 323). Over 500,000 women die each year (1,370 each *day*) from causes related to pregnancy and childbirth. Of the 140 million births occurring each year, almost 120 million are in developing countries. In Westernized cultures, however, the lifetime risk of dying of pregnancy-related causes is estimated at 1:1,750, a very low probability. So, I still insist that to use this kind of reasoning to promote oral contraceptive use for westernized women is inappropriate. On the other hand, if the mortality estimates cited here are correct, the risk of dying from pregnancy is very real in developing countries. The benefit from hormone contraceptive use for these women is life; the risk without contraceptives is death. The World Health Organization estimates that from 1990 to the year 2000, some seven million women will die in childbirth, with the majority of these deaths occurring in developing countries.

I know now that assessment of risk versus benefit related to hormone methods of contraception, and hormone use at menopause for relief of symptoms, needs to be based on a clear understanding of a woman's socio/cultural/political situation—not feminist rhetoric, personal bias, prejudice, or someone else's personal value system.

With regard to menopause, I have lived through the decades of estrogen-alone replacement, followed by combination hormone replacement. I have disagreed with physician and nurse practitioner colleagues who claim that the disease-preventing benefits of hormone use outweigh any harms. I do not oppose hormone use for pre- or postmenopausal women. For women who have been made *hormone-deficient,* either by surgery, radiation, or drugs, hormone replacement is an absolute necessity. It is also a viable option for some women who cannot tolerate the changes associated with menopause. For these women, menopausal symptoms such as hot flashes and mood swings are intolerable. They interfere with activities of daily living, affecting communication abilities and the quality of a woman's interpersonal relationships. For these women, the benefits of hormone use are relief of symptoms and the ability to get on with their lives.

I disagree with my nurse and medical colleagues regarding hormone replacement in the assignment of disease status to menopause, whether explicit or implicit, and the eagerness to prescribe hormones to all postmenopausal women based upon an unsubstantiated ideology that equates menopause with disease. Menopause, specifically, has become medicalized. The widespread belief that menopausal women are estrogen-deficient resulted in increased estrogen use during the 1970s. Estrogen, subsequently, was found to be causally linked to an increased rate of uterine cancer. The rationale given to women in support of estrogen during this time was that it would prevent diseases such as cancer of the uterus and breast, and heart disease, in addition to maintaining a woman's "femininity and sexuality forever." The cancer scare of the 1970s has resulted in a decrease in hormone use by women, despite researchers' claims that combination hormone therapy (estrogen and progesterone together) is safe.

For now, the phenomenon of "medicalizing" menopause appears to be confined to Westernized, developed countries. Only recently has information been generated on the experience of menopause in other cultures. According to Yewoubdar Beyene, for women in the Yucatan, a developing country, menopause is an event to celebrate. The reason? These women have either been pregnant or lactating their entire menstrual lives. Menopause, for them, is not viewed as a time of loss or disease. Rather, it is a time to be "young and free" (Beyene, 1989, p.123).

During the past three decades, hysterectomy and breast cancer rates in the United States have increased. It is astonishing to realize how many gynecological surgeons recommended to women patients that they be castrated—to submit to a bilateral oophorectomy (removal of both ovaries)—when their uterus was removed, to protect them from developing ovarian cancer. This view was made explicit for women identified at high risk of developing ovarian cancer at a recent NIH (National Institutes of Health) Consensus Conference on ovarian cancer. It is even more astonishing to realize that women agree to have the procedure done, believing that if they do not, their risk of developing ovarian cancer increases dramatically. Removal of perfectly normal ovaries is unnecessary mutilation and abuse of women. In early 1993, the media publicized this issue quite widely, advising women to obtain a second opinion when hysterectomy with ovary removal was recommended. As a result of this publicity, the hysterectomy rate has decreased somewhat.

Unfortunately, the situation has not changed for the better with breast cancer. Over the past two decades, the risk of breast cancer has increased from 1:14 to 1:8 in a woman's lifetime. I am especially concerned about this, since just being a woman increases my personal risk of developing breast cancer. Rather than preventing and understanding cancer, or winning the war against breast cancer and its causes, we have not made much headway. Everyone who reads this book either has felt or will feel the impact of this disease, either in the death of a family member or a friend to the disease. During the summer of 1995, three women I know, one a former student in her thirties, another a former research assistant, and the third a colleague's mother, a woman in her sixties, were diagnosed with breast cancer in advanced stages. Perhaps we would have made more progress in understanding the cause of breast cancer if as many research dollars in the past had gone to study it as were spent to cure heart disease and AIDS in men. As a scientist, I have long disagreed with my medical and research colleagues who claim that the risks associated with steroid hormones related to initiation or promotion of breast cancer is either minimal or nonexistent. Breast tissue is hormone-responsive tissue, and to deny that hormones are not in some way causally linked with the increase in breast cancer is to deny the reality of the mechanism of hormone action at the cell-molecular level. Women have been exposed to hormones since the 1960s, either in oral contraceptives to prevent pregnancy, in estrogen or hormone replacement to treat menopausal symptoms, or in the prevention of menopause-associated diseases. It is illogical to think that hormones are not involved in breast cancer just because we do not have enough scientific proof. What is it about women that makes scientists and physicians insist that women need to take hormones? Do they want to kill women off? Or are these scientists and physicians practicing paternalism at its highest level, believing that they are protecting women from death and disease through their efforts? There is something wrong with this picture. What is wrong is the overarching belief we have placed in scientific results, and our refusal to believe that such results can work against a particular segment of society. My journey into women's health research was one of consciousness-raising, shock, and disbelief at what has happened to women in the name of health care.

Chapter 1

Ann's Journey
into Women's Health Research

This is my voice. It is my journey. Throughout the past two decades, my research has been directed at establishing woman-centered science as verifiable and valid, both to the scientific community and the public at large. I have listened to women and I have listened to myself. The most important thing I have learned is that what we have to say, as women, is not only worth saying, but saying it and being heard provides a way to achieve control of our lives. Through years of listening to women and recording their voices, I and other woman-centered researchers have begun, albeit quite modestly, to fill in the gaps related to the full spectrum of human experiences and perception. Without that spectrum, we have no hope for achieving a balanced or healthy society that so many claim to seek.

My journey into women's health research has been hand-in-hand with other women who have volunteered their stories, and unselfishly consented to have a variety of measurements made of their bodies and substances within their bodies. As a researcher, I am less comfortable in 1995 than I was in 1971 when my journey began. Along the way, I and others were to discover that all steroid hormones, including the sex steroid hormones estrogen and progesterone, interact with a receptor inside target cells. After a hormone binds with the intracellular receptor, it forms a "hormone-receptor" complex, which then translocates (moves inside) into the cell nucleus. In the nucleus, this complex then binds to the genome, deoxyribonucleic acid (DNA). In the early days of research on steroid hormones, we learned that the sex hormones did two things. When an estrogen-receptor complex bound with a DNA receptor in the uterus (the DNA is now referred to as the nuclear receptor), the cells were instructed to divide and increase in number. As long as estrogen was present, the process of cell division would continue. This is the reason the lining of the uterus, that is, the endometrium, increases in size premenstrually. Following ovulation, progesterone stops uterine cell division, and, also acting via the nuclear or DNA receptor, transforms the uterine lining into a structure that is hospitable for implanting a developing blastocyst (a hollow ball of cells that has formed from repeated cell divisions if an egg has been fertilized). However, if no pregnancy occurs, the cells lining the endometrium are shed. The shedding of endometrial cells and fluid is a process very familiar to women: menstruation.

I also learned that in order for uterine cells (and breast cells, too) to increase in number and do the things necessary for cells to stay alive, whether related to menstrual cycle events, pre-pregnancy, or lactation, the sex steroids had to perform another function: they had to induce the synthesis of proteins, growth factors, or growth-inhibiting factors. Certain of these growth factors have been suspected as playing critical roles in cancer promotion. I learned that the processes initiated by the sex hormones could be induced, whether or not the hormones were those made within a woman's body (which, by definition is termed *endogenous*), or were taken in pill, patch, or implant form (*exogenous*). At that time, I wondered whether differences in metabolic processes were initiated if the hormone was naturally synthesized in a woman's body versus the exogenous agent, since hormones made in a woman's body were regulated by a complex feedback mechanism. I discovered that the processes involved in regulating endogenous hormones were not the same as those when hormones were taken exogenously. Rather than interacting almost exclusively with reproductive target tissue, these agents interact with a variety of body cells, and they are metabolized slowly. I also discovered that when exogenous hormones are taken by mouth, as will be described later, they deliver a large dose of drug to the liver (in medical terminology this is referred to as a *bolus*), initiating a variety of unnatural metabolic activities. Knowing this helped explain the many side effects related to pill use.

The liver is the center of metabolism in the body. It is the major detoxification organ, the control center for clotting and bleeding, and for regulating sugar and fat metabolism. When blood glucose is at dangerously low levels, the liver can begin, through the stress response, to mobilize mechanisms to convert fat and protein into glucose. Much of this is accomplished through hormonal induction of specific enzymes. Thus, when a large concentration of steroid hormone reaches the liver through taking a pill, the liver responds via the hormone receptor mechanism. It does not matter that the steroid hormone bathing liver cells, i.e., estrogen, is not a hormone that normally activates liver cells, such as those involved in regulating glucose metabolism. Because estrogen resembles cortisol, the hormone that stimulates the liver receptor, the receptor is tricked. In other words, the liver cell receptor recognizes estrogen as a steroid. If enough estrogen is present (and there is, since a bolus of the hormone has been taken by mouth in pill form), it will bind with the liver cell receptor. The binding may not be of the high quality it would be with cortisol (in technical terminology, this is referred to as *high affinity* and/or *specificity*), but may be enough to initiate some metabolic processes (Martin et al., 1985, pp. 559-561). The bottom line here is that processes may be initiated which are undesirable, and, for the most part, unwanted: water retention, pseudo-diabetes, headaches, altered fat metabolism, clotting, etc.

All steroids, not just estrogen and progesterone, are potent initiators and/or regulators of metabolic events. Knowing that naturally synthesized hormones were under rather carefully controlled regulatory mechanisms, and that steroids taken in pill or patch form were not under the same kind of regulation, made me uneasy and cautious about enthusiastic endorsements for hormone replacement. But I am getting ahead of myself. It was a series of events unrelated to hormones that led me to women's health research.

When I began doctoral study in 1971, I did not view the world through the lens of a feminist women's health researcher. I was a nurse who had an opportunity to pursue graduate work through a federally funded program. Several things happened during graduate study that changed my worldview. Had it not been for the women's movement and the vision of certain nursing leaders during the early days of the second wave of feminism, the opportunity for me to pursue doctoral study might not have been possible. The writings and criticisms of early feminists, which made explicit the absence of women in science and research as generators of knowledge, helped nurse leaders establish a predoctoral fellowship program for nurses. As Sue Rosser and others have made clear, the choice of problems that are studied is determined by a powerful group of researchers who, in essence, establish a national research agenda to define what is worthy of study and who is best qualified to study the problems. At the time I entered graduate school, I was ignorant of the fact that most of the research done in the health sciences and/or on women's health was done by the dominant, powerful group in our society—those who were white, middle class, and male. The dominant paradigm used to study women was disease-oriented, and incorporated a masculinist societal bias that regarded women as weak and inferior beings.

In 1977 these negative attitudes about women and biases in research were challenged. I am very proud to have been one of a few women in the health professions who gathered in Chicago with a select group of researchers to organize the Society for Menstrual Cycle Research. This gathering occurred almost a decade before national task forces on women's health issues were convened. The menstrual cycle researchers met in order to provide a much-needed forum for presentation of papers, the raising of issues related to the unequal distribution of federal research dollars, and an opportunity to discuss issues related to gender bias and the absence of woman-centered research on menstruation and menopause. These research-ers early on questioned the validity of previously reported research findings on menstruating women, on the grounds that the findings were based on sexist myths and stereotypes. They raised as issues the biases inherent in research designs, flaws in methodology, and the faulty conclusions drawn from such research, which promoted and perpetuated negative stereotypes of menstrual and menopausal women. Drs. Alice Dan and Effie Graham, at the University of Illinois, coordinated this conference, which was the first of many, and the beginning of an important and powerful research pres-ence—one that continues to gain momentum. Today, women's menstrual, reproductive, and menopausal issues are national research priorities. The Society for Menstrual Cycle Research will celebrate its twentieth anniversary in 1997. Alice Dan will coordi-nate the conference in Chicago, the theme of which will be to examine what gains have been made regarding bias and flaws in research, the questions of whether women's health and research in the area has really progressed, and, if women have made gains, what may have been lost along the way?

THE JOURNEY

My entry into women's health research was rather circuitous. I had returned to graduate school in 1971 to pursue study toward a doctoral degree. At this time my primary interest was *not* in women's health. I was a nurse with a master's degree, teaching medical-surgical nursing in a baccalaureate nursing program. It was my plan to return to school to learn the skills necessary to become a research scientist. As a teacher of nursing, I found myself uneasy in the clinical arena, raising many questions about nursing practice related to intravenous water and electrolyte replacement therapy in sick people. As I worked with students caring for critically ill patients, I realized that the life of these patients in many instances depended upon the nurse who was responsible for carrying out orders related to fluid replacement therapy. In the 1970s no scientifically based practice guidelines were available to assist nurses in understanding the physiology and biochemistry of intravenous fluid replacement. In other words, I wanted to know what it meant to the patient when a nurse assisted in a fluid replacement. Bottles of intravenous solutions contained water and sugar and sometimes substances called electrolytes, such as sodium, potassium, and other inorganic ions. My goal in returning to graduate school was to understand what these substances did when administered to sick people. My ultimate goal was to develop practice guidelines for nursing.

It is important to realize that in the 1970s when I returned to school, there were no doctoral programs in nursing for nurses wanting to pursue a doctor of philosophy degree. And, at this time only a few nurses held doctorates, which had been earned in other disciplines, such as education. This should not be too surprising, since nursing for a long time had aligned itself with medical practice, and had neither carved out a niche for itself nor greatly differentiated its practice from medicine. This situation began to change in the 1960s. Nursing leaders were beginning to develop nursing theory, and declared that nursing care needed to be based upon the application of scientifically generated knowledge. To increase the number of doctorally prepared nurses who could conduct the kind of science required to make the discipline respectable, a "Nurse Scientist Fellowship Program" was approved by Congress to support nurses who wished to pursue doctorates. Since there were no doctoral programs in nursing, these research opportunities were offered in fields other than nursing. My interest in researching the metabolism of water and electrolytes led me to apply to the Nurse Scientist Training Program, and I was accepted as a predoctoral trainee in biology.

At age 40, I began graduate work. Had I known then that peri-menopause could begin in my late thirties or early forties, I might not have been so eager to make a major life change decision that meant leaving a secure teaching position and moving across the country. Even though I would turn 41 in March, my concerns were not related to the functioning of my reproductive system or menopause. Rather, at 40 years of age I was a healthy, regularly menstruating woman. My major concern was whether I was really smart enough to be successful in school. (This is one of many hang-ups that women have–whether they really can succeed. "Could I," I wondered, "compete with the younger students?") In 1971, I was what is referred to now as a "nontraditional student." Nontraditional in the 1970s meant that you were older, and, "What are you doing in graduate school?" I discovered that older students, particularly older students who were female and nurses, were not enthusiastically welcomed by some faculty. I was totally unprepared for the sexism and ageism that were alive and well on the campus.

The biology department assigned an advisor to work with me on program planning and to serve as a mentor. This individual took little interest in me or my ideas, and through words and actions, he questioned my ability to succeed. He accused me of not being able to have written an article on fluid and electrolyte therapy which was published in the *American Journal of Nursing* (1970). The material in that article was the result of my curiosity, as well as uneasiness about the lack of research-based information on water and electrolyte metabolism. I was very proud of that article; it was being read and used by clinicians. It was the result of months of library research and consultation with experts at the medical center where I was employed. After reading the article, my advisor said, "This article is too good to have been written by a nurse. Who really wrote it?"

Each time I scheduled an advisement meeting, I was discouraged from progressing in the program and urged to pursue another, less demanding field. "Biology," I was told, "is not as easy as nursing." My student nurse scientist peers, enrolled in programs in other fields, suggested that I discuss these issues with the department chair. I did. The department chair was sympathetic, saying that my advisor was not so bad, that he sometimes said things he did not mean, and that he (the chair) would not intervene in the situation; I should try to work it out. I found out that there was no working it out at any level in the university, not even the graduate school.

I was ready to leave graduate school when another professor of biology, Ivan Lytle (an advisor to two of my nurse scientist students), suggested that I explore my research ideas with faculty in the animal physiology department. Ivan had a joint appointment in biology and animal physiology. With his assistance, I contacted Dr. Tom Wegner, and Dr. Gary Stott, the department chair. The reception by these two men was overwhelmingly positive. Tom subsequently became my academic advisor and chair of my dissertation committee. Ivan Lytle continued as my friend and mentor until his untimely death from cancer.

The precise direction my research in water and electrolyte metabolism would take remained unclear. At this time I continued to conceptualize research problems from a nursing perspective, e.g., what could I study related to water and electrolyte balance that would be applicable in an acute care clinical area? Fortunately, it did not take long after transferring to my new department to make that choice. Each semester students were required to enroll in a departmental seminar. What this meant was that each one of us had to assume responsibility for presenting one seminar related to the theme identified for that semester. The topic for discussion during the first seminar was reproductive physiology. Great, I thought; I could increase my knowledge of water and electrolyte metabolism by presenting a seminar on the fluid changes associated with mammalian pregnancy. I already knew from my nursing background, and from caring for pregnant women, that women increased body water during pregnancy. This was also true for other animals.

During the course of my library research on the topic, I discovered that while much documentation on water volume increase during the first trimester (first three months) of pregnancy was available, exactly when (timing) and how the water volume changes were initiated (mechanism) was speculative. Was it possible, I wondered, for the fluid changes to be initiated prior to pregnancy–during the estrus cycle in animals and during the menstrual cycle in humans? As I read the human physiology literature, I discovered that little was written about the interface between the menstrual cycle and the pregnancy cycle as related to fluid volume changes.

Reviewing the menstrual cycle literature in preparation for that seminar was a mind-boggling event. As I read, I was overwhelmed by the negative attitudes expressed in the literature about menstruating women and the horrible sick ways women were supposed to change during the premenstrual phase of the cycle. I was a menstruating women; the authors of the articles I read were talking about me and other women in demeaning and derogatory ways. Menstruating women were said to suffer from affective and somatic symptoms–particularly so during the premenstruum. In the 1970s this was called *premenstrual tension*. Water retention and abdominal bloating were frequent complaints, as were inability to concentrate, irritability, mood swings, pain, etc. Women during the premenstrual phase of the cycle were characterized as out of control, with some even being capable of committing murder during this time. Causative physiological agents of premenstrual distress were explored on the basis of the complaints women presented to physicians. It was the empirical treatment of complaints–weight gain, bloating, breast tenderness, and irritability–that generated one pathophysiological explanation for premenstrual distress: edema, which is a pathological increase in total body water. Women were said to suffer from premenstrual edema. Treatment of the condition was aimed at alleviating water retention by prescribing diuretics and instructing women to decrease their intake of salt.

I began to realize that the research reports I read (with the exception of some of the emerging feminist research on the menstrual cycle) were mostly based on stereotypes about women and how they are expected to behave. In the 1970s, to question the assumptions on which research was based was to question the very heart of the science that I was being taught. Yet, I had to question. Science, as a social system, was not value-free, and the contemporary reports about menstruating women were no more than a reflection of the dominant beliefs held by our society about menstruating women. What, then, is premenstrual tension? Does it really exist, or is it a figment of someone's imagination? If women have it, what causes it? What causes women to bloat, to be irritable, to suffer headaches, to become, so to speak, transformed into a different person for at least one week out of each month? The search for answers to these questions meant reviewing the literature on the endocrinology (hormonal) and biochemistry (metabolism) of the menstrual cycle. This also meant reviewing literature on ovulation (what caused the egg to leave the follicle, a place in which it had been resting since intrauterine gestation?), which necessitated reviewing the scientific literature on menstrual cycle changes to uncover specifics: How much fluid did women accumulate premenstrually and what mechanisms were involved? What was the purpose of this increase in fluid volume? What really was menstruation? It was defined in the medical literature as the shedding of the uterine endometrium, a failed pregnancy. I had menstruated for almost 25 years. Yet, even with that many years of experience, not to mention my nursing background, I really did not understand what caused the uterine endometrium to shed. What was the composition of menstrual blood? Why did (could) women bleed from the uterus and not bleed elsewhere? Genia Pauli-Haddon describes a woman during the menstrual phase of the cycle as "the body that bleeds but is not wounded" (1993, p. 129).

Many details related to mechanisms of action were not well understood. I began to appreciate how intimate the relationship was between the brain, ovaries, and uterus in women, and that even though we knew a lot, many of the regulatory details remained fuzzy, such as what causes the regression (decay and death) of the corpus luteum (the mature postovulatory follicle that had contained the egg) after a period of seven or eight days? What causes menstruation? What is the precise mechanism of feedback control at the level of the brain? Of course, in the 1990s, we are much more enlightened about regulatory control mechanisms. But this does not mean that we respect them to any greater degree.

I realized that regulation of the menstrual cycle was anything but simple–too many mechanisms were not understood. This did not stop the scientists who developed and advocated contraceptive drugs and devices from interrupting these processes in women. Viewing women through a sexist lens, these researchers concluded that it was more logical to stop ovulation in women, a once-a-month event, than to interfere with spermatogenesis, an ongoing process in men. Events associated with ovulation are quite complex, perhaps more than those associated with spermatogenesis. If both mechanisms were fully understood, infertile couples in the 1990s would not have to experience multiple failures of fertilization and/or implantation as they attempt to become pregnant through *in vitro* fertilization procedures.

In the early 1970s, little was known at the cell-molecular level about how the sex steroids estrogen and progesterone work to promote ovulation, prepare the uterus, or sustain a pregnancy. The work of O'Malley and Schrader, and many others, which described the genomic mechanism of action would not be published until later. It occurred to me that any alteration or manipulation of the female reproductive system, such as occurred when a woman took oral contraceptives or used an intrauterine device (IUD), would interfere with, and thus alter, finely-tuned regulatory control mechanisms. What might result from either short- or long-term perturbations of the reproductive system? The high praise for effectiveness and unsubstantiated claims of low risk by pill and IUD users was worrisome. Not all of the mechanisms related to the menstrual cycle were understood; however, it was the female's physiology that was being manipulated with drugs and devices, based by and large on unsubstantiated assumptions about how reproductive processes were regulated, and on the high value attributed to the man's role in reproduction.

I knew enough about research methodology to appreciate that when an agent was experimental, human use of that drug or product had to await controlled clinical trials. Human use related to oral contraceptive use and IUDs concerned women, not men. When females were used as experimental subjects to test for side effects of oral contraceptives, often, according to Sue Rosser (1989), they were not treated as fully human. In a study on pill use related to nervousness and depression, one investigator gave dummy pills to women who went to his clinic specifically in order to obtain oral contraceptives to prevent pregnancy. None of the women were told that they were participating in research or that they were receiving a placebo (sugar pill) (Rosser, 1989, p.129). When I raised this ethical issue related to human experimentation and the sexism inherent in the research protocols carried out to validate the safety of the pill, the male scientists I consulted did not view these concerns as bona fide issues.

Incredible as it seems, I completed that first seminar, but was never again to view the world of research or read a research report in the same way. At the conclusion of the seminar, I advanced a hypothesis based upon a new view: The changes women experienced during the premenstrual phase of the menstrual cycle were normal, not a sign of pathology. I argued from an endocrinological normative perspective that the changes were hormonally induced, and that it was imperative that a pregnant female increase body water to ensure a healthy, successful pregnancy. I suggested also that the mechanisms which initiated body water increase occurred in the postovulatory phase of the menstrual cycle. In other words, during the luteal (premenstrual) phase of the cycle, these changes, rather than being interpreted as signs of a disease, could be thought of as the body's way of preparing for pregnancy—indirect indicators that hormonally induced prepregnancy physiological adjustment mechanisms had occurred. I argued this position from work reported in the literature to understand the phenomenon of premenstrual edema.

Initially, premenstrual edema formation was thought to be due to the salt-retaining effects of endogenous progesterone. This hypothesis emerged out of animal experiments in which progesterone was identified as a salt-retaining hormone. Research on humans, however, established a natriuretic (salt-losing) action for progesterone. Extrapolating this finding to women, researchers hypothesized that a luteal phase progesterone increase in women induced salt loss. This resulted in a compensatory hypersecretion of aldosterone, an adrenal steroid hormone that regulates salt in the body.

It seemed reasonable to hypothesize that the somatic (bodily) and psychic changes occurring during the premenstrual phase of the cycle were due to progesterone's ability to antagonize, and thus diminish, the effects of aldosterone to retain salt. As salt left the body, so did water. Premenstrual edema could be due to the rebound ability of aldosterone hormone to overcome progesterone's antagonism. As salt was retained, other hormonal mechanisms were initiated to retain water in order to dilute the high concentration of salt in the blood.

Theoretically speaking, a woman may conceive, but she is not "pregnant" until the blastocyst, the ball of cells that has formed from the union of the sperm and the egg, has implanted in the uterus. Knowing this, I thought it was logical to assume that mammals, in general, would not wait until conception to initiate mechanisms critical to ensuring implantation and nurturing of the embryo. From an evolutionary perspective, it is possible that the increase in body water is a trait that was selected for as mammals evolved. Having in place the capacity to increase the delivery of nutrients and the removal of waste products of metabolism from a growing conceptus/embryo would ensure the potential for maximal growth and survival. Fluid volume increases in other parts of the body, such as abdomen and breasts, is explainable by drawing upon the evolutionary biology concept of *pleiotropy*. In other words, retaining desirable traits, those that have been selected to ensure survival of the species, sometimes necessitates paying a price. Along with the desirable trait selected for (intrauterine gestation) are unwanted effects of water retention in other tissues. In this case, the organism obtains the survival benefit associated with a protected pregnancy and an increase in total fluid volume to nourish the developing fetus via an increased capacity to carry more water and nutrients in the blood. Phenotypically (which means the way the gene is expressed, how we look, or what happens in our body), the survival benefits are enhanced for the fetus; for the woman, however, the host for the developing fetus, the changes are experienced bodywide, and are not viewed as a benefit.

This theory was and still is hypothetical. The explanation I advanced, however, served two purposes. First, it allowed me to reconceptualize the changes that occurred premenstrually into a normative framework for women. Specifically, the changes women experienced were not premenstrual at all. Rather, more correctly, they were the expression of prepregnancy changes. Second, following this first seminar, I changed my research focus from understanding the pathophysiology of water and electrolyte metabolism in illness, to the physiology of the mechanism(s) that initiated premenstrual changes in healthy women.

And so, in 1972 my research career in women's health began.

The change in research focus was also a philosophical turning point. I had begun the process of reconceptualizing events associated with women's menstrual and reproductive lives. As indicated, a basic assumption underpinning my doctoral research was that a premenstrual increase in body water was not only normal but necessary to support a pregnancy. I had hypothesized that the water volume change was hormonally mediated, and that the change was probably related to aldosterone, the steroid hormone that regulated sodium metabolism in the body and thus, indirectly, water balance. Based on what was known about the structure of steroid hormones, all possessing the same four-membered ring, I hypothesized that high levels of progesterone during the luteal phase of the menstrual cycle were antagonistic to the sodium-retaining effects of aldosterone. If this occurred, one would expect to measure first a decrease in aldosterone during the luteal phase of the cycle, then an increase in order to overcome the antagonism of progesterone. To test this hypothesis, I measured the concentration of both of these hormones in the blood of women. Measurement of blood steroids was possible using a newly developed laboratory method: radioimmunoassay.

In the course of my laboratory work, which involved analyzing blood samples of 20 women during one menstrual cycle, I made an important finding—one that would benefit me personally at a later time. I observed that there were some days when doing the hormone assays that I could get little repeatability when running the standards which, simply, are known concentrations of the hormone being measured. After several months of rather discouraging, erratic results, despite following the procedures as outlined, and having to dispose of several days' work, I stopped the analyses. It was back to the library to review the steroid chemistry radioimmunoassay literature. An article by Guy Abraham, a pioneer in hormone assay research and now known for his work on premenstrual syndrome (PMS), provided the insight needed. In that article Abraham said: "The condition of the technician will affect the assay" (1974, p. 25). What Abraham meant by this statement was that all steroids have the capacity to diffuse, to emanate or leak from the human body through the skin and the mucous membranes. The most compelling words of wisdom in Abraham's article, however, were that all pregnant women, as well as women in the luteal phase of their menstrual cycles, should be prohibited from entering any laboratory where steroid hormones are being measured. The potential for assay contamination from high levels of the sex steroid hormones in pregnant women (by diffusing through the skin and the mucous membranes into the environment) was incredibly high. For women technicians in their prime reproductive years, Abraham's advice was to put on a mask, gown, and gloves when running hormone assays during all phases of the menstrual cycle. Similar precautions were advised for male technicians who were assaying for low levels of testosterone.

What an important lesson to learn: that during the luteal phase of my menstrual cycle, I had been contaminating my assays. As a result of this discovery, I washed all glassware, scrubbed the walls of the lab, and had no further problems with the assays if I took the proper precautions.

In order to know when I was in the most assay-contaminating phase of my cycle (the luteal phase), I began keeping a record of my menstrual starts and stops, as well as when I perceived ovulation to occur. It was not unusual to know when I was ovulating as I experienced a bit of pain midway through my cycle. This phenomenon is called *mittelschmerz*. I continued to keep my menstrual record long after finishing the hormone assays. It was informative to see how the cycle interval as well as bleeding interval varied from cycle to cycle, and how the pattern of bleeding changed as I approached menopause.

Abraham's advice also made me think about an old wives' tale I had heard, claiming that women who lived together (especially women college students cloistered in dormitories), would cycle together. Women still talk about this phenomenon, which is called *menstrual synchrony*. To date, little serious research has been conducted on this phenomenon.

How much each one of us unknowingly affects or is affected by the hormonal output of others, male and female, would be a most interesting project to pursue. Much is known about pheromones, sex attractant steroid hormones found in animals other than humans. These pheromones are powerful indicators that the female is physiologically ready to breed. Winnifred Cutler, working at the Athena Institute for Women's Wellness Research, thinks that we are not so far evolved from our animal heritage that a similar effect is operational in humans. Dr. Cutler believes that a substance, which she has defined as "essence," found in the sweat of humans, performs a similar sexual function for humans (Vigoda, 1993). If a laboratory technician can contaminate an assay from his or her endogenous sources of hormones, surely our hormones must have an effect upon others with whom we live and work. Women, during the luteal phase of the cycle, synthesize large quantities of estrogen and progesterone. During pregnancy progesterone hormone in a woman's blood is ten times the concentration found in the blood during the luteal phase of the menstrual cycle.

Since discovering this bit of information, I have wondered how much of what we observe as family friction and/or dysfunction might be attributable to a mother and daughter cycling together, affecting each other, and affecting the father if there is a father in the home, or how much the hormonal output of the male affects the female, or vice versa. For years the focus in menstrual cycle research has been to study the changes in the female premenstrually. Perhaps it is the male's response to female hormones that needs to be studied in order to understand the dynamic interplay of hormone changes and effects of these changes?

That humans are affected by exogenous (external to the body) sources of hormones is documented in the literature. In the 1960s and early 1970s, when diethylstilbestrol (DES, an estrogen-like drug) was being fed to farm animals to increase the percent of fat in the meat, men who worked in plants where DES was manufactured developed breast tissue (gynecomastia); they also became impotent. The same phenomenon was observed in men in the early days of extracting estrogens from the urine of pregnant mares.

ONWARD

In March of 1976 I defended my dissertation. It took five years to take the courses–chemistries through steroid biochemistry, mathematics through calculus, advanced physiology and research methods, selected laboratory methodologies–and to complete my research. My nursing background was good, but it did not prepare me for a change in disciplines. Many times I have reflected about what I had to do in order to fulfill the requirements for the PhD in another discipline. It would have been easier to complete a degree in nursing since I would be building on the knowledge base of the discipline. But in the 1960s and 1970s, there were no doctoral programs in the United States in nursing (in 1995 there are more than 60!). I was not alone, however. Many nurses earned doctorates in disciplines other than nursing. I have also reflected many times on the impact this has had on the direction the profession has taken. But then, that, too, is another story.

The findings of my doctoral research supported my hypothesis: there was a statistically significant luteal phase increase in the concentration of the hormone aldosterone, as well as a statistically significant luteal phase time-lag correlation between progesterone and aldosterone. A time-lag correlation between the two hormones provided data supporting the hypothesis that progesterone antagonized aldosterone's function to reabsorb salt, (Voda, 1980). Initially, I postulated that this would result in a loss of salt and water. To overcome this loss in body water as well as salt, aldosterone would have to be secreted in larger amounts than were normal in order to overcome the antagonistic effect of progesterone. Thus, the increase in aldosterone, following the same pattern as progesterone, albeit later (the time lag), during the luteal phase of the cycle would result in sodium reabsorption, and indirectly, water reabsorption. That many women crave salty foods during the premenstruum fits with the aldosterone hypothesis. The importance of a significant time-lag correlation between the two hormones led me to believe that this could be the mechanism which initiated the fluid volume increase of pregnancy, albeit physically and temporally, being located during the luteal phase of the menstrual cycle.

Whether or not the mechanism described here is the one that initiates the fluid volume increase of pregnancy has yet to be resolved. It does provide a normative framework for understanding premenstrual changes and/or reconceptualizing them as normal and necessary prepregnancy changes.

MY MENOPAUSAL JOURNEY

Midway through my doctoral program, I experienced my first hot flash. This was in 1974 at 44 years of age. The flashes occurred infrequently for the next six years, confined mostly to the hours of sleep. A review of my menstrual calendar indicates that I experienced menopause on October 7, 1981. I was 51 years old. Yet, I had experienced hot flashes for seven years prior to menopause; I am still experiencing hot flashes, mild as they are, triggered mostly by a glass of wine, stress, a warm environment, or upon awakening in the morning.

Had I not kept a record of my menstruations, I would not have known with any certainty when I had become menopausal. I had not menstruated from October 1981 to October 1982. By definition, a woman is not menopausal until she has gone one year without a menstrual bleed or show of any kind. Had I menstruated, or even spotted at any time during this period of time, say at the tenth or eleventh month, I would have had to wait another 12 months from the time I had menstruated in order to be defined as menopausal.

But menopausal I am, and glad of it. In October of 1995, as mentioned, I was 14 years past menopause. The hot flashes, when they occur now, are warm and gentle, like a caress from an old friend. However, this friend was not always so kind and gentle. Around menopause, for a period of about two years, the intensity and frequency of the flashes during day and night increased almost exponentially from what it had been.

But, I was to discover that my hot flash experience was similar to that of women I have studied. In 1977 I was funded by the National Institutes of Health to study the menopausal hot flash. I was shocked to learn that virtually no research had been done on the phenomenon. Yet it was, and still is, the most widely treated symptom of menopause, whether with over-the-counter agents or with estrogen hormone. I found through my research, working with women in Arizona and Minnesota, that hot flashes occur more often than not, pre- *and* perimenopausally. And, like my own experience, they can occur for years prior to menopause and years following menopause. They are not debilitating for most women; instead, they are more a darn nuisance and/or an inconvenience.

I found also that these women experienced hot flashes postmenopausally, albeit at a lowered level of intensity and frequency. This finding debunks a common medical myth related to hot flashes, as well as other changes: namely, that if you take hormones for a couple of years prior to menopause, you will experience menopause without a symptom. I learned from the women that shortly after hormones are stopped, the hot flashes return. And how they return! Taking hormones merely postpones the inevitable. The hot flash, how to track it, and how to cope with it, is described in more detail in Chapter 11. The hot flash tools, body diagrams, and diary are described in Section IV, "Keeping Records and Keeping in Touch."

In 1980 I was awarded another research grant to continue work on the hot flash as well as other menopausal changes, such as changes in body composition. Shortly after menopause, I began to notice certain changes in my body shape and size. I had always been a well-proportioned woman, not fat, no pot belly, no painful enlarged breasts during my menstrual cycles, no weight gain other than that normally experienced by most women premenstrually. At menopause it became noticeable that blouses did not fit the way they used to. That is, while my body weight had remained stable, my upper body appeared to be getting bigger, my waist thicker. Blouses fit like those drawn for the character in the Smilin' Jack cartoon, who, because of an increased amount of upper body fat, kept popping buttons off of his shirt. As a result, his shirt was always gaping open (and, as my sister Vicki reminded me, there was always a chicken there to catch the button). Well, much to my chagrin, I observed that a change had occurred in my upper body too, which necessitated a size larger blouse and/or shirt. My breasts had increased in size! Now, for some women, this may be the answer to a lifelong prayer. It was not for me. Work with other women led me to discover that changes in body composition were not unusual in postmenopausal women.

THE JOURNEY CONTINUES

In 1984 I assumed the Directorship of the Menstruation Reproductive History (MRH) Program, which was renamed The Tremin Trust by the first director of the program, Dr. Alan E. Treloar. The words of the women participants of The Tremin Trust will be heard throughout the book. Since acquiring the MRH program, a yearly survey has been revised and expanded so as to incorporate a more focused, woman-centered approach to research. The research program is discussed in Chapter 4. In collaboration with Dr. Phyllis K. Mansfield, a special survey and special menstrual bleeding calendar with a rating scale are mailed yearly to a group of midlife Tremin Trust participants and other women. This ongoing research is designed to chart the participants' passage to menopause, and most particularly, to document how the pattern of menstrual bleeding changes premenopausally. Information on menstrual bleeding changes are presented in Chapter 12.

LIFE ENERGY

As in any journey, I have discovered from working with women that to successfully travel the reproductive life journey of a woman from first bleed to the last, necessary preparations must be made, i.e., keeping records and keeping in touch, and precautions must be taken to avoid certain obstacles, such as having inaccurate information. Along life's journey, the transitions through and beyond menarche and menopause are perhaps the most confusing, demanding, and yet rewarding of life's experiences. At those times, a dramatic redirection of a woman's life energy occurs.

I believe that life energy had its origins with the origins of the universe itself. Through space and time it has moved toward the moment when it is actualized, or brought into being, or an altered state of being, at the forming of an ovum with the message of life recorded on the DNA in that ovum. It continues beyond the life journey of a single person, through the process of reproduction, and through other processes at a person's death. Visualizing life energy as a spiraling line that has extended from an infinite or nearly infinite past and continues to extend into what appears to be an infinite future, there then is the axis, the center point of that line, which is found to be within the womb of woman. From this perspective of human life, the womb is not merely the place where gestation of human life occurs, or merely the focal point of reproductive and productive life energy, or simply the womb itself. Conceptually and physiologically, it is the central cosm in which and out of which all other levels and cosms flow—worlds within worlds, the center of the universe.

Women often describe this part of life's journey, and the channeling of life energy, as the opening and closing of a series of doors, doors that lead to several rooms which are occupied for varying periods of time. The first door to open after birth is the door to childhood, and it is also the first door that must be closed. Once physical growth and development and puberty are completed, life energy is redirected to meet menstrual and reproductive demands. As the door to childhood closes, a woman finds herself in a hallway with doors that open into two rooms; one is the menstrual room, the other the pregnancy room. Many women in Westernized cultures spend many years in the menstrual room, sometimes 30 years or more, depending upon the number of times the pregnancy door had been opened. Other women, in the Yucatan for example, spend little time in the menstrual room and almost all of their reproductive life in the pregnancy room. For these women, menstruation is an infrequent visitor. Some women may spend little time in either the menstrual or pregnancy rooms because of misdirected energy or insufficient energy to meet demands related to reproduction. For example, women with exercise-induced amenorrhea spend less time in the menstrual room than do women who have had a hysterectomy. Since the advent of hormone treatments, we now find some postmenopausal women increasing the time spent in the menstrual room if menstruation is prolonged through hormone use.

When a woman stays in the menstrual room, some life energy is dedicated to preparing for pregnancy, no matter if that pregnancy does not occur. When it does not, menstruation commences, the uterine lining is shed, and, before the last cell and blood are gone, new sources of life energy are channeled into the next menstrual cycle to prepare the body for pregnancy. The cyclic nature of these prepregnancy menstrual changes are predictable, periodic, and familiar to women. In this context, I believe, as do others, that biology is destiny, in the sense that it is females, not males, who are destined genetically to ovulate, gestate, lactate, and menstruate. Each one of these biological functions is energy demanding.

A woman may choose to open and close the menstrual and pregnancy doors many times during a lifetime. Or a woman may choose never to open the pregnancy door. These women, infertile women, males—all of us on this planet—however, will have spent some time in the pregnancy room. All humans, male and female, spend vary-ing amounts of time inside the body of a woman who is pregnant with them. During this occupancy, a primordial ball of genetic DNA was transformed into tissues, tissues into organ systems, organ sys-tems into the creation of a new life. Margaret Mead wrote that for a female, this occupancy means spending time in the womb of a person who is like her instead of a person who is different from her—a womb within a womb (1977). For a male, this nine-month intrauterine experience means being in the body of an alien, a person who is different endocrinologically, kinesthetically, and in every other way. According to Genia Pauli-Haddon, when males first question "Who am I?," it is answered with the awareness "I am different from the person who gave me birth" (1993, p. 29). Alien or not, males do get to spend time, albeit of short tenure, in the pregnancy room. Following birth, however, they can never return to this room, at least in the physical and biological sense that women do. Knowing this must affect them in some way. In other words, they can never fully understand the changes that occur within the woman—mentally and physically—as a life-creating pro-cess progresses. Men must feel disconnected from this process, and thus, they must feel some insecurity and uncertainty.

Ultimately, women must close the door to menstrual and repro-ductive life. The message to bring closure to the process was written while the woman was a fetus in her own mother's womb. It has been known for a good number of years that women possess a finite number of healthy ova that can be ovulated. Menopause signals the exhaustion of that finite supply. At menopause women redirect life's energy into the next room, postmenopause and beyond. Prior to menopause, a great deal of energy is consumed while closing down menstrual/reproductive processes. Body cells that had been bathed in sex hormones for more than 30 years now react to the absence of these substances. For a while, life energy is directed toward coping with the cellular stress being experienced by hor-mone withdrawal.

Once the menstrual door is closed, unlike the situation with men, no life energy *ever* again needs to be channeled to support menstrual and/or reproductive events, unless, as mentioned, these events have been artificially prolonged with hormones and/or high technology attempts to induce pregnancy via *in vitro* fertilization.

Many women during the course of their menstrual life have referred to the menstrual cycle and menstruation as a "curse." This is particularly true, I suppose, if a great deal of time was spent in the menstrual room and one experienced PMS. I spent 35 years in the menstrual room. For me and for many of the women in The Tremin Trust Research Program, it is a great relief to have closed the door to that room. But pity the poor men who never bring closure to reproductive life, who constantly throughout their adult years must direct life energy to make sperm—trapped in sperm rooms for the totality of their postpubertal lives! For men, spermatogenesis may diminish somewhat with aging, but, unlike women and menopause, there is no closure to the process.

And so, I wonder: Is menstruation *really* a curse, or a blessing in disguise?

Chapter 2

The Egging of the Sperm

The myth of conception: In sexual reproduction, the egg is passive, the sperm is active. The sperm fertilizes the egg.

On March 21, 1930, my mother gave birth to me. And when she did, my journey toward menopause had already begun. Sometime during menopause, theoretically, I had ovulated my last egg. The last journey to wombworld had been taken. Most of the eggs in my ovaries never took this journey; they remained in ovarian follicles which, from about the fifth month of fetal age, would spontaneously degenerate. I learned that while around seven million eggs resided in my ovaries at five months of age (while a fetus in my mother's uterus), the number would decrease to about 900,000 at age seven, and to about 300,000 at menarche. Even though most of the eggs in my ovaries at birth would never be ovulated, for the few that were, the opportunity existed to produce a new human, to create a new life.

THE BEGINNING

Within the womb of a woman pregnant with a female child is the womb of that child. Within the ovaries of that unborn child are all of

---

The title of this chapter was created in 1988 and presented in a paper "The Egging of the Sperm and Other Knowledge for a New Decade" at the April 7, 1990, New England Women's Studies Conference, University of Rhode Island. The presentation of that paper related to "egg" and "sperm" preceded publication of Emily Martin's "The Egg and the Sperm," which was published in *Signs*, 16:3, University of Chicago Press, Chicago, IL. Any similarity to Martin's published work is purely coincidental.

the ova or eggs needed to someday create a new human. A woman giving birth to a woman who will birth a human—generations and regenerations. It is within woman where the potential to reproduce human life exists. The creation of a new life in humans, by definition, is achieved through the process of sexual reproduction. Under normal and natural circumstances, the first step in the process occurs when an ovulated egg fuses with a sperm within the fallopian tubes of a woman's body. Until recently, this process has been referred to as fertilization, i.e., a sperm fertilizes an egg.

In some distant age, when life on earth was new and simple, and only found in the invisible single cells of immortal microscopic things, these single-cell creatures reproduced, as do amoeba, by dividing themselves and becoming two, again and again. In fact, the amoeba of today may be the very same creatures of that long-ago past. The expanse of time, expenditure of energy, and alterations in the environment provided some with changes, and eventually mutated forms developed that no longer reproduce by cell division; these new single-cell life forms reproduced sexually. Some cells were distinctly male or female. The male formed sperm and the female formed eggs. When the egg and sperm were joined, the product of their reproduction was more of their kind. As Lynn Margulis describes the situation, "Human sexuality seems more than a wondrous accident, born of a kind of original sin among protozoans" (Nash, 1992, p. 47). Nonetheless, sexual reproduction was an exciting and important development because with its advent, again, depending upon whom one reads, came the opportunity for greater diversity and for tremendously increased reproductive activity, both of which opened the way for richer and more profuse mutation among species. And so began the journey of life.

Sex is not essential, however, to reproduction. Nature follows more than one script; not every animal or plant species has two sexes. And, as far as anyone knows, organisms that reproduce through cell division do not die in the same way as organisms that reproduce sexually. Theoretically, those that reproduce through cell division, if maintained in an ideal environment, would continue to divide and live forever. Sexually reproductive organisms age and eventually die, no matter how ideal their environment. Consequently, it is likely that death entered the world riding on the back of sexual reproduction. That this may also seem a curse accompanying a blessing is only so until one realizes that this is nature's way of protecting its new species. If it had been otherwise, intense reproductive activity of sexual beings would have caused overpopulation of the planet much sooner than the situation that confronts humankind currently. Overpopulation would have brought an end to the species and to any possibility of reproduction and mutation for the evolution of life.

Ages upon ages passed, and life evolved from one-celled organisms to more complex creatures, all moving step-by-step toward the eventual emergence of Homo sapiens and other life forms that share the world with us today. With the evolution of warm-blooded animals (mammals) came the mechanisms of estrus and menstrual cycles, intrauterine gestation, and hormonal regulation of sexual reproduction.

This account of life, its origins and its death, is far from being the only one, and is hardly complete, giving only a glimpse of what may have been. In every account, however, there emerges the awareness that humans are sexual, reproductive beings and, for better or for worse, it is this activity that has brought humankind to where it is now.

An examination of histories, cultures, and science makes it clear that the central burden for sexual reproduction in humans rests firmly upon the female of the species. Yet, as noted previously, through the ages, women, rather than being praised and rewarded for this life-giving function, have suffered repeated degradation and invalidation regarding the reproductive function of their bodies. From the beginning of recorded history, we have accounts of the maze of rites and superstitions and misconceptions regarding menstruation/reproduction.

Related to human sexual reproduction, the traditional or patriarchal view of the female body has been that of a passive vessel, as matter upon which a male acts to create a new human. This view has perpetuated a diminished and devalued view of the role of the female in the process. In the patriarchal view, according to Genia Pauli-Haddon, it is inevitable and correct that masculine triumphs over feminine. Progress is defined as penetrating new frontiers, claiming new territories, movement toward goals, etc. The ideal is to make successively upward progress. This ideal, Pauli-Haddon argues, has been projected onto nature in the theory of evolution, which attributes to man the characteristic of being the superior being. The patriarchal worldview has been humankind's collective story, told over and over. Its theme resonates in fairy tales, religion, and in the scientific method of generating new knowledge (p. 11). Its theme generated the view of the female body as a passive vessel in which, in sexual reproduction, the sperm is active and fertilizes a passive female egg.

In antiquity, neither sperm nor egg had been identified, nor fertilization imagined. To explain reproduction, Hippocrates speculated that both the female and the male produced seed, though the male seed was viewed as stronger and it was thought that it probably contained a miniature human. Later, when the microscope was invented and sperm were examined, some scientists were convinced that contained within the sperm head was the body of a tiny man.

Most early scientists and philosophers believed that women, when compared to men, were deficient. Aristotle viewed women as being in an arrested state of development since they did not possess enough vital heat, that is, the heat necessary to concoct, to transform menstrual blood into semen. In procreation, semen took on a sacred character. It was believed that males, through semen, infused dead matter (passive menstrual blood) so that it could grow into a human. Even though much later semen was identified as sperm, it too was viewed as the vital spark of life. The value attributed to semen/sperm by Aristotle and the devaluation of women in sexual reproduction ushered in an era of sperm idolatry, one that continues today.

The makers of our myth (the egg is passive; the sperm is active; the sperm fertilizes the egg) were scientists who perpetuated Aristotelian beliefs about the value of semen and maleness, and Darwinian, Victorian stereotypes of evolution in the name of scientific discourse. According to Bleier (1984), within this paradigm, passive behavior was defined as feminine, while active, or goal-oriented behavior, as identified by Pauli-Haddon, is masculine. Within this paradigm, it is the masculine that is valued; the feminine is not. The stereotype is firmly in place regardless of whether scientists are observing behavior in animals, algae, bacteria, people, or sperm. Consequently, spermatogenesis in males, because it is an active, ongoing process, has been more valued than ovulation in females, a one-time event in the menstrual cycle. This view of sexual reproduction, coupled with sperm idolatry, is the underpinning of fertility control methods being developed for and used almost exclusively by women.

In the 1990s, fewer U.S. tax dollars are being spent to understand the cellular mechanisms that regulate sexual reproduction. The focus of these efforts, until recently, has been exclusively on the mechanism of action of steroid hormones and control of ovulation. Research on male contraception is poorly funded.

CONCEPTION

The traditional patriarchal view of fertilization and conception suggests that females do very little of importance in the process of sexual reproduction. In reality, however, fertilization is a highly complex process, an intricate series of steps, which begins when a sperm is able to successfully attach to an egg's thick extracellular coat. No sperm swim directly through a woman's cervix into the uterus and on into the fallopian tubes to fertilize an egg unless important changes have occurred in cervical mucus. Sperm would flagellate in a non-goal-directed manner and perish. Sperm so-directed to an egg must undergo certain reactions that are induced and controlled by the egg before fertilization can occur.

Fertilization is a fusion process, the joining of sperm and egg. Following fertilization, cell division begins. From one cell, two cells (the zygote) are formed, then four, and so on. At this time, however, a woman is not yet pregnant; no special maternal arrangements have been made to support the zygote. To be able to divide, the zygote needs only to be in a progestational fluid environment. Progesterone is made and secreted from the corpus luteum of the ovary. Progesterone also acts to transform the lining of the uterus into a vascular, spongy surface that is suitable to nurture the growing organism.

By the time the eight-cell-stage of division has occurred, the embryonic structure contains more than 1,000 kinds of protein. Thereafter, only the quantity, not the variety, of protein increases.

All of this has been achieved while a woman is in a prepregnant condition.

Approximately four days following fertilization, the cluster of dividing cells is now about 32 or 64 cells and is referred to as a blastocyst, which, as has been defined, is a nearly hollow ball of cells. When the blastocyst reaches the uterus, the stage corresponds to about day 19 or 20 of the menstrual cycle. Five days following fertilization, about 120 cells are contained in the human blastocyst. At this point, however, the developing embryo continues to be free-floating, without a placenta, and independent of any maternal source of nutrition or hormonal stimulation of cell division. Once the blastocyst safely reaches the uterus, it needs to quickly make arrangements to implant (which means to embed itself into the uterus). Implantation has been facilitated by the maternal synthesis of estrogen, which early on in the menstrual cycle stimulated the uterine endometrium to proliferate and to become rich in blood vessels.

Implantation of the blastocyst in the wall of the uterus has been described as a remarkable process, one that is invasive in order for human embryonic tissue to come in contact with maternal blood. Once implantation has been accomplished, the blastocyst cells, from which the embryo, the fetus, and the placenta develop, can be described as "parasitic" on the woman. By the twentieth day of the cycle, a progesterone-primed uterus has become a highly vascular, spongy "nest," ready to accept, nurture, and protect the developing organism. The pattern for a new life has become established.

If there is no sperm to fuse with an egg, or no egg to fuse with a sperm, as is the case with a woman who uses oral contraceptives for birth control, or there is an inhospitable environment for the dividing ball of cells, as is the case with a woman who uses an intrauterine device (IUD), or a chemical or mechanical barrier such as a condom or chemical foam prevents sperm from entering the uterus, blocking sperm travel to the fallopian tubes, pregnancy will not occur. If a woman conceives and implantation is successful, pregnancy, a nine month intrauterine period of fetal growth and development, begins.

During the period of intrauterine gestation, embryonic and fetal growth and development are dependent upon the ability of the maternal organism to tolerate as well as sustain and nourish the parasitic organism within the uterus. Pregnancy in mammals acts much as a graft does, bringing into direct contact the tissues of two genetically distinct individuals. Why a fetus escapes rejection by the mother's immune system remains a mystery even today.

What is most incredible about the process of ovulation and conception is the fact that the formation of that pregnant woman's egg, the egg that fused with a sperm, occurred while she was an unborn fetus within her own mother's womb. Within that waiting ovum, recorded upon a spiraling strand of DNA, is one-half of the design that will become another human. As we consider the heritage of the genes upon which the DNA message is recorded, we learn that the message, at least in part, has been there for ages, within each ancestral generation, waiting for the moment when it would take the first step toward being. We learn that the message within the egg as well as the messages in all body cells were programmed for expression at a later date. Some messages function to mature the woman or man, some promote conception, some sustain pregnancy, and others bring closure to some processes, such as stopping bone growth at puberty and menopause in women.

The ancestral message to bring closure to the reproductive process in women was inscribed upon fusion of paternal sperm and maternal egg, and that first cell division, waiting until menopause for transcription.

Menopause began at conception.

Certain environmental factors may affect when these life messages are expressed. By and large, however, what is expressed in the form of menstruation, ovulation, conception, pregnancy, lactation, menopause, and even premenstrual changes are phenotypic (what we see in terms of bodily appearance, or metabolic activities) manifestations of our ancestral heritage. Evolutionary biologists would argue that these characteristics were selected to ensure survival of the human species. Yet, they are not totally understood. The means by which sexual reproduction occurs in mammals is fundamental to the maintenance of human life. Survival of the species depends upon the female's ability to express the appropriate ancestral messages, which means preparing for pregnancy (via the menstrual cycle) and facilitating intrauterine gestation if conception occurs.

We know now that in females, many biological events precede the fusion of egg and sperm. These events must occur in a precise order–selection and development of one follicle, ovulation, corpus luteum maintenance, cyclic changes in the endometrium, species-specific cellular recognition between sperm and egg, and intracellular and intercellular fusions. Additionally, enzyme-catalyzed reactions begin in the egg at the time of a woman's conception and continue throughout menstrual and reproductive life. All these processes depend upon precise coordination and control of a variety of hormones from the brain and the ovary, as well as the ability of reproductive target tissue to respond to hormone stimulation. Research during the last decade has contributed much toward understanding the menstrual and pregnancy cycles. Perhaps the most important contribution has been an increasing appreciation of the complexity that characterizes the regulation of these cycles.

FERTILIZATION: THE MYTH

We have been taught, and those of us who teach this material have taught it at one time or another, that the dominant actor in the book of life is the sperm; one sperm fertilizes and activates one egg. As mentioned, the traditional view advanced is: The egg is passive, and the sperm is active. The story, as it appears in texts, reads something like the following (the emphasis is mine):

The sperm fertilizes the egg. Following ejaculation (during penis-in-vagina intercourse), sperm at first tumble along in seminal fluid through a mucous-lined cervical opening into the uterus. The first phase of the journey means traversing a uterus not yet hospitable to having tadpole-like foreign objects in it. Once in the uterus, sperm become active, swishing tails, swimming toward the area where an egg may be waiting. Sperm with weak tails and small heads become weaker in a turbulent, contracting uterus, and falter, unable to turn the corner into the fallopian tubes. Sperm that swim into the tube now flagellate, driven by the vision of a fat, passive egg waiting patiently to be fertilized. So far, however, sperm have not yet had to use their heads. Brute strength provided by a flagellating tail has been the only requirement to gain access to the ciliated road to the egg. Swimming up the tube, a group of sperm "break away" to take the lead in the race. Swimming is now more forceful and coordinated; only a few thousand sperm get this far. Suddenly, the zona pellucida comes into view, the thick extracellular coat that surrounds the soft, round, sleeping, beautiful egg.

At the periphery of the zona pellucida, tail wagging stops; sperm must now use their "heads" to reach the egg. To fertilize, they must penetrate, slice their way through the zona pellucida before it hardens. At this point, it is the brightest as well as the strongest of sperm that survive. It will take more than a flagellating tail to penetrate the zona pellucida. Penetration requires that sperm recognize and bind with specific sites on the zona; the fit must be like a key in a lock. The price a sperm must pay to bind with, to unlock the zona pellucida, is to "lose its head." Nonetheless, headfirst and steadfast, the victorious sperm convulse and contort as they penetrate. But sadly, only one sperm out of the many can fertilize the egg. Fertilization means activating the egg. Only one sperm will feel the egg's embrace. Only one will conquer. For the rest, to have come this far and not penetrate, means death.

At the egg membrane, the victorious sperm fuses with the egg. Arms reach out from the egg to embrace the champion. The sperm is gently drawn into the egg in the embrace, and the egg is activated. *The sperm has fertilized the egg!* Cell division begins.

What would we do without sperm?

FERTILIZATION: THE REALITY

Fertilization is a cell fusion process, one that occurs between two gametes, one maternal, one paternal, each one containing one-half of the number of chromosomes which characterize the body cells of a species. Prior to fertilization, unlike the fictional account I just wrote, which portrays a passive egg waiting for an active sperm, metabolic activity within the egg has been substantial. An excellent review article by Paul Wassarman, published in *Science*, describes the prefertilization activity of both egg and sperm as occurring in six phases. The contemporary scientific view of "fusion" as presented by Wassarman (1987) is summarized as follows:

1. *Attachment.* In this first phase, there is a loose, nonspecific association between sperm and egg at the surface of the egg's

thick extracellular coat, called the zona pellucida (ZP). The function of the ZP is to form a protective barrier around the egg. It has several important functions, the most important of which is to facilitate entry of sperm and to prevent a lethal condition called "polyspermy" (which means entry of additional sperm into the egg) from occurring.

2. *Binding.* Sperm which have attached to the ZP bind with sperm receptors (which, technically, are called ZP receptors or ZP3), which are present in the ZP. Sperm also bind with a complementary egg-binding protein on the sperm plasma membrane. This binding is species-specific. Thus, the ZP plays a significant role in restricting interspecies fertilization. In mice, as many as 1,500 sperm were observed to bind with a single mouse egg ZP. To fully bind, however, sperm must recognize some molecular features of ZP3 receptors in a species-specific manner. Each ZP contains about a billion copies of ZP3. These receptors were synthesized and secreted along with other receptors by ovarian oocytes at puberty. At ovulation, when the egg has matured, production of ZP3 receptors has fallen to very low levels. Binding is not complete unless an egg-binding protein associated with the sperm-head plasma membrane is present. Binding is necessary in order to initiate the acrosome reaction in the sperm.

3. *The acrosome reaction.* The acrosome is a membrane-bound, lysosome-like structure (which is a bag that releases its contents). It is located in the anterior (upper) region of the sperm head, above the nucleus and below the plasma membrane. According to Wassarman, for bound sperm to penetrate the ZP and fuse with egg-plasma membrane, they must complete the acrosome reaction. Since mouse sperm have been observed to complete the reaction after binding to the ZP, it is now thought that a component of ZP induces the reaction which involves fusion of sperm plasma and outer acrosomal membranes. As a result, acrosomal contents are released, and the inner acrosomal membrane, with its membranes, is exposed.

4. *Sperm penetration of ZP.* After the acrosome reaction, sperm make their way through the ZP. Penetration is accomplished by limited dissolving (proteolysis) of the ZP.

5. *Sperm-egg fusion.* Once through the ZP, sperm can make contact with, adhere to, and fuse with an egg. The plasma membrane of the sperm head fuses with the egg-plasma membrane. Once fused, egg-plasma membrane-bound microvilli (armlike projections) cluster tightly around and interdigitate over the sperm head. As the microvilli are resorbed, a sperm is drawn into the egg in a process similar to "cell drinking." Incorporation of a sperm within the egg is thought to be by contraction of actin and myosin fibrils (similar to the process that occurs in contracting muscle). It is the fusion of one sperm with one egg that prevents fusion of additional sperm, thus avoiding polyspermy. Prevention of polyspermy is thought to be achieved through a rapid and transient change in the electrical potential of the membrane.

6. *Egg activation.* Following fusion of sperm and egg, embryonic development begins. Fusion induces what is called a cortical reaction, which then induces the zona reaction. Cortical granules are small, membrane-bound, lysosome-like granules that occupy a region of egg cytoplasm just beneath the plasma membrane. Mouse eggs contain several thousand of these granules. These granules are thought to fuse with the plasma membrane. Fusion results in the release of cortical granules and enzymes into perivitelline space. These granules then enter the ZP to induce the zona reaction minutes after fertilization. The zona reaction consists of a hardening of the ZP, resulting in a loss of ability to bind sperm. These changes are thought to constitute a backup mechanism, that is, a slower block to polyspermy.

Based upon the foregoing, perhaps a more conceptually correct definition of fertilization arises—*the egging of the sperm!* However, it is not my intent to make fertilization a dirty word. The word is indeed appropriate if used properly. It needs to convey the message that two gametes, one ova from a female of the species and one sperm from a male of the species, have fused. The intent here has been to demythify as well as demystify the high value attributed to sperm in human sexual reproduction.

Wassarman's view of the events that lead to fertilization refute ideas about egg passivity, sperm dominance, and the Aristotelian view that woman is in an arrested stage of development. Clearly, the instructive review by Wassarman suggests that it is the female of the species who has developed to the very highest level. It is the female who carries the ancestral genetic messages that make life possible, and who allows the sperm to penetrate, to fuse. It is within the female where all human life begins and where the power to "reproduce" the species exists. It is the egg that prepares for and selects a sperm. It is the female who ovulates, gestates, and lactates, not the male. It is the female who has a life within a life which reproduces life, not the male. No man can duplicate the nourishing, life-giving functions of a woman's womb. In reality, it is perhaps more likely that it is the female who is the norm in the book of life, rather than the male. Knowing that it is the female of the species who has fewer gametes (ova) available than the male who can continually produce sperm, why do the ovaries of the female (the site of the waiting ovum with the ancestral message), and the uterus (the organ that nurtures the conceptus and the growing fetus for nine months), continue to be the focus of contraceptive research which is designed to manipulate and alter the normal function of these organs?

CONTRACEPTION:
TRICKING THE EGG AND THE SPERM

In 1990, 13.8 million women in the United States and 60 million worldwide used steroidal oral contraceptives for birth control. The first concerns over the safety and health risks to women using these drugs were raised in the mid-1970s. Widespread use of oral contraceptives prompted Hellman, then newly elected President of the American Gynecological Society, in his 1975 keynote address, to suggest that a therapeutic dilemma had reared its head in medicine. For the first time in recorded history, said Hellman, healthy people are taking potent drugs voluntarily over a long period for an objective other than controlling disease (1975, p. 335). The "well" people Hellman referred to were young women of reproductive age.

The first warnings about possible side effects from oral contraceptive use emerged from the United Kingdom, where an increased risk of heart attack and circulatory problems was observed (Beral, 1976). This study, which reported on 200,000 woman-years of pill use, suggested that differences in death rate from diseases of the circulatory system between those who have at any time used oral contraceptives and those who have never done so was 20 per 100,000 women per year, an increase of one death per 5,000 oral contraceptive users per year. Advocates of the hormonal method of contraception maintained that risks connected with its use were small and insignificant when compared with the risks associated with pregnancy. In Chapter 1, I discussed this aspect of risk versus benefit, indicating that the benefit of pill use may in fact override the risks, depending upon the nation and the culture of the women concerned.

Based upon the risk/benefit criteria developed in the early 1970s, oral contraceptives are declared extremely safe for young women, even though a variety of disadvantages and some serious side effects are associated with their use. For example, after more than two decades of pill use, circulatory disorders, identified in the 1970s as serious complications, are just as risky for women pill users in the 1990s, with the risk of heart disease increasing in women hormone users older than 35 who smoke. All of the known side effects associated with oral contraceptives are contained in a "patient package insert" included with each prescription.

ORAL CONTRACEPTIVES AND CANCER

Whether or not the hormone-like drugs in oral contraceptives cause cancer has been a source of continuing debate, particularly because of the known long latency period that is possible between exposure to a carcinogen (a substance that can cause cancer) and clinical manifestations of cancer. An example of the temporal aspects of cancer latency tragically surfaced years after some women in the 1940s and 1950s took the drug diethylstilbestrol (DES), a synthetic estrogen-like compound, to prevent miscarriages. Women exposed to the drug while in their mothers' wombs 10 to 20 years later developed cancer of the vagina, miscarried when pregnant, experienced ectopic (out of the womb) pregnancies, and/or birthed premature babies. Another example of latency between time of carcinogen exposure and clinical appearance of cancer is the increased rate of breast cancer in the women who took DES to prevent miscarrying. Twenty years had to elapse before the rate of breast cancer was observed to increase in these women when compared to women who had not taken DES.

As the twenty-first century rushes toward us, proponents of hormonal methods of contraception are very excited about six new progesterone-only approaches to birth control. These methods offer protection from pregnancy for periods ranging from three months, via injection of Depo-Provera, to up to five years with the new implant, Norplant. Norplant involves a minor surgical procedure to implant small silicone tubes beneath the surface of the skin. These tubes contain the progestin levonorgestrel, which periodically enters (diffuses into) the systemic circulation.

Of great concern is whether or not breast cancer will be latently expressed in any specific group of women oral contraceptive users, for example, progestin-only users, users prior to first-term pregnancy, users with fibrocystic breast disease, users whose breast cancer was diagnosed at a young age or premenopausally, or long-term oral contraceptive users. During almost three decades of oral contraceptive use, the incidence of breast cancer in general has increased steadily, with the most dramatic increase occurring over the last five years. About 11,700 women under age 40 are diagnosed with breast cancer each year. Breast cancer in these women is a different and more aggressive disease than that which develops in older women. More younger than older women are apt to choose a hormonal method of contraception. Younger women have been identified as at risk for breast cancer if they began pill use before age 20 and if they were on the pill for ten years or more. The connection between pill use and breast cancer in young women is alarming.

Methods of birth control that have been developed in contemporary society are said to reflect the technological state of development of a society, but not necessarily the evolution of an advanced civilization in which there is major concern for the safety of all individuals. The World Health Organization definition of health makes clear that everyone has a fundamental right to the highest attainable standard of health without distinction of one's race, religion, sex, politics, or socioeconomic status. Whether women who use drugs and devices and surgical means to prevent conception enjoy the highest attainable standard of health is questionable. No male oral contraceptive has been marketed to stop spermatogenesis, although one, gossypol, has been developed, but it is viewed as risky because of undesirable side effects, such as impotence or slow return of fertility. And no internal device, similar to the IUD for women, has been developed for implantation within the testes, spermatic cord, or penis. Vaccines and drugs are being studied. In 1976, the proportion of male and female surgical sterilizations was about equal. By 1982, the percentage of female sterilizations had increased more than vasectomies even though vasectomy in men is a simpler and less risky procedure.

I have wondered for some time whether a higher standard of health has been established for males. Will they, in the future, be willing to alter their reproductive physiology as women now do with invasive drugs and devices to control fertility? If women continue to assume all of the risks associated with birth control, what are the short-term as well as the long-term implications, whether for women's reproductive capability, and thus, survival of the human species, or for women's health in general? Are we at risk of fulfilling Margaret Atwood's compelling and chilling fictional and futuristic story of how societal institutions, to include sexual reproduction of the species, were restructured following widespread environmental pollution, drug use, and various other abuses? In Atwood's *The Handmaid's Tale*, a small group of powerful men controlled the society. Only a small group of women escaped the effects of pollution on fertility. These women were used as breeding stock to maintain the society.

Contraceptives developed for women, based upon an assumption that spermatogenesis is more important than the totality of woman's contributions to the process of sexual reproduction, may make Atwood's *Tale* more truthful than fiction. In fact, we may be closer than we think. It will be unfortunate indeed if, in the end, we learn that the scientists who created the drugs and devices for use by women have instead created problems related to women's health, not the well-intended solution.

In 1990 the Food and Drug Administration (FDA) instructed manufacturers to revise labeling for oral contraceptive products to reflect current scientific opinion that the benefits associated with the pill for contraception for healthy nonsmoking women over 40 may outweigh the possible risks. Even though the FDA acknowledged that an increased risk of cardiovascular disease could be linked with oral contraceptive use, the same criteria of risk to health and life associated with pregnancy are used to argue in support of pill use.

At a 1990 Contraceptive Technology conference, no paper presented discussed new methods of fertility control for men. In fact, the opening paper at this conference was titled "New Technologies in Contraception–Norplant Implants." It is a progesterone drug which, when implanted under a woman's skin provides contraceptive action for almost five years. Reproductive engineers described the implant as the most exciting contraceptive prospect since the pill.

In 1993, Norplant was approved by the FDA for contraceptive use in U.S. women.

SECTION II.
THE MENSTRUAL CYCLE

To understand menopause, the closure of menstrual life, it is first necessary to understand the events that precede it: conception and fertilization, menarche, the menstrual cycle, and menstruation. Women are genetically programmed to begin and end menstruations. Over a period of 30-plus years, a woman's body undergoes periodic changes, directed specifically toward conception, the union of sperm and egg. If no union occurs, the uterine lining is shed and the cycle begins anew. Until recently, knowledge of the menstrual cycle was generated mainly through myth and folklore, or research based upon faulty assumptions which implied that during the premenstrual phase of the cycle, women were unstable, out of control, and needed treatment ranging from drugs to psychotherapy. Each source of information has had its own unique impact on how the menstrual cycle is viewed today, and each is discussed in the sections that follow.

Indeed, there is no denying that the menstrual cycle is a hormonal event. A woman no sooner stops menstruating, and she is already days into the next series of hormonal fluctuations. Menstruation is also a periodic and bloody event, but it is not as regular as the lunar cycle, and the quality of the bleeding changes from menarche to menopause. Each aspect of the cycle, whether the beginning or the end, is surrounded by its own unique batch of myths and misconceptions, resulting in confusion for women and clinicians alike. In this section, the basic information necessary to understand the menstrual cycle, with the pregnancy cycle and the phenomenon of menstruation as a biological process, is presented. The events that resulted in the medicalization of menstrual/reproductive phenomena are also discussed.

If the menstrual cycle is viewed as a medical and/or pathological event, it is no surprise to find that this same view extends into menopause. Instead of now having to deal with wild and/or excessive amounts of hormones circulating in the body, at menopause women are faced with the prospect of disease as these same hormone levels wane.

As indicated elsewhere, as women, we're damned if we do, and damned if we don't—menstruate, that is.

Chapter 3

The Menstrual Cycle
as a Hormonal Event

Among the normal phenomena of a woman's life is the recurring cycle of potential motherhood. Every three or four weeks a new ovum, or egg, matures in the ovary and undergoes certain chemical changes which send into the blood a substance called a hormone—a messenger—stimulating the mucous membrane of the womb into making its velvet pile longer and softer and its nutrient juices more abundant in readiness for the ovum. The same stimulus causes the whole organism to make ready for a new life. The phenomenon as a whole is a physiological function and should be accompanied by a sense of well-being and comfort as in the exercise of any other function, such as digestion or muscular activity. Only too often, however, it is dreaded as an unmitigated disaster, a time for giving up work or fun and going to bed with a hot water bottle until the worst is over. (Jackson and Salisbury, 1921, pp. 305-306)

Almost one-half of a woman's life is spent in a body that is in a constant, regulated state of change as a result of cyclic fluctuations in a variety of hormones. Estrogen and progesterone are the primary sex hormones synthesized in a woman's body by the ovaries and released into the circulation. During prime reproductive years, the concentration of these hormones in the blood rises and falls cyclically with the phases of the menstrual cycle. To fully understand the menstrual cycle, its various phases, and menstruation requires first that we return to wombworld.

GENETIC SEX

Every month from the time of sexual maturation (puberty), as beautifully described by Jackson and Salisbury, the human female prepares for a possible pregnancy. Both males and females at puberty enter what has been defined as the period of "genital" sex. The key event in the female at this time is the development of an egg or ovum (or oocyte). In the male, it is the development of sperm. These differences in sexual function between males and females depend on whether or not the male contributes an X or a Y chromosome at the time of fusion of sperm and egg. (As discussed in Chapter 2, both sperm and egg must undergo certain reactions in order for fusion to occur, and recent evidence puts the egg in the driver's seat related to control, and shows that it is the egg that is most active, not the sperm, in the formation of a new life.)

If, on the union of the sperm and egg, the contribution from the father is a Y chromosome, the offspring will be a genetic male. At the time of puberty, this individual will have functional male gonads (testes) and will be a "genital" male. If the combination is two X chromosomes, the offspring will be a genetic female. And, likewise, at puberty, this individual will have functional female gonads (ovaries).

DEVELOPMENT OF OVA (EGGS)

As early as about the sixth week of embryonic age in the genetic female, about 2,000 amoeba-like germ cells (which are precursors to the eggs) migrate from a specialized region of the embryo (the yolk sac specifically) with a full set of chromosomes—23 from the female ova and 23 from the male sperm—to a "genetic" female's ovary. After the eighth week of embryonic development, the number of germ cells in the ovary increase exponentially through cell division. At five months postconception, the developing genetic female, now defined as a "fetus," has about seven *million* eggs (oocytes), which are now contained in follicles. From this time onward, the follicles will begin a degenerative process, so that at birth between 500,000 and two million oocytes remain (depending on who you read). At menarche, it is estimated that 300,000-400,000 oocytes remain, and most of these eggs in follicles are destined for spontaneous degeneration. At menopause only a few remain. Why the destructive process is so pernicious is unknown. The process of degeneration continues during childhood, adolescence, and throughout the reproductive years. Only an occasional egg actually ovulates, and when one does, selection appears to be random.

Let's look at a few examples. If a woman experiences menarche at around age 12 and menopause at age 50, she has the potential of ovulating on average 12 times for each of the 38 years. This would mean the possibility of 456 ovulations. The work of Vollman informs us that until about age 21 or 22, and between ages 40 and 50, about 20 percent of the menstrual cycles are anovulatory (meaning that no egg is released). On average, then, a woman could ovulate *less than 400 times* during a menstrual life of 38 years.

From the thousands of primary follicles formed while *in utero*, a few develop when circulating levels of FSH start to rise prepubertally. The work of Sherman and Korenman provides evidence that the rise in FSH begins years before puberty. At menarche, the onset of the first genital bleed, certain structural and functional changes have occurred in the brain, the ovary, and the uterus, which now commence operation to initiate menstrual cyclicity.

MENSTRUAL CYCLE PHASES

Generally, the menstrual cycle, for purposes of discussion, is divided into phases. I have chosen to discuss it in terms of the following four phases: follicular, ovulatory, luteal, and menstrual. Each phase as an endocrine event will be discussed separately. An understanding of menstrual cycle endocrinology is critical if one is to understand the changes that occur normally during each cycle, how to monitor the cyclic changes, and how the cycle is manipulated with steroid contraceptives, devices, and hormone replacement at menopause.

Follicular or Proliferative Phase, Days 6 to 14

This phase is also referred to as the proliferative phase of the uterine endometrium. Understanding this phase of the cycle is basic to understanding the rationale for treating menopausal women with hormone replacement—a combination of progesterone and estrogen hormone.

During the menstrual phase of the cycle, new follicles in the ovary have begun to mature. Under the influence of follicle stimulating hormone, which is synthesized and secreted from the anterior pituitary gland at the base of the brain, several follicles on the ovary begin to increase in size; some reach one millimeter.

To illustrate the size of a 1 mm follicle, the following example is provided. The length of 1 cm (centimeter) is: _____. There are 10 mm in 1 cm. Therefore, if you divide the 1 cm line into 10 equal parts, 1 part would represent the size of the follicle.

However, most of the follicles do not reach this size; they grow to a diameter of about one-half to one millimeter, and then become atretic, that is, they degenerate and die. Why some follicles are selected for development and some are not is not known. Was the decision for follicle development made in the previous cycle a so-called priming effect? Or, more plausibly (in terms of the best chance for species survival), was the selection process purely chance–with nothing predetermined? The current hypothesis regarding which follicle is selected is that the first follicle that is able to respond to FSH achieves an early lead, not because of its size, but because it is able to synthesize and secrete estrogens. During the phase of follicular development, there is little change in the blood level of the ovarian hormones, estrogen and progesterone. The follicles need to reach a certain level of maturation before an appreciable amount of hormone synthesis occurs. Also, developing follicles will not reach full size or synthesize estrogen until luteotrophic hormone (LH), the other trophic hormone synthesized in the pituitary gland, is introduced, which is between days 9 and 13 of the cycle.

The second event to occur during the follicular phase of the cycle is *steroidogenesis*, an endocrinological term which means synthesis of steroids. In this case, estrogen now is synthesized in the follicles. As the follicular synthesis of estrogen commences, one follicle becomes more sensitive to FSH and continues to increase in size.

As estrogen synthesis increases, the concentration of the hormones increases in the blood. The uterus responds to increasing levels of estrogen by renewing the endometrium, the lining of the uterus, which had been shed during the previous menstruation. The changes in the uterus initiate what is referred to in the literature as the *proliferative phase* of the endometrial cycle. Regeneration of the endometrium may begin as early as the first few days after menstruation. As estrogen is synthesized in the ovarian follicle, the effect is to promote endometrial cell division, which increases the number of cells. The important point here is that as long as estrogen is present, the uterine cells will continue to divide and increase in number. Estrogen's job is to build up that uterine endometrium. If progesterone is not present, the cells in the uterus will keep dividing and increasing in number.

Under normal conditions, during prime reproductive years, as estrogen levels continue to rise, they function as a negative feedback mechanism at the level of the hypothalamus and the anterior pituitary to suppress the secretion of brain hormones (releasing and trophic hormones). Critical to this phase is the suppression of FSH. About midcycle, say day 14 (and here one needs to pick a magic number because the number of days women spend in this phase of the cycle varies), degenerative changes occur in the collagen of the follicular cell membrane to weaken this area of the cell. These changes must occur if the egg is to be released from the follicle in the process referred to as ovulation. The reader is referred to the *Textbook of Medical Physiology* (Guyton, 1986), *Human Reproduction* (Hafez, 1980), and *The Physiology of Reproduction* (Segal, 1974) for further reading.

Ovulatory Phase

During the ovulatory phase, the egg, or oocyte, bursts from the rupture point, i.e., the weakened area in the membrane, in a cascade of follicular cells and fluid. Prior to ovulation, however, several hormonal events must occur. First, estrogen must increase rapidly, then drop precipitously. The rise and fall of estrogen is critical because it is the increase in estrogen concentration that induces the release of luteotrophic hormone (also referred to as the LH surge) from the anterior pituitary gland at the base of the brain. The LH surge is also accompanied by an increase in FSH. Following the LH surge, more steroidogenesis occurs; that is, progesterone synthesis in the follicle increases quite dramatically. In the meantime, the released egg is swept from the surface of the ovary by the undulating open end of the fallopian tube. At this point, the egg, unlike the sperm, has its full complement of 46 chromosomes. The process of reduction division (meiosis, also called *nuclear arrest*), which had begun in fetal life and which was suspended for many years, now commences. Extrusion of the first polar body occurs, carrying the haploid (half the number of chromosomes). Then the remaining 23 chromosomes replicate once more. Only after a sperm contacts the egg is a second polar body expelled, which ensures that the egg now has 23 chromosomes to combine with the 23 chromosomes of the sperm. The process of nuclear arrest, that is, suspended reduction division, may range from 10 years before the first egg is ovulated (around puberty) to 40 years, when the last ovulation occurs at age 50 or 51.

Unlike women, men do not experience a midlife closure to reproductive life. They continue to make sperm until old age. In fact, there is an unending supply of sperm in the universe; one only needs to think about the millions of sperm contained in the ejaculate of a reproductively mature male to confirm this notion. In contrast, the number of eggs a female will ever have to ovulate is fixed, and was genetically predetermined at the time of conception. As mentioned, of the total number of eggs available at birth, great losses will occur between the time of fetal life and menarche. No research-based data are available which document the temporal trajectory of egg loss, or the metabolic transformation that occurs with age. If these data were available, we would understand why some women in their late thirties and forties, who have chosen to postpone conception have difficulty conceiving. The longer one postpones child-bearing, the greater the number of eggs lost, and the greater the number of years the egg(s) remain in a state of nuclear arrest.

When ovulation occurs, according to observations, from 5 to 10 milliliters of fluid (about one-third of an ounce) is extruded with the egg. Throughout the follicular and ovulatory phases, the uterine endometrium continues to be estrogen-dominated and continues to proliferate. Once ovulation occurs, the follicle is transformed into a yellow body, which, in reproductive endocrinological terms is called *the corpus luteum*. We now enter the luteal phase of the menstrual cycle.

Luteal Phase

During the luteal phase, the cells surrounding the follicle increase in size. They resemble yellow containers because of a pigment called *lutein*, which is characteristic of a structure called the corpus luteum. The follicle has been transformed into the corpus luteum; it is the structure that maintains pregnancy should fusion of sperm and egg occur. Then other structural changes occur. First, the corpus luteum increases in size. Then capillaries form and penetrate the cavity. If conception does not occur, about 10 or 12 days after ovulation the capillaries begin to regress (shrink). Ovulation is necessary for survival of the corpus luteum and progesterone synthesis.

During the luteal phase, estrogen secretion increases. However, the dominant sex hormone of this phase is progesterone, which is antagonistic to estrogen—in simple terms, it stops the division and rapid growth of uterine cells. Progesterone transforms the uterus into a secretory structure, one that promotes implantation of the conceptus into the uterus, and ensures that the uterine physiology is appropriate to nourish the implanted conceptus. (Knowing that estrogen is antagonized by progesterone during the normal menstrual cycle is the reason a progestin is added to estrogen replacement for menopausal women with a uterus.) Under the influence of progesterone, glycogen (sugar) storage of the uterus increases and tissue is now ready to supply much-needed energy in the form of glucose to the conceptus (now called the blastocyst, that is, a ball of cells). If there is no blastocyst to implant, the corpus luteum regresses. Estrogen and progesterone reach their highest concentrations during the midpoint of the luteal cycle. Both FSH and LH are inhibited through negative feedback of high estrogen and progesterone. If conception occurs, and blastocyst implantation is successful, pregnancy ensues. A hormone synthesized in the newly developing organism (which shortly after implantation is referred to as the embryo), human chorionic gonadotrophin (HCG) now becomes the trophic hormone to maintain corpus luteum function until the placenta is mature enough to assume the synthesis of estrogen and progesterone.

If there is no pregnancy, the corpus luteum is not able to synthesize hormones, levels of estrogen and progesterone decline, and menstruation (the discharge of endometrial cells, fluid, blood, and quite possibly an ova in nuclear arrest) commences. As menstruation begins, a new cycle is also beginning with the secretion of FSH and LH from the anterior pituitary gland (Hafez, 1980; Segal, 1974).

Menstrual Phase

In ancient times, menstrual blood set women apart from men in mysterious, magical ways. Menstrual blood flowed, but women were not disabled from such blood loss, nor did they die. Today, most people know that menstruation is not a sign of supernatural power. At a medical, scientific level, it has been characterized as a sterile inflammatory reaction, a reaction that both cleanses and protects the uterus. As progesterone and estrogen hormone levels decrease during the postovulatory phase of the cycle, blood, fluid and endometrial tissue are shed.

Menstruation is the shedding of the uterine endometrium. As a human phenomenon, the cellular mechanisms that combine to produce a menstrual discharge (cells, blood, fluid) are poorly understood. If hormone synthesis, initiated in the luteal phase of the cycle, is not maintained, endometrial tissue, which had been proliferating during the follicular phase of the cycle and then was transformed into a secretory glandular structure during the luteal phase, regresses at a rate that is parallel to a decrease in blood levels of the sex hormones.

For one to two days preceding menstruation, the endometrium is characterized by increased signs of cell injury, cell depletion, and signs of intracellular resorption and reorganization. It is injury to blood vessels via kinking and vasoconstriction that causes red blood cells to suffuse (moisten) the endometrium to cause menstruation. The endometrium has been observed to shed in layers, a result of interstitial hemorrhage (which means bleeding from the spaces between cells), which lifts a dissolving layer of tissue from cells in the underlying endometrium. Conceptualizing menstruation as a "shedding" provides support for the concept that menstrual bleeding serves as a cleansing function. Hence, a by-product of cleansing is bleeding. As each shedding layer is removed from its underlying tissue, the previously connecting vessels are torn apart and left to bleed until some mechanism induces hemostasis, which means "stopping of bleeding." What most people do not realize is that *most* of the endometrial buildup, which includes fluid and cellular material(s), is resorbed. Technically, the endometrial buildup that is shed, and that is commonly referred to as menstruation, is "menstrual discharge." On average, the material that is shed accounts for about one-fourth of the total amount of endometrial buildup, which is about 26 milliliters of fluid (about equal to one fluid ounce). This estimate of loss is appropriate for healthy women in prime reproductive years when the system is mature, and for women who experience regular ovulatory menstrual cycles. However, whether the same resorptive process occurs as women make the transition to menopause when the bleeding pattern changes is unknown. There is reason to believe that the efficiency of the resorptive and bleeding processes changes since a common complaint of perimenopausal women is heavy bleeding, sometimes with blood that gushes and with the passing of clots.

The absolute temporal parameters of the duration of the bleeding interval are yet to be established. Alan Treloar's research on menstrual interval informs us that at age 20, the central 90 percent of all menstrual intervals recorded could be expected to fall between 22.1 and 38.4 days. He also cautioned that what is true on average may be anything but true in the individual experience. From this perspective, it appears that Grahn's (1993) theoretical position that the lunar and menstrual cycles are synchronized is premature. What does it mean to women whose bleed onsets do not synchronize with the lunar cycle?

A continuing lack of research-based information on menstrual cycle interval and menstrual blood is due to several factors. First, even though tampons and "sanitary" napkins are openly advertised on TV and in magazines, there are unspoken taboos about menstruation. According to Root (1992), women first and foremost view menstruation as a burden. Manufacturers of feminine care products view it as a dirty process that needs sanitizing. Women do not identify with menstruation as a within-the-body experience. Root discovered that women described menstruation as an outside-of-the-body experience, that is, *"It came last night, and it was painful; it is a curse."* These attitudes of shame, secrecy, burden, etc., carry over into society in general. To provide a personal example, when Dr. Phyllis Mansfield and I applied for funding to study the components of menstrual blood (which meant collecting used menstrual pads and tampons) in order to document how the pattern of menstruation changes premenopausally, while not outrightly disapproved on scientific grounds, we were not given a great deal of encouragement to resubmit our research proposal.

If menstruation is kept hidden, secret, or as something to be avoided, it will be next to impossible to collect the data needed in order to dispel myths—that there exists synchrony between the lunar and menstrual cycle; that menstruation rids the uterus of pathogens; that women who take oral contraceptives can regulate bleeding, etc. The schedules for oral contraceptive use are based on the myth of regularity of the 28- to 29-day menstrual cycle. Taking the pill lets women menstruate (and so they still feel feminine, like a woman), without large amounts of messy bleeding or pain, and without having the expense of purchasing tampons and pads of various absorbencies. Women on the pill are led to believe that they are now able to regulate the menstrual cycle, and indeed, when they stop taking the pill, they do induce a bleed. What women do not realize is that in place of regulating pregnancy and menstrual bleeding, they have *de*regulated their reproductive endocrinology. They have, in effect, turned off the brain control center. They continually flood their bodies with estrogen and progesterone. And in so doing, they may be increasing their risk of breast cancer and other diseases.

We can hypothesize, poeticize, romanticize, even exorcise about the meaning of menstruation to society, and the function of menstruation for a woman. While such rhetoric makes for interesting reading, what is needed are studies grounded in the reality of woman's experience, studies that continue Treloar's work related to documenting the menstrual interval, and studies that describe the nature of the bleeding process and the bleeding interval. Neither researchers nor clinicians agree on the defining characteristics associated with a menstrual interval or a bleed. Is a spot a bleed? Is a spot, followed by nothing, then a spot, and then gushing bleeding for three days a normal menstrual bleed? Is a light bleed of 17 days, a normal bleed? Is passing of clots with bleeding normal? We do not have the answers to these questions. And because we do not, the risk to women's health increases, since any departure from the mythical 28-day cycle, with a five- to seven-day bleed, is viewed as a dysfunctional cycle or dysfunctional bleeding that needs to be treated. Dr. Mansfield and I, and other menstrual cycle researchers, are working on this problem of definition. More detailed discussion on how the pattern of menstrual bleeding (discharge) changes is found in Chapter 12.

Chapter 4

The Menstrual Cycle
as a Periodic Event

The onset of menstruation is evidence that control mechanisms and the reproductive system have reached a certain stage of development. Contrary to current beliefs, we do not know exactly when, following menarche that ovulation occurs on a regular basis. Treloar (1967) and Vollman (1977) documented that women do not establish typical or regular menstrual cycles immediately. In fact, full maturation of the reproductive system, as shown by a regularity in menstrual cycle interval (from start of one bleed to start of another), is not complete until around age 23 or 24, about a decade beyond the time of the first menstruation. Until full sexual maturity is reached, a high percentage of menstrual cycles are said to be anovulatory, which means that ovulation has not occurred. Equating menstruation with ovulation and assuming that if a woman menstruates that she also ovulates is a common misunderstanding of menstrual cycle function.

MENARCHE, THE FIRST BLEED

Menarche is the first menstrual bleed. It is also a time of sexual maturation for females, which may also be correctly referred to as puberty. On average, menarche occurs between 12.8 and 13.2 years of age. Prior to menarche, certain body changes occur: gain in height and weight, development of secondary sex characteristics (breast bud development), and growth of pubic and underarm hair. Internally, changes are also occurring. Most important for reproductive purposes is the maturation of the ovaries and the uterus. Menarche may occur any time between ages 9 and 16.

Prepubertal growth and development does not occur without accompanying morphological changes in the structure and shape of the body. Tanner (1973, 1978) documented body composition changes that occur as part of the growth and development of pubescent males and females. Generally, between the ages of 11 and 16 years, the female breasts achieve their full development. This development is hypothesized to occur as a result of changes in fat metabolism. Development of the rounded mature female proportions, the typical feminine figure, is due to fat deposits on the hips, extending down into the thighs midway between the knee and the tip of the thigh bone, the buttocks, the inner arms and the lateral aspects of the back of the arms. Fat is also deposited in the middle of the back, below the neck. The reader is referred to Golub (1992) for additional information of prepubertal growth and development.

MENARCHE AND THE IMPORTANCE OF FAT

Whether or not a critical amount of body fat is really necessary and/or is the trigger for menarche is still controversial. The need to maintain a balance between a certain percent of body fat (25 to 30 percent) and lean body mass or muscle tissue is important throughout the life of a woman. Frisch and McArthur suggested that the percent of body fat in females was strongly correlated to normal growth and sexual and reproductive development. They found that the onset and maintenance of regular menstrual function in women was dependent upon maintenance of a minimum weight for height, which, apparently, is representative of a critical fat storage (Frisch and McArthur, 1974). The reason is that it takes a tremendous amount of energy to grow, develop, and mature the reproductive system, and then to maintain that system for the next 35-plus years. Metabolically, fat per gram yields the greatest amount of energy in calories, around 9 calories per gram, versus 4 calories for glucose. Malnutrition, specifically undernutrition, is known to delay sexual development in both boys and girls. This relationship has also been demonstrated in other mammals. Overnutrition, as in the case of obesity (excessive body fat), is also implicated in altered reproductive function. The risks to the reproductive system due to obesity will be explained more fully in the chapter on menopause. For now, however, keep in mind that it has been known since the 1960s that obese women were at high risk for developing uterine cancer. The reason is that fatty tissue has the ability to synthesize estrogen. This estrogen is not the estrogen that is dominant during menstrual life but it does have the capability of binding with estrogen receptors, and can stimulate target tissue. The synthesis of estrogen in "extra gonadal tissue" (fatty tissue) is a lifelong process, beginning in childhood, and improving with age in both sexes. The mechanism of extra gonadal estrogen synthesis, and the benefits of such a mechanism, will be discussed more fully later. For now, it appears that we need work similar to that of Frisch and MacArthur on the menopausal end of the menstrual cycle, to see if there is indeed a correlation between time of closure of menstrual life and a woman's percent body fat.

Undernutrition during menstrual/reproductive years, like overnutrition, alters reproductive function in human females. This information is of extreme importance since more and more prepubertal girls are engaged in strenuous athletic competition. And, while parents and coaches of these girls may not consider the girls "malnourished," they have, with respect to normal development and puberty, changed their critical ratio of fat to lean tissue (e.g., less than 24 percent).

In another study, Frisch (1981) questioned whether intense exercise delayed menarche and amenorrhea in athletes. She also asked, do late maturers choose to be athletes? Frisch studied 21 college swimmers and 17 runners with a mean age of 19.1 years. The mean age of menarche of all of the athletes was 13.9 years, later than that for the population in general, at 12.8 years. When Frisch examined the mean menarcheal age of the 18 athletes who began training before menarche, the age was 15.1 years. The mean age of menarche for the athletes who went into training after they experienced their first menstrual period was 12.8 years, similar to the age of menarche for the general population. For each year a premenarcheal girl was in athletic training, menarche was delayed, on average by five months, and only 17 of the women had regular cycles. Of women who were postmenarcheal and trained athletes, 60 percent had regular menstrual periods, 40 percent were irregular, but none were amenorrheic. The effects of athletic training also resulted in the building of muscle mass, not fat, and in fact, resulted in subsequent inability to deposit the body fat characteristic of normal prepubertal development.

The moral of the fat story is: too little fat as a prepubertal child can delay menarche; too little fat as a postpubescent adolescent can delay reproductive maturation; too much fat at premenopause may prolong menstrual life.

The relationship between the amount of body fat in women, sexual maturation, and pathology at menopause, is an area that has received an increased amount of investigation, in large part due to the increased numbers of young girls in athletics. With prepubertal girls, as mentioned, the delay in sexual or reproductive maturation may result in a delay of menarche. In postmenarcheal girls, it may manifest itself in amenorrhea (no periods). This has been established from studies done on women gymnasts. The specific cause of delayed maturation and/or amenorrhea is due to a reversal of the body fat to lean tissue ratio.

There is also much attention and concern over the importance of maintenance of normal body fat due to the obsessive preoccupation in our society to be thin. In the past several decades the incidence of anorexia nervosa (inability to eat) and bulimorexia (the ingesting and subsequent vomiting or purging of huge amounts of food) has increased. These two conditions also result in delayed menarche, menstrual period irregularity, amenorrhea, and/or early menopause. In fact, some young women use these methods not just to be thin, but for contraceptive purposes as well.

Maintenance of a normal percent of body fat throughout menstrual life has other implications for women as they approach menopause. Amenorrhea due to low body fat during prime reproductive years, the years between 23 and 35 when menstrual cycles are preponderantly ovulatory, can deprive a woman of years of estrogen and progesterone. Amenorrhea and early menopause increases the risk of developing osteoporosis, which is thinning of bones, increasing the risk of fractures.

In novels and in folklore, menarche is described as a stressful time for some young women. As an example, Colleen McCullough, in her novel *The Thorn Birds*, creates the character of Meggie, dramatizing the experience of menarche as a significant turning point, as well as a time when Meggie begins to question what is happening in her body. McCullough wrote:

Just before Meggie's fifteenth birthday, as the summer heat was building up toward its stupefying peak, she noticed brown, streaky stains on her drawers. After a day or two they went away, but six weeks later they came back and her shame turned to terror. The first time she had thought them signs of a dirty bottom, thus her mortification, but in their second appearance they became unmistakably blood. She had no idea where the blood was coming from, but assumed it was her bottom. The slow hemorrhage was gone three days later, and did not recur for over two months; her furtive washing of the drawers had gone unnoticed, for she did most of the laundry anyway. The next attack brought pain, the first non-bilious rigors of her life. And the bleeding was worse, far worse. She stole some of the twins' discarded diapers and tried to bind herself under her drawers, terrified the blood would come through. (pp. 158-159)

For Meggie, as for many real, living women, a mystery had come into her life. Eventually she found the answers to her questions. She found them from a man, Father Ralph. Fortunately, he understood and answered her with compassion and supportive, validating calm. Undoubtedly, life has played out such scenes time and time again. Just as undoubtedly life has played other, less fortunate scenes. For generations, the questions women have asked about menstruation too often and too traditionally have been ignored as being either the product of "something in the head," or, if the questions were heard, the symptoms described were diagnosed as the result of disease, deficiency, and even depravity. Men, particularly, have been provided with an easy out from confronting a reality separate and different from their own. No doubt many, if not most, men actually believed their pontifications, believed so strongly in fact that women began to believe it themselves. Consequently, scientists and physicians have provided answers to questions about menarche, menstrual, and reproductive issues, but they are not necessarily the answers women need.

A question I am asked over and over again has to do with the "regularity" of menstrual bleeds following menarche. "What does regular mean? How will I know if my cycle is normal?" Once menarche occurs, an almost universal assumption is that menstrual bleeds will issue forth in a regular manner, that is, about every 28 days, and that a girl, now turned woman, is fertile once she starts to menstruate. This assumption is based upon the belief that at menarche a woman's reproductive system is mature.

Is it?

NORMAL PATTERN OF MENSTRUAL CYCLES

The normal postmenarcheal menstrual cycle pattern is characterized by irregularities in cycles, with long intervals between cycles being the *rule* rather than the exception, and a high probability that many cycles are anovulatory. I will discuss later why it is important to monitor and record menarche and subsequent menstruations in order to infer the maturity level of a woman's reproductive system. This information is especially important to have when making decisions about sexual activity, reproduction, and whether and how to contracept.

Once a woman reaches reproductive system maturity, in her twenties, the menstrual cycle pattern, unless altered through oral contraceptives, intrauterine devices, athletic activity, malnutrition, or pregnancy, will be repeated with some regularity until she reaches her forties. Most cycles are ovulatory during this period until the transition to menopause begins, when the pattern again changes, often resembling more the pattern of menstrual cycles of postmenarche.

We would not have information on the normal patterning of menstrual cycle intervals on U.S. women if it were not for the vision and curiosity of one man, Dr. Alan E. Treloar, the first director of The Tremin Trust Research Program on Women's Health (formerly known as the Menstruation Reproductive History Program). Alan had the courage to challenge traditional science and its paradigms. Listening to women, he was sensitive to their concerns about menstruation. Contrary to evidence available in the 1930s, Alan suggested that "regularity," as applied to the menstrual cycle, was a vague term, one that should not be taken literally to mean "without variation." Alan postulated that there was no such thing as an average cycle. Rather, he felt confident that if a large-scale study could be done, the results would show that not only was duration of menstrual interval between bleeds different from one woman to another, but that they would vary for each individual woman from menstruation to menstruation.

In the 1930s, when Alan made these pronouncements, I had just been born. At this time, there were no large-scale, long-term studies of menstruation and menopause. In fact, the words themselves were hardly spoken except in doctors' offices and medical books. Yet, in 1932, Alan, while on faculty at the University of Minnesota, recognized the need for such a study and took action. Three years later, the Menstruation and Reproductive History Program (MRH) began its first survey. In 1984, 50 years after its inception, and following Alan's retirement, the program found a home at the University of Utah.

REMEMBRANCES OF THINGS PAST: ANN'S VOICE

July 16, 1983, Salt Lake City, Utah

Stacy, Suresh, and I were in the laboratory working to debug the analysis program. Perhaps a few years ago I might have said to myself, "What am I doing here?" But, I knew what I was doing on that weekend in July. Hopefully, the problem with the computer would be the last problem to solve related to data analyses on the hot flash research. For several months, the computer had been infested with problems that sometimes made me want to pull my hair out; it also was a scary experience to have so much of the information we had obtained on hot flash trapped in an electronic box whose lifeline was a power cord plugged into a wall outlet.

Standing there beside Suresh and Stacey, both of whom had worked with me for several years, recalling the many men and women who have worked with me and have unselfishly given of their time and energy to find answers to questions I asked and those asked by other women, there was no question why we were there. And there was no doubt that the problems with the data analysis program would be solved.

I left the laboratory and walked to my office on the fifth floor. From that office I could see far beyond the smokestack of Kennecott Copper, adjacent to Interstate 80 and the Great Salt Lake. It was a clear day, and it was even possible to see the etchings of ancient Lake Bonneville on the distant Oquirrh Mountains to the west.

For a moment I reflected upon my own discovery journey into women's health, back to questions that I thought were mine, only to find out that my questions about menstruation were the questions asked not only by many women, but questions asked by Alan in the early 1930s. I thought a moment of Stacey and Suresh, working hard on a weekend, time they might rather have spent hiking in the Wasatch Mountains. It was late when we left. The computer program was debugged, and our analyses were run. I looked at the work that waited for me. I knew there would be a long night ahead. I did not realize at that time how many more of them would await me in the future. The following year the University of Utah acquired Alan's research program. At Alan's request, the program was renamed The Tremin Trust; "Tre" for Treloar, and "min" for Minnesota, and I was appointed the second director.

December 28, 1989, Salt Lake City, Utah

All 1,364 envelopes were stuffed with the annual mailing of The Tremin Trust Research Program. Everything had gone smoothly this year. Not so in past years. As I looked at the envelopes in boxes, ready to go to the mail room, I recalled the sequence of events that preceded the acquisition of the research program in 1984. On that table, in that box, were the names and addresses of the women who continued on as "active" participants of Alan's MRH Program. Some of these women had been recording events related to menstruation, pregnancy, births, deaths, illnesses, surgeries, menopause, etc., since enrollment in the 1930s.

I first met Alan at the 1979 Society for Menstrual Cycle Research Conference on Menopause in Tucson, Arizona, which I coordinated with Myra Dinnerstein and Sherry O'Donnell. Alan was one of our invited speakers. It was at the Tucson conference that Alan began discussions with me and other menstrual cycle researchers about locating a home for the MRH research program. He had recently retired from teaching and research after a long and distinguished career at the University of Minnesota.

ALAN'S STORY

An Australian by birth, Alan immigrated to the United States at age 26 to study the chemistry of wheat and flour. Travel to Minnesota was by way of three western provinces of Canada, to glean what he could in that wheat-growing area. On arrival at the University of Minnesota campus in St. Paul, Alan, according to his own words, *"braced for the first contacts with advisors in agricultural biochemistry and cereal chemistry."* He expressed a desire to include biometry in his studies. One of his advisor's intimate friends, J. Arthur Harris, head of the Botany Department on the Minneapolis campus, had introduced biometry to the University as a major research tool. During the 1929/30 academic year, Alan served as a research assistant to Dr. Harris. Early in April of 1930, Harris became ill with abdominal complaints (intestinal blockage?). In those days, antibiotics were just ideas in the minds of very few researchers. Surgery was recommended as the only recourse for Harris' ailment. Sadly, about a week after diagnosis, Alan wrote in his diary: *"Harris died and three months later I was appointed head of biometry at the University of Minnesota."*

Alan acknowledged that his rudimentary knowledge of biochemistry was not in any way an adequate substitute in teaching for Harris' wide-ranging experience within the natural sciences. Bewildered by this, he decided that hope lay in the possibility of illustrating points to be made if the human body was used as the object of reference. Alan admitted that his knowledge of the medical sciences was probably less than that in biochemistry. However, he felt confident because he had the experience of Harris to draw upon. All departments in the university could learn how Harris approached the interpretation of assembled data. Alan felt that they could all learn together. But he also realized that he needed to carve out his own area of research. When he uncovered data Harris had painstakingly transcribed from hospital records on length and weight of newborn infants of various nationalities, Alan decided to investigate duration of pregnancy as a variable of interest, independently of Harris' investigation. As a result, his academic interest in menstrual and reproductive events, as a scientist began. His curiosity about menstruation, however, as he described in his diary began as a boy in Australia. If Meggie, the main character in Colleen McCullough's *The Thorn Birds,* needed Father Ralph to explain the mystery of menstruation to her, pity the poor boy who, neither experiencing the event nor understanding it, had no one to turn to. Alan was such a boy, and wrote the following in his diary.

Alan's Remembrances of Things Past (Australia, Early 1900s)

A boy with five brothers in a family lacking daughters with their matching effects in obscure ways is apt to develop some imbalances in his perceptions of life. I had heard that girls of high school age are prone to periodic malaise, that there is something about bleeding at such times that I did not then understand, and that it was unforgivable to inquire openly about such matters.

When of high school age myself, our home in Sydney provided residence for a mature woman, Edith, who, when free of other engagements, served as a companion to my mother. She also worked in a large department store in the city. On one occasion I embarrassed her in the laundry where I discovered her secretly washing a piece of toweling still stained pink in places; she continued her task of their removal. Smugly pretending not to notice, I disappeared from the area. However, this bit of information fitted together with others in mind. It was my introduction to a subject that was to command a great deal of attention later in life, and set the direction of my research.

Prior to the late 1890s, diapers, mostly of flannel, were used to collect menstrual flow. Some women pinned these homemade devices as a diaper, while others folded them into pads to be pinned to underclothing. These diapers and towels were washed and reused. In 1921, the pad manufactured by Kotex became the first to be marketed as a sanitary pad. In 1936, Tampax (now known as Tambrands, Inc.) marketed the first internal tampon. Alan would not be too surprised to learn that the next challenge facing menstruating women, according to Dr. Barbara Czerwinski (1991), a menstrual cycle researcher at the University of Texas, Houston, is how to handle menstruation in space. If in this century the United States establishes a permanent human presence in space on a space station, moon colony, etc., midcentury humans (men and women) will take part in an exploratory trip to Mars from the moon. Before flying off into space, according to Czerwinski, plans needed to be made for space travel, and personal hygiene information on women needed to be obtained. Women were found to be capable of handling weightlessness, and did not have any particular problems in space because of menstruation. Menstruation was evaluated as a normal physiological function. It appears that the major problem to be solved will be how to dispose of tampons; Czerwinski found that 20 of 21 female candidates interviewed for an astronaut position were found to use tampons exclusively.

Alan's Voice Continues (St. Paul, MN, 1920s)

During the spring of 1929, after Dr. Harris' secretary (Molly, to her intimates) and I had pledged our troth, I arrived at Molly's residence as usual on a Sunday afternoon, to find her not much interested in the usual walk or drive, but looking rather pale and forlorn. It was not long before she excused herself and retired to an adjoining room and closed the door. Mystified, I pretended to read a magazine, having little interest under the circumstances. It was not long before sounds like moaning came from that room, and her mother responded to the signal. All alert, I dared to ask, "What is the matter?" The response that Molly was having "her period" was followed by more audible groans, which I felt obliged to investigate for myself. There on the bed was my betrothed, writhing in agony as I looked on helplessly. I withdrew, enveloped in a cloud of ignorance. To me, a period was a punctuation mark. But the clouds cleared a little, and my suggestion that I return whence I had come was appreciated as I left for another abode.

I had witnessed in a dramatic way a case of discomfort attending the menstrual flow. The medics had a word for it: dysmenorrhea. In Molly's case, because of its severity (for which drugs could be prescribed), the best solution recommended was to "get married." This was according to much medical opinion. In this case, marriage was in the offing, but I was to learn in time that here, as elsewhere, a fancy word was just cover for "sweeping a problem under the rug."

Early the next morning I was in the main library of the university, searching for more information about what I had seen the day before. I learned what the word dysmenorrhea meant: painful menstruation! *At this point, I resolved to make feminine genital bleeding my major research interest. And yes, Molly and I were married.*

In the spring of 1934 an attractive young lady, Esther Doerr, came to my office for advice with respect to her wish to proceed toward a Master of Science degree in Biometry. An opportunity thus presented itself for me to engage in a research project to which I had been looking forward for a long time. Esther's intellectual qualifications made her a very acceptable candidate for an advanced degree. I dared to present to her the problem of defining the human menstrual cycle in quantitative terms, based on recorded facts, to serve the best of scientific purposes. Recovering from a minor shock, she expressed a willingness to attempt the task. So was born a project in research that is still being pursued.

Our first objective was to see if young university women would be willing to keep accurate records of their menstrual flows, and let her have those records at the end of a year, for objective study. Responsibility for designing the record materials became primarily mine, although my senior assistant, Dr. Borghild Gunstad, contributed equally to accomplishing the goal. We soon had a specially designed card printed and enrollment forms ready for Esther to proceed with her part.

The card shown in Figure 4.1 (a sample from 1938) is referred to as the Menstrual Calendar Card, and continues to be used today by menstruating Tremin Trust Participants. The card has also been used by many other menstrual cycle researchers.

Meantime, our need for an appropriate sponsor had been resolved when Dr. Ruth Boynton, Director of the University Health Service, encouragingly agreed to act in that capacity. All students were met as groups, in person, by Esther (in sororities and physical education classes). She explained to the students that if the prevalent notion that menstruation occurred "regularly every 28 days" was true, then that should be established as fact; and if the notion was false, the truth should be ascertained and made available to all concerned.

Well over 1,000 students accepted Esther's invitation to study the card and form, with the result that their enrollment followed. In order that the study should be free at this stage of unnecessary extra problems, enrollment was restricted to single women—very few students in those days were married.

We expected some loss due to lapse of interest right away, when initial curiosity had been satisfied, and further defection after the extra effort involved became obstructive in some way. Rather than being disappointed with the return of 526 completed cards for the first year, we felt fortunate to have had about 50 percent success in the first try. Gratitude for this quickly turned to excitement as detailed examination showed no sign of any faked circlings of dates, as well as no sign of

FIGURE 4.1. 1938 Menstrual Calendar Card

UNIVERSITY OF MINNESOTA STUDENT'S' HEALTH SERVICE—MENTAL HISTORY STUDY

Please circle dates of onset and cessation of flow, joining them by a line passing through all days in the flow period.

C. No

Calendar year   1938   only

JANUARY
1 2 3 4 5 6 7 8 9 10 11 12 13 14 15 16 17 18 19 20 21 22 23 24 25 26 27 28

FEBRUARY
29 30 31 1 2 3 4 5 6 7 8 9 10 11 12 13 14 15 16 17 18 19 20 21 22 23 24 25

MARCH
26 27 28 1 2 3 4 5 6 7 8 9 10 11 12 13 14 15 16 17 18 19 20 21 22 23 24

APRIL
25 26 27 28 29 30 31 1 2 3 4 5 6 7 8 9 10 11 12 13 14 15 16 17 18 19 20 21

MAY
22 23 24 25 26 27 28 29 30 1 2 3 4 5 6 7 8 9 10 11 12 13 14 15 16 17 18 19

JUNE
20 21 22 23 24 25 26 27 28 29 30 31 1 2 3 4 5 6 7 8 9 10 11 12 13 14 15 16

JULY
17 18 19 20 21 22 23 24 25 26 27 28 29 30 1 2 3 4 5 6 7 8 9 10 11 12 13 14 15 16

AUGUST
15 16 17 18 19 20 21 22 23 24 25 26 27 28 29 30 31 1 2 3 4 5 6 7 8 9 10 11

SEPTEMBER
12 13 14 15 16 17 18 19 20 21 22 23 24 25 26 27 28 29 30 31 1 2 3 4 5 6 7 8

OCTOBER
9 10 11 12 13 14 15 16 17 18 19 20 21 22 23 24 25 26 27 28 29 30 1 2 3 4 5 6

NOVEMBER
7 8 9 10 11 12 13 14 15 16 17 18 19 20 21 22 23 24 25 26 27 28 29 30 1 2 3

DECEMBER
4 5 6 7 8 9 10 11 12 13 14 15 16 17 18 19 20 21 22 23 24 25 26 27 28 29 30 1

2 3 4 5 6 7 8 9 10 11 12 13 14 15 16 17 18 19 20 21 22 23 24 25 26 27 28 29 30 31

any straight line of onset dates to indicate regularity in any history, let alone a vertical line to indicate a 28-day regularity.

Provision of record cards for 1936 assured both participants and staff of a second year of data to compare with the first, and further examine the source of information for its consistency over time. There remained no doubt whatever in our minds but that the data were fully reliable, and that we were in a position not only to demonstrate a myth, but to replace it with facts of considerable dependability. We felt that two years' data from only a relatively small sample of university women might not have the necessary impact to upset long-held notions. Addition of many more cases over several years seemed most desirable, very fortunately, to Dr. Ruth Boynton.

A physical examination at the health service was required in those days of alertness of the university authorities to protect students from contagious diseases, especially tuberculosis and others that might be carried by persons apparently in good health. Ruth approved a plan to present the menstrual study opportunity to women students at the end of their physicals. The yield of enrollments each admission period was not high, but by keeping at it for three years, we secured enough new entrants to call a halt to that effort. The student loss at the end of the first year was high, and more normal losses occurred at the end and during each year, so our total enrollment of persistent recorders among these students was not much above 2,500, including the pilot members.

And did we find regularity in the menstrual cycle? Anything but! Variation so clearly characterized every history that we wondered how the word "regular" had come to be applied—not only that, but so firmly entrenched. As biometricians, we were prone to define a term like regular in a strictly mathematical sense, as straight lines of circled onset dates, which never appeared on the cards as we studied them individually and in great numbers each new year. Surely, if we were persistent enough in assembling data, we could convince those who were apt to regard the menstrual cycle as "regular" as the superlative of falsehood. We had a battle ahead of us if we chose to continue, and with that prospect clearly defined, we chose to go ahead.

And go ahead they did. Three decades later, in the 1960s, a new student group was recruited in order to identify whether or not variation in the menstrual cycle occurred over time. This time, however, enrollment of participants was done through the mail, since health examinations were performed by family physicians. The three-year recruitment effort resulted in 1,367 women.

In 1965, 1,000 Alaskan women and girls were enrolled to provide data on whether or not seasonal variations, such as the widely varying length of the solar day, influenced the menstrual cycle. All menstruating Eskimo, Aleut, and Indian women residing in nine rural villages located in the Yukon-Kuskokwin delta region of southwestern Alaska were invited to participate in the study. Later, native women in two larger commercial centers, Bethel and Barrow, were enrolled to augment the village women. After enrollment of the native women, 170 Caucasian women were enrolled in order to achieve a suitable study population and enable a closer comparison with data from the villages.

In 1967, the first research article resulting from analyses of recorded menstruation start-and-stop records kept by the 1930s panel was published in the *International Journal of Fertility*. The research reported in this article is now acclaimed as a classic by menstrual and reproductive researchers. The findings reported in this article have been overlooked by authors of medical, nursing, and other related texts, or disregarded, since the menstrual cycle continues to be defined as a regular, temporal event—namely, an event that occurs every 28 days. This belief has been institutionalized for women on the pill who have a fail-safe 28-day menstrual cycle. Women take the pill for 21 days, stop, and are off for seven days to induce a bleed. Menstrual regularity is cited as an advantage when clinicians inform women regarding risks and benefits of pill use. The concept of regularity extends into menopause as well. Women on combination hormone treatment, on estrogen and progestin, also take two hormones, just as women on the pill do, in order to have "regular" bleeds.

Let us return to Alan's findings, as reported in the 1967 article. Through the calendar year 1961, the number of person-years of menstrual history that had been recorded was 25,825 (2,702 participants who had recorded 275,947 menstrual intervals). Analyses of these data reinforced for Alan that the menstrual cycle was anything but regular. He observed that from about seven years postmenarche, the variability in menstrual interval decreased gradually until about age

20, at which time a period of *relative* stability prevailed. The analyses of menstrual interval data demonstrated clearly that over a period spanning almost 40 years, two decades, from age 21 to 39 inclusive, were the most stable. Even so, they, too, were characterized by variability in menstrual interval duration among and between women. The variability in the menstrual experience is summarized in a graph from the original article (Figure 4.2), and Table 4.1 displays in numerical form the selected percentiles for the distribution of menstrual interval by age in three zones of experience.

At menarche (in Figure 4.2, this is the beginning of menstrual year zero, or "0"), 5 percent of the menstrual intervals (duration in days between bleeds) were observed to be 18.3 days or less. Following the zero line upward on the graph, on average, 25 percent of these post-menarcheal menstrual intervals were 24.6 days or less. Continuing upward to the 50 percent line, this line is interpreted to mean that, on average, 50 percent of the menstrual intervals were less than 29.1 days in duration, and 50 percent were greater than 29.1 days. Proceeding upward to the 95 percent line, at menarche, on average, 5 percent of the intervals were estimated to be longer than 83.1 days, or 95 percent were less than this duration between bleeds. The range in menstrual duration between bleeds, then, postmenarche, is substantial: 18.3 days and lower between bleed onsets at the lower end, and more than 83 days at the upper end.

The data in Figure 4.2 also show the wide range of variability in menstrual onsets throughout menstrual life. If one follows the horizontal line on the graph from menstrual year zero (0) at menarche, to two years later, menstrual year 02, and moves upward along the menstrual year 02 line, all values for menstrual interval duration have decreased substantially from year zero, albeit still exhibiting variability. Moving along the graph to the right, at each menstrual year from year 02 onward, menstrual interval duration continues to decrease until, at about menstrual year 07, when, generally speaking, they approach the recorded patterns for women at chronological age 20.

Alan and his colleagues decided to categorize the data as "menstrual year," "chronological age," and "premenopausal year." As such, the data displayed in the graph are divided into these three zones. An examination of the middle zone, ages 20 to 40, labeled "chronological age" on the graph, indicates that on average women can expect to experience about 20 years of relative regularity of menstrual intervals before the transition to menopause begins. Variability in menstruation onset from one bleed to the next decreased from chronological age 20 to 40. This general trend is shown in the middle section of the graph. To appreciate fully the data displayed in this zone, one needs to follow the lines for the chronological ages 20 and 40 upward to the 95 percent line. Alan cautioned, however, that one needs always to keep in mind that what is true on the average may be anything but true in the individual experience.

Moving along on the horizontal line now to the third zone, premenopausal year, the graph indicates that on average, the change in duration of menstrual interval is rapid, and attains more extreme values, albeit inversely, than the postmenarcheal variation, continuing until menopause. Transition to menopause, the closure of menstrual bleeding, appears to occur more slowly in terms of time to reach the end point, when compared with the data on the graph for menarche. For example, on average, about seven years are required from menarche to reach the stable, normal middle zone pattern of menstrual interval. What is important to keep in mind as one examines data in the third zone on the graph is that as women make the transition to menopause, they pass from the most stable and regular years in duration between menstrual bleeds, to a period which is dominated by more variability than that found in either the menstrual or chronological zones. Alan and colleagues concluded from this observation that increasing variability in menstrual interval, with long durations between bleeds, premenopausally, could be considered normal.

That women smoothly make the transition from the comparative regularity of the "middle life" years between 20 and 40 over a period of many years for both the postmenarcheal and premenopausal experience may be new information to many. In fact, an examination of the data in the graph and the table suggests that the transition to menopause appears to be very much a mirror image of the menarcheal pattern of change in menstrual interval, again keeping in mind the temporal differences in the two zones, seven versus eight years.

A plot of menstrual intervals of one woman who recorded menstruations on the MRH Menstrual Calendar Card, from time of enrollment in the program until menopause is shown in Figure 4.3.

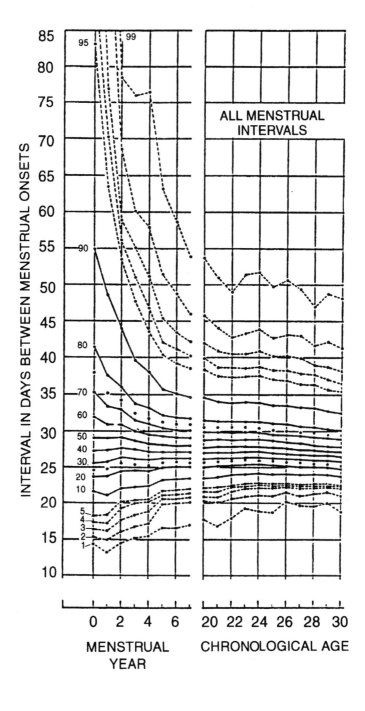

FIGURE 4.2. Contours for the Frequency Distribution of All Menstrual Intervals in Three Zones of Experience

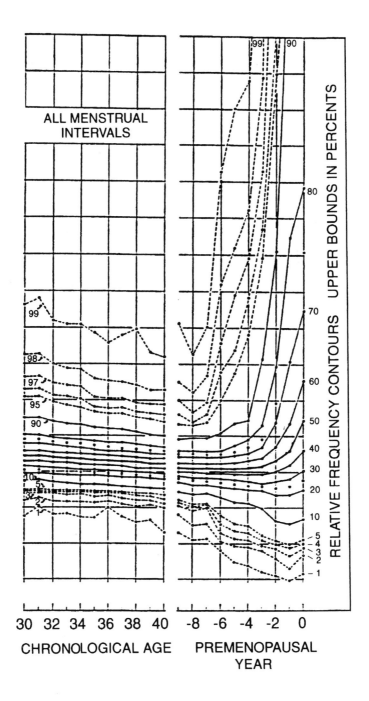

ALL MENSTRUAL
INTERVALS

UPPER BOUNDS IN PERCENTS

RELATIVE FREQUENCY CONTOURS

99
98
97
95
90

10
5

1

99   90

80

70

60

50

40

30

20

10

5
4
3
2
1

30 32 34 36 38 40

CHRONOLOGICAL AGE

-8 -6 -4 -2   0

PREMENOPAUSAL
YEAR

TABLE 4.1. Selected Percentiles for the Distribution of Menstrual Interval by Age in Three Zones of Experience for All Subjects Collectively

Age Scale	Year	Number of Intervals	Percentiles						
			5	10	25 (Q₁)	50 (median)	75 (Q₂)	90	95
Postmenarche	0	522	18.3	21.6	24.6	29.1	38.0	54.9	83.1
	1	2,080	18.4	21.1	24.8	29.1	35.2	48.6	63.5
	2	2,435	20.2	22.0	25.6	29.2	34.3	44.0	53.5
	3	2,546	20.4	22.2	25.4	28.7	32.5	39.6	47.7
	4	3,157	20.6	22.4	25.3	28.3	31.8	38.1	43.6
	5	4,909	21.7	23.3	25.7	28.2	31.3	35.8	40.4
	6	7,097	21.8	23.4	25.8	28.0	31.0	35.1	39.2
	7	9,488	22.0	23.5	25.7	28.1	31.0	34.7	38.6
Chronologic	20	4,928	22.1	23.5	25.7	27.8	30.6	34.6	38.4
	21	8,692	22.2	23.7	25.8	27.9	30.6	34.0	37.5
	22	10,968	22.5	24.0	25.9	27.9	30.6	33.9	37.4
	23	11,259	22.7	24.1	26.1	27.9	30.6	34.0	37.5
	24	10,904	22.8	24.2	26.0	27.9	30.5	33.9	37.6
	25	10,548	22.7	24.1	25.9	27.8	30.2	33.6	37.1
	26	10,055	22.7	24.1	25.7	27.7	30.1	33.6	36.9
	27	9,734	22.6	24.0	25.7	27.5	29.9	33.3	36.4
	28	9,585	22.7	24.1	25.6	27.4	29.8	33.2	36.4
	29	9,426	22.7	24.0	25.5	27.3	29.6	32.8	35.7
	30	9,255	22.5	23.8	25.3	27.2	29.5	32.5	35.4
	31	9,100	22.6	23.9	25.3	27.2	29.5	32.6	35.5
	32	9,286	22.4	23.6	25.1	27.0	29.2	32.0	34.8
	33	9,340	22.4	23.4	25.0	26.9	29.0	31.7	34.3
	34	9,259	22.4	23.3	24.9	26.8	28.9	31.6	34.0
	35	9,278	22.3	23.3	24.9	26.7	28.7	31.2	33.4
	36	8,957	22.3	23.2	24.8	26.6	28.4	31.0	33.2
	37	8,970	22.2	23.0	24.7	26.5	28.3	30.9	33.2
	38	8,863	22.1	22.9	24.6	26.4	28.2	30.6	32.7
	39	8,412	22.0	22.8	24.5	26.2	28.0	30.2	32.4
	40	8,393	21.8	22.7	24.4	26.2	27.9	30.1	32.0
Premenopause	−9	1,451	21.1	22.3	24.1	25.6	27.5	29.6	31.7
	−8	1,462	20.5	21.9	23.8	25.5	27.5	29.7	31.5
	−7	1,462	20.6	22.0	23.7	25.5	27.4	29.7	31.9
	−6	1,502	18.9	21.4	23.5	25.5	27.5	30.4	35.1
	−5	1,551	17.8	20.8	23.3	25.5	27.8	31.8	38.8
	−4	1,505	17.5	20.6	23.1	25.6	28.4	32.2	44.2
	−3	1,439	16.2	19.9	23.0	25.8	29.6	40.8	54.7
	−2	1,274	15.4	18.2	22.8	26.6	34.7	55.5	80.0
	−1	915	14.9	17.8	23.0	27.9	48.2		
	0	360	15.6	18.4	23.9	32.2	55.4		

FIGURE 4.3. A Complete History of Menstrual Intervals from Menarche to Menopause

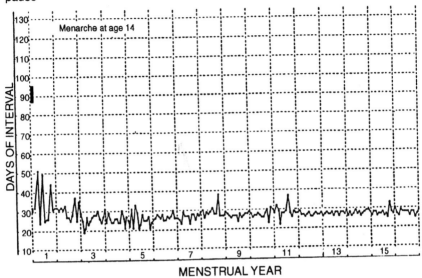

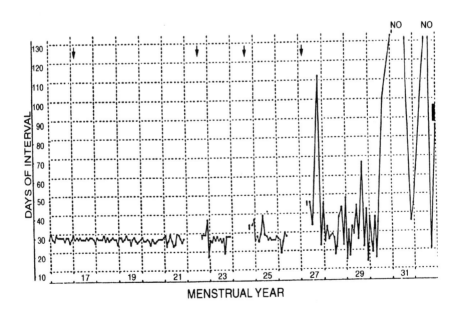

What factors contribute to the variability in menstrual interval among women and within individual women is not known. Certainly, the status of a woman's health, as well as stress level, has the potential to affect menstruation onset. Related to the stress factor, when practicing nursing, it was not unusual for me to hear young women patients who had just had surgery say, "My period started and it wasn't due for another week!" Certainly, nutrition and body fat, as mentioned previously, are important factors. Root did an extensive review of the literature to identify whether there was an association between life events as stressors that could affect menstrual outcome. She cautioned that linear causality is probably an inappropriate assumption (Root, 1992). Yet, most menstrual studies rely upon alterations in menstrual cycle duration to support that stress affects a woman's cycle.

Two studies, discussed by Root, showed clear evidence of hormonal and/or anatomical affects associated with stress. In one instance, a physician in London during World War II examined the endometrial tissue of women who had been close to bomb explosions and who had become amenorrheic. The pathologist's report indicated that endometrial development in these women had been arrested. In another situation, frequent blood hormone assays were done on two women admitted to a hospital to evaluate the effect of hospitalization on the menstrual cycle. In both women, hormone levels indicated that ovulation was delayed until the women were released from hospital.

Until we have more information on factors that affect menstrual interval, it is important to keep Alan's words in mind: *"Did we find regularity in the menstrual cycle? Anything but! Variation so clearly characterized every history that we wondered how the word regular had come to be applied."*

Instructions on how to record menstrual interval using Alan's Menstrual Calendar Card are included in Section IV, Keeping Records and Keeping in Touch.

MENSTRUATION WHILE ON ORAL CONTRACEPTIVES

Using contraceptives too early, whether through chemical or mechanical means (the pill, IUD, sterilization, progesterone implants, etc.) increases health risks for young women. These risks to health are compounded if the reproductive system has not yet reached complete maturity. Interference in the normal process of growth and development of the reproductive system could delay maturation (delay menarche, or delay onset of regular periods), prevent normal growth and development of reproductive target tissue (this will be discussed in more detail in Chapter 16, "Estrogen and Hormone Treatment: Cancer Risks"), and increase the risk for developing a chronic disease. For example, current research on the risk of breast cancer with oral contraceptive use suggests the possibility of a minimally increased risk among women ages 20 to 24.

Presently, a woman who wishes to use oral contraceptives, which are a combination of estrogen and progesterone, must consult a physician or nurse practitioner and undergo a physical examination. An attempt to sell oral contraceptives over the counter recently met with defeat. The issue, according to Planned Parenthood Federation of America, is not safety. Rather, the concern is that little is known about what motivates people to use birth control, and at what cost. Some scientists believe that birth control pills are safe, and are the most effective way to prevent pregnancy. Selling them over the counter, without a prescription, would be the easiest way for the greatest number of women to obtain them, and it would give women more control over their own health. Self-care advocates believe that easy availability would help to break up what is perceived as a physician monopoly on providing health care to women. An official of Population Action International, a family planning organization with an overseas focus, believes that women can and do take the pill correctly, without having to go to a doctor. Yet, safety *is* an issue. The National Women's Health Network opposed having the pill sold over the counter. Long an advocate for the safety of products and drugs marketed and targeted for women, Cynthia Pearson, then the Network's Program Director, stated that the major reason the network opposed selling oral contraceptives over the counter is the growing evidence related to the increasing risk for breast cancer in young women who start on the pill before age 20, and stay on it for long periods (Neus, 1993).

Related to young women and oral contraceptive use, the one question clinicians ask most frequently of the editors of *Contraceptive Technology* is: When can a young teenager start taking birth control pills? Of course, "teenager" here translates into "young woman," not "young man." The answer provided by the Hatcher group is that,

> Ideally, one would like young teenagers to have from six to twelve regular periods before they start pills. However, if a young teenager is already having sexual intercourse, the medical and social risks of pregnancy probably exceed the risks of her taking OCs, even if she has not started having menstrual periods. (Hatcher et al., 1990, p. 250)

No information is available to indicate that it is safe for a prepubescent female to take oral contraceptives other than that which relates to estrogen and growth of long bones. The estrogen found in current low-dose oral contraceptives does not appear to limit height due to premature closure of the epiphyses (ends of long bones that promotes growth of bones).

The menstrual bleed that pill users experience is not a natural bleed; it is one that has been induced as a result of endogenous hormones. A pill-induced bleed is brought about by withdrawing estrogen and progesterone contained in the oral contraceptive. The concentration of the two sex hormones, as well as the kind of progestogenic agent contained in the pill, varies. The concentration of the hormones is much lower than it was when the pill was first marketed in the 1960s. No matter. The mechanism of action is the same: Oral contraceptives are designed to prevent ovulation. Preventing ovulation prevents conception. Preventing conception means preventing pregnancy. Preventing ovulation means that the normal function of the menstrual cycle has been altered, that is, follicle stimulating hormone and luteinizing hormone (LH), normally secreted from the anterior pituitary gland, are suppressed. Prevention of ovulation is primarily due to the estrogenic component of the pill. The progestogenic effects change the consistency of the cervical mucus, which impedes sperm transport, transforming the endometrium into a hostile environment in the event that breakthrough ovulation and fertilization occur. The most immediate and expected effect of the pill, then, is the disturbance in the hypothalamic-pituitary-ovarian function. In other words, the normal feedback mechanism of regulation of the menstrual cycle *by the brain* has been shut down.

Earlier I expressed concerns related to long-term health implications for women who use oral contraceptives. In the early days of high-dose oral contraceptives, women pill users developed a syndrome, "post-pill galactorrhea and amenorrhea" (PPGA). These women lactated, and they were amenorrheic. The hypothesis advanced to explain why women developed this condition was that certain cells in the area of the anterior pituitary gland (a gland located at the base of the brain) had atrophied (shrunk). It took four to five years for women who experienced the PPGA syndrome to resume normal menstrual and reproductive function. Dr. Carl Djerassi, sometimes called the "father of the pill," and whom I met while at Stanford, praises the pill if for no other reason than it has taught people that reversible contraception can be separated from coitus by a method that, for the first time, permits the woman to decide whether and how to control fertility.

Pill users, whether postmenarcheal or premenopausal, experience a menstrual bleed. The onset is predictable because bleeding is induced when drugs are withdrawn. In the new low-dose oral contraceptives, the pills are color coded to indicate the concentration of the drugs in each pill. In Triphasil, manufactured by Wyeth-Ayerst Laboratories, for the 28-day regimen, pill colors range from brown, white, light yellow, and green, and a woman takes one color-coded pill a day. In each brown pill, taken for six days, the concentration of the progestogenic agent, levonorgestrel, is 0.050 milligrams (mg), and the estrogen, ethinyl estradiol, is 0.30 mg. In each of five white tablets, the concentration of levonorgestrel increases to 0.075 mg, and the estrogen is 0.04 mg. In the ten light yellow tablets, the concentration of the progestogenic agent increases to 0.125 mg, while the estrogen decreases further to 0.030 mg. The last seven green tablets contain inert ingredients. It is during the green-pill-taking regimen that withdrawal bleeding occurs. The regularity, predictability, and decrease in volume of menstrual bleeding obtained with pill use receives high praise from women pill users.

MENSTRUATION WHILE ON
PROGESTOGENIC-ONLY AGENTS

Recently, two long-acting progestogenic agents were approved for preventing pregnancy. In December of 1990 the FDA approved

Norplant (trade name for a long-acting [five-year] contraceptive device manufactured also by Wyeth-Ayerst Laboratories in the United States), which contains the progestogenic agent levonorgestrel. This device, unlike the pill, must be surgically implanted under the skin to function as a long-acting contraceptive. Once implanted under the skin of a woman's upper arm, the drug diffuses into the body through six flexible capsules. The major benefit attributed to Norplant is that a woman is afforded contraceptive protection for five years; she does not need to take a pill every day, and she does not need to worry about getting pregnant if she forgets to take the pill. The major disadvantage associated with the progestogenic agent in Norplant, and other progestogenic-only methods of birth control, is the alteration in bleeding pattern that occurs. A woman may have prolonged menstrual bleeding, spotting between periods, or scanty or no menstrual discharge at all.

In March 1993, a second progestogenic agent, medroxyprogesterone acetate (Depo Provera), was approved by the FDA as an injectable contraceptive. The recommended dose of the drug is 150 mg, administered every three months. A major disadvantage associated with this agent, as with Norplant, is menstrual bleeding irregularities. Side effects associated with the drug use vary from woman to woman and include prolonged bleeding at first, followed by spotting between periods, and culminating in no bleeds at all (amenorrhea). To bleed or not to bleed when using progestogenic-only agents is a real concern for women. Even though women participants in The Tremin Trust Research Program describe menstruation as a nuisance, they worry when their bleed is late, has stopped, or has changed in interval or duration. Menstrual bleeding is viewed as a very important part of being a woman. Contraceptive methods designed to eliminate menstruation were developed by scientists who had little idea about the meaning of menstruation in the lives of women. Similarly, I am reminded of an article written by a Canadian colleague, Anne Rochon-Ford (1986). In Canada in 1985, Upjohn Canada, the manufacturers of Depo Provera, requested approval to use the drug as an injectable contraceptive. Despite widespread doubts about its safety, the Canadian Department of Health and Welfare indicated that they would approve it for use in Canada. A spokesman in support of the drug said that it was culturally acceptable to say that menstruation is a nuisance—women taking the drug need to be taught that it is not unhealthy for their genitals to be in a dormant state, just like they were when they were nine or ten years old.

Of course it is unhealthy for a woman's genitals to be in a dormant stage. It would be unhealthy for men, as well. The comment made by this bureaucrat is based in gender bias, and it is pretty outspoken evidence of the value placed upon a male's gonads and the ability to constantly produce sperm, and the lesser value for woman's monthly production of hormones, which induce ovulation and the potential to create a new life. This gender bias permeates North American society. For example, in 1992, a repeat sex offender in Texas pleaded with a judge to arrange castration rather than a prison sentence. The judge was agreeable with the man's request, but had to reconsider the decision when no doctor could be found who would agree to do the surgery (Associated Press, 1992).

In 1992 the USFDA reported that long-term use of progestogenic-only drugs did not prevent demineralization of bones.

Chapter 5

The Menstrual Cycle as a Medical Event

Menstruation is a natural, healthy cleansing of the uterus. Technically, it is one phase of the menstrual cycle. It is the shedding of the uterine endometrium in a process referred to as a *sterile* inflammatory reaction. Approximately once a month for 30 to 35 years of reproductive life, the menstrual cycle repeats itself. During the span of 26 to 30 days during prime reproductive years, all menstrual cycle activities are coordinated to promote ovulation and changes in the uterine lining to ensure successful implantation of the developing ball of cells that resulted from the fusion of egg and sperm. If there is no conception, the concentration of estrogen and progesterone falls, and menstruation begins. (Menstruation, as a physiological process, is discussed more fully in the chapter on changes in premenopausal bleeding patterns.)

As menstruation begins, gonadotrophic hormones, follicle stimulating hormone, and luteinizing hormone begin to increase in concentration in the blood. Before one cycle has ended, another has begun.

Primitive people did not have this kind of information or understanding of menstruation. Because of this, there was no greater fear than that held about the power associated with menstrual blood. Today, menstrual blood is no longer feared in most societies. Instead, the fear has been replaced by PMS. In 1983 Lauersen and Stukane dedicated their book to the five million silent sufferers of PMS, women in the dark about the severe hormonal imbalance that affects them ten days each month. PMS had become the curse of menstruation.

It is tempting to think that today the veil of ignorance surrounding menstruation and menstrual blood has been lifted. For example, menstrual tampons and pads are now advertised in magazines and on TV (although with the red color replaced with blue on a pad or tampon), and the products are no longer sold packaged in brown paper. That menstrual tampons and pads were marketed was no small achievement; as a result, women have many choices related to sanitary or feminine hygiene products and they no longer need suffer with menstrual cramps. Drugs such as Prēmsyn and ibuprofen are available by prescription or over the counter to relieve premenstrual distress. In the course of collecting data on the premenopausal bleeding study (as well as collecting used products, I should add), Phyllis Mansfield and I discovered that women maximized their potential to choose: 32 women used a total of 46 different feminine hygiene products over the course of three menstrual cycles.

In the not-too-distant past, however, women were burned at the stake for incidents that happened in their communities coincident with their menstrual bleed (Delaney, Lupton, and Toth, 1988, p. 42). The disastrous effects of menstruating women on men, cows, gardens, bees, milk, and wine are analogous to the evil effects of witchcraft as it was understood by the ancient church and state in Europe. Inquisitors were urged to look to a woman when witchcraft was suspected in a neighborhood, because woman was perceived as more carnal than man. The authors of *The Curse* suggest substituting menstrual blood for carnal. They cite the *Malleus Maleficarum* (hammer of witches) as the handbook of witch-hunting, setting forth a documented link between attitudes toward women's bodies and their persecution and burning of witches at the stake. Today we no longer believe that menstruating women are responsible for societal problems. Menstruating women are no longer secluded in menstrual huts; indeed, menstruation has become an out-of-the-closet phenomenon. PMS posters, Hallmark Shoebox greeting cards, calendars, and lapel buttons publicly declare the emotional lability and instability of premenstrual women. A widely circulated poster reads: "Beware, I have premenstrual tension; I am armed and dangerous!" A Shoebox card reads: "You always have a smile on your face; don't you ever get your period?"

That women experience certain changes premenstrually, such as irritability, decreased activity, fatigue, decrease in concentration, headache, bloat, weight gain, food cravings, etc., has been well documented.

Lange critiqued Aristotle's biology of reproduction theory as grounded in the differences between males and females and their ability to "concoct," that is, in the ability to produce semen and menstrual blood. The female concoction was viewed as a less refined concoction than semen; it had no sperm. It was a greater amount of vital heat in men that enabled them to concoct semen. Females were unable to concoct this higher-level substance, and were viewed as weaker than men because they possessed less "vital heat" (Lange, 1983). It followed then that if women were *weaker* than men, they were also *inferior* to men. And, since reproductive processes of gestation and birthing occurred in an inferior person, these functions were declared as inferior as well as animalistic–less than human.

Sigmund Freud contributed much to perpetuating the myth of male dominance over women in contemporary times when he wrote that women were defective because they lacked a penis, implying that biology shapes behavior, and anatomy is destiny. In other words, men and women were destined by their dissimilar bodies to develop different needs and abilities, and to play distinctive roles in life.

Robinson, in 1917, resonated Aristotle's theory as he described the secretion of fluids associated with orgasm:

> The culmination of the act of sexual intercourse is called the orgasm. It is the moment at which the pleasurable sensation is at its highest point, the body experiences a thrill, there is a spasmodic contraction in the genital organs, and there is a secretion of fluid from the genital glands and mucous membranes. This fluid in women is not a vital fluid like the semen in man; it is merely mucus . . . (p. 183).

In 1907 Stall's anatomy-as-destiny advice to young men, writing in *What a Young Husband Ought to Know*, focused on the differences in the anatomy of the bony pelvis:

> In man this structure is simply to subserve the purposes of strength and motion. In woman this bony basin, which forms the lower part of the body, has an additional purpose of special importance. At her side the hip-bones form the highest points, and from these the pelvis slopes down until in front it forms a

comparatively narrow rim called the pubic arch. This change of
form in woman is designed to adapt her body to become the
first cradle of her children, and in the fullness of time, to permit
the easy transit of a new being into the outer world. In preparing woman for maternity, God has thus equipped her with such
physical adaptation as is suited to the carrying of her temporary
burden, while at the same time affording protection for the
hidden life within, thus fitting the physical frame of woman to
the mother-nature with which He has endowed her . . . God has,
with like wisdom, adapted man in all of his physical endow-
ments to become the shield and defender of woman. He is to be
her protection and her defense. His fiercer visage, his broader
shoulders, his more masculine frame, all speak clearly of the
divine purpose. (pp. 33-34)

If a woman's body was to be the first cradle for the unborn child,
then the woman's arms were to be the second. Stall recommended
to young men that the first thing they need in life is a wife: "No
woman who is weak and sickly and nervous is fitted to be a wife,
and much less a mother" (Stall, 1904, p. 186).

The descriptions of woman as weak and sickly, and man as
strong, are grounded in differences in sexual function in which man
is used as the standard. The differences, however, are not sexual at
all. They are gender based. Sex means maleness or femaleness. Sex
is genetically determined. Gender means masculinity or femininity;
gender is a psychological term that describes thoughts, feelings, and
behaviors expected of the sexes. Gender is socially and culturally
constructed; it defines what is feminine and what is masculine, and
these definitions have arisen out of the differences between the
sexes in terms of reproductive function. Fausto-Sterling (1985)
believes it is the difference in reproductive function between men
and women that has placed women in the eyes of medicine in a
naturally diseased state. Contrary to current belief, a woman's
menstrual cycle is not an added burden that men do not have. It is
instead a normal female biological function. The menstrual cycle
does not make woman less than man; it creates and regulates the
conditions and the environment that make intrauterine gestation
possible. It is humanity's link with generations past and future.

Gena Corea (1985) believes that because of the menstrual cycle, woman has a continuous reproductive experience, which involves sexual intercourse, conception, growth of the fetus, and birth of a child nine months later. From this perspective, a woman is indeed the biological cradle of the human species. As such, woman—unlike man—has an enduring genetic continuity with the human species. In fact, this continuity is more than feminist rhetoric. A research team at Wayne State University discovered that a mother carries in her blood a little piece of every baby she has had. The researchers discovered this when they found Y chromosomes in women who were pregnant with females, but who had birthed males previously. The cells are immature white blood cells. One woman who was not pregnant, but who had birthed her last boy 27 years previously, was found to carry the fetal marker (the Y chromosome). The researchers are sure that cells of female babies are also left behind; however, it is just easier right now to track the Y chromosome (*Detroit News*, July 3, 1996). Corea presents a compelling argument to support that it is separation from the reproductive experience that mobilized man to control woman and to try to make the reproductive experience his own through creating a variety of reproductive technologies for use solely by women, and also medicalizing all events associated with a woman's reproductive life. It is a fact that men do not gestate, lactate, or menstruate. Thus, using man as the standard, these particular functions associated with female biology cannot be viewed as normal since man's only reproductive functions are the making of sperm and impregnation.

MEDICALIZATION OF THE MENSTRUAL CYCLE

Lander (1988) believes that medicalization of the menstrual cycle has been made explicit in the form of the gynecologist. In other words, woman is thought of as so defective that she requires a medical specialty. Enter the theory of the defective woman. Victorian medicine presented women as inherently vulnerable to sickness, and we continue to struggle with the medical mythology of women as "sick": the weaker sex, the imperfect sex, i.e., the sex with the lesser quality of vital fluids. "The man who does not know sick women does not know women" wrote Mitchell in 1888.

Women's problems were subsequently defined as being rooted in their biology. That women internalized an image of themselves as deviant and inherently sick was seized upon by medicine. Stripped of their own sense of self to define inner reality, women turned to medicine seeking answers, and willfully submitted to interventions.

Lander thinks medicine has the power to instill enormous anxieties or bring enormous relief. It all depends on whether a physician contradicts or validates a woman's own experience. For example, when medicine progressed from the view that menstrual cramps and menopause were "psychosomatic" to one that provided a biological explanation for them, women felt enormous relief. In the early 1980s, the changes experienced by women premenstrually were diagnosed as PMS, a disease in need of treatment. This validation popularized PMS, resulting in an outpouring of testimony from women who self-diagnosed a variety of conditions as PMS. In 1982 PMS was declared "the disease of the year." That this view was grounded in reality was made explicit in the first sentence written in Lever and Brush's 1981 book *Premenstrual Tension*, to wit: "Millions of women suffer from it." Written on the cover of Lauersen and Stukane's book in bold print was the following:

> Over 5 million women are in the dark about a severe hormonal imbalance affecting them ten days out of every month. They are frightened by violent fluctuations in mood, depression, and weight gain, and they don't know what's causing them. It is one of the greatest medical and political controversies of our time.

More than a decade of publicity and media hype regarding PMS has revived old stereotypes, such as "Women are sick, weak, and hysterical"; "Women are victims of their hormones"; and "Biology is destiny." Of course women menstruate. This does not mean, however, that because they perform this function they are any less healthy or human than men.

In 1931, R. T. Frank described a group of women who experienced varying degrees of discomfort preceding the onset of menstruation. Frank, however, viewed this discomfort as normal. It was outside of the context of normalcy in which Frank identified a class of patients in whom grave systemic disorders were manifest during the premenstrual period. These women were experiencing severe premenstrual tension. Clinical or medical interest in menstrual cycle physiology was at first generated by the varied complaints women presented to physicians during their premenstruum. These complaints, defined by Frank as premenstrual tension, were resurrected in 1982 as "Premenstrual Syndrome" (PMS).

PREMENSTRUAL SYNDROME

It is an understatement to say that considerable attention has been given to the study of psychophysiological aspects of the menstrual cycle. Since the resurrection of Frank's model of premenstrual tension in 1982, the legacy from more than a decade of publicity and media hype concerning PMS has revived the old stereotype about women: Biology was destiny for suffering, illness, and disease during the menstrual cycle. In short, the woman with PMS emerged as the prototype for all menstruating women.

What causes PMS? Fluctuating levels of estrogen and progesterone were first thought to be the cause of the disease. Then diet, stress, vitamin deficiencies or excesses, etc. You name it, and you will find it linked to the more than 150 signs and symptoms associated with PMS. Katharina Dalton (1983), an English physician, was the first clinician who tried to cure PMS with progesterone. Dalton believed that PMS was due to progesterone deficiency. She replaced progesterone in her PMS patients and had variable success with the treatment. Hormones are still considered to be implicated in PMS; exactly how they cause PMS remains unclear. The widespread publicity of PMS has had some undesirable consequences. According to William Keye (1988), a PMS researcher, a demand for care and treatment has come before a thorough understanding of PMS has been reached. The same concern applies to menopause. Throughout the 1980s and into the 1990s, women believed that their bodies at menopause had become reservoirs for disease and decay. The view of menopause as an "endocrinopathy" has resulted in thousands of women demanding treatment, although a thorough understanding of the changes associated with the menopausal transition and postmenopausal years has not been reached.

PMS, however, is a disease. What most women experience during the premenstruum is not PMS; rather, they are experiencing "premenstrual changes," changes described by R. T. Frank as normal. As described in Chapter 3, these premenstrual changes are hormonally initiated. As the concentration of estrogen and progesterone fluctuate during the menstrual cycle, women experience mood changes, from a midcycle high to flattened affect premenstrually, they retain water, they bloat, they may be irritable, breasts may be tender, concentration sometimes is impaired, and appetite changes to the point of craving certain foods, particularly salty foods, etc.

Since the early 1980s there has been a continuing interest in PMS by a variety of individuals—laypersons, lawyers, politicians (as will be described later), bureaucrats, etc. As mentioned, the search for a PMS cure has focused on alterations, deficiencies, or excesses of organic or inorganic bodily substances. According to Linda Gannon (1985), hormone deficiencies or excesses have been favorite avenues of investigation. An excess of premenstrual hormones was the origin of a "raging hormone hypothesis" advanced by Frank and later used by Edgar Berman, a physician member of the Democratic Party's Committee on National Priorities who was also Vice President Hubert Humphrey's physician. In 1970 Berman remarked to a female member of Congress: "Even a Congresswoman must defer to scientific truths . . . there just are physical and psychological inhibitants that limit a female's potential." Berman went on to demean midlife/menopausal woman, stating that he "would rather have a John F. Kennedy making decisions about the Cuban missile crisis than a female of the same age who might be subject to the curious mental aberrations characteristic of the age group." The full text of Berman's message is contained in a letter to the editor in *The New York Times*, July 26, 1970.

Recently, the increasing involvement and success of women in politics has been attributed to an "unmasking" effect of testosterone by menopause. According to Dr. Stephanie Riger, Professor of psychology at the University of Illinois, a few scientific studies report finding a relationship between elevated testosterone levels and women in positions of dominance. However, it is not clear from such studies whether testosterone is a cause or effect of the social position. Riger questioned whether men's interest in politics is related also to high testosterone levels. If so, she said that we should expect that older men, in whom testosterone levels are declining, should also be less interested in politics. Of course, this is not so. Riger contends that biological explanations for human action tend to focus on women, their hormones, their menstruations, and, now at menopause, their lack of female hormones and an increase in male hormones (Hedrick, 1992).

The Berman incident gave feminists the opportunity to refute assumptions that questioned women's competence in positions of leadership, whether they be menstruating or menopausal. The incident was partly responsible for sparking research on the menstrual cycle. The Society for Menstrual Cycle Research (SMCR), as mentioned, was organized in 1979. The research and activities of members of the SMCR, as well as others, brought the menstrual cycle and PMS more clearly into focus. For better or for worse, PMS became a household word. It still is.

The fallout from research directed at disproving the raging-hormone hypothesis has had both positive and negative implications for women. I again asked, "What did we lose compared to what was gained?" The gain, according to William Keye, has been to validate for a small number of women (about 5 percent) that PMS is real and it is debilitating. The loss is acceptance of the assumption that all women will experience PMS sometime in their life. The net effect of the PMS debate has been to strengthen the woman-as-defective, raging-hormone hypothesis: Not only are women incapacitated premenstrually, but they are also extremely dangerous.

Perhaps the most alarming consequence of the raging-hormone hypothesis arose when PMS was used as a defense to justify murder. In 1980 Katharina Dalton claimed that one of her clients, Sandie Smith, was suffering from PMS when she murdered a barmaid. This incident was just what proponents of the raging-hormone hypothesis were waiting for. Subsequently, the manufacture and sale of PMS-focused products became a burgeoning industry. In 1986, the American Psychiatric Association (APA) began discussions on whether or not to include in the *Diagnostic and Statistical Manual of Mental Disorders* (referred to as the DSM III-R) a diagnostic category for premenstrual "emotional trauma." Professional women have seldom been as united as they were on this issue. Nine professional organizations went on record as opposed to including the diagnosis. Ultimately, the premenstrual diagnosis was not adopted. In its place, however, a diagnostic category, "late luteal phase disorder" (LLPD), was included in the appendix to the diagnostic manual. Karen DeCrow, then President of the National Organization for Women, warned that the LLPD diagnosis was a "disaster waiting to happen." DeCrow said, "If one scintilla of evidence existed to support that women are impaired mentally, all women would be excluded from politics, government, and business." (1990, personal communication).

The controversy regarding the DSM III-R diagnostic category and the implications of such categorization for menstruating women places women as well as researchers in a dilemma. If women admit to premenstrual physical and mood changes, how will this admission be interpreted by others? Will it be used in support of the raging-hormone hypothesis? Early on Sommer (1983) cautioned that if PMS is a function of women's reproductive physiology, then theoretically, any menstruating woman would have an excuse for irrational behavior.

As a researcher, I am less expert on menstruation and premenstrual changes than some of my SMCR colleagues. As a woman, however, it is a different story. I menstruated for 37 years and experienced premenstrual changes for many of those years. Did I spend 37 years in a diseased and sick body? Certainly not. I was creative, and I did not go crazy. I did not commit murder. I earned a doctorate during my premenopausal/menstrual years—perhaps *that* was a little crazy?

My colleague Jan Root (1992) has important insights on the PMS/normal menstrual cycle changes issue. She begins by examining the word "syndrome." What is a syndrome? By definition, according to the *International Dictionary of Medicine and Biology* (1986, p. 2782), a syndrome is an aggregate of signs and symptoms considered to constitute the characteristics of a morbid entity, that is, a disease state. Premenstrual syndrome, according to this definition, then, is a morbid entity, a disease, associated with the premenstrual phase of the menstrual cycle. A "disease," by definition, is a condition that impairs normal physiological functioning. Rudolph Moos, a pioneer in menstrual cycle research as well as creator of the Menstrual Distress Questionnaire (MDQ), describes PMS as an aggregate of 150 signs and symptoms (1968). Popular books on PMS cite statistics claiming that 75 percent of all women experience some of the PMS symptomatology during their menstrual life. Current estimates suggest that less than 5 percent of the population experience PMS. However, if even some of the symptoms attributed to the syndrome are experienced by the majority of menstruating women, can the experience be characterized as abnormal on this basis and, thus, described as a disease?

At this point we need to ask, who is describing and defining what is happening in women's bodies? As indicated previously, no man has ever menstruated, yet by and large it has been men who have been describing and defining what is normal for women and what is not normal, based upon man's view of woman's reproductive biology, using man as the standard. If a premenstrual change is problematic for a women, does this imply that the problem is an indication of something abnormal? Root argues that a process that is problematic does not have to be abnormal. Furthermore, whether menstruation or premenstrual changes are problematic is not the issue. The issue is "normalcy," and how assumptions of normalcy define what is thought to be disease. Physical states can be both normal and problematic. For example, many of the physical changes that accompany menopause and aging are both normal and, for some women, problematic. According to Root, the PMS model is flawed since it operates from an implicit assumption that a woman's condition when she is not menstruating or about to menstruate is her normal condition. The PMS model is based on the assumption that women, like men, exist in a physiologically steady state. Women, however, do not exist in a physiologically steady state (at least women in Westernized cultures who have chosen not to spend most of their time in the pregnancy room). Nor do men. Women are always in one phase or another of the menstrual cycle. To be a cycling woman is normal. To experience changes with each phase of the cycle is also normal.

Root claims that the PMS model is effective in providing a framework from which to discuss certain problematic aspects of the menstrual cycle. William Keye agrees, the PMS model does work for women in that it formally legitimatizes problematic aspects of the menstrual cycle experienced by some women that previously were denied. However, to label as problematic any premenstrual change is to risk being diagnosed with PMS. Viewing PMS from this framework, only women who do not experience premenstrual changes are considered free of disease. Thus, the PMS model supports the concept that noncyclicity is normal for women. In other words, women should function as men are perceived to function biologically and not experience monthly cyclic changes. Indiscriminately applying the PMS construct to all women implicitly labels women as diseased. I have labeled this the "M&M Theory of the Defective Woman." Women are sickly and diseased because of their reproductive biology for their entire reproductive life, from menarche to menopause.

PREMENSTRUAL CHANGES

In Chapter 1, I introduced my doctoral research on premenstrual changes. A basic assumption underpinning the study was that physical and effective changes were a normal and necessary part of a woman's biological functioning. The cause of the changes was hypothesized to be an increase in body water–in technical terms, an increase in circulating plasma volume–which was hormonally mediated. This assumption was based on two important pieces of information: (1) all pregnant women increase total body water, and (2) the menstrual cycle and pregnancy cycle are closely related. I concluded that premenstrual changes were not only normal but necessary to fulfill the demands that would be incumbent upon the maternal organism if a pregnancy did occur. In other words, women do not prepare biologically for pregnancy the moment they conceive. This would be too late to have certain backup mechanisms in place–such as the uterine changes that need to occur in order to ensure a successful implantation of the blastocyst. One of the most important changes that must occur, other than transforming the uterine endometrium into a "soft, velvety pile," is the increase in total body circulating volume. The time at which a woman becomes pregnant is when the blastocyst implants in the uterus. At this time, a woman's body needs to be ready to deliver needed nutrients to the developing embryo as well as have the capacity to carry away and detoxify waste products of embryonic metabolism.

PREMENSTRUAL FLUID RETENTION

Two investigators, MacDonald and Good (1992), observed the onset of body water increase to occur in the menstrual cycle, after ovulation, a time which coincided closely, but not exactly, with conception. No wonder premenstrual fluid retention is one of the most frequently reported symptoms of the menstrual cycle. Any increase in total body water, whether or not a woman is pregnant, affects the functioning of all body cells, primarily due to a transitory dilutional effect. (For example, if you put a teaspoon of sugar into a glass and fill it half full, you will taste a certain sweetness. If the glass is now filled to the rim with water, the sweetness will be diminished; the concentration of the sugar has been diluted by about 50 percent.) I proposed that an increase in body water premenstrually diluted the concentration of body salt. A specific concentration of salt in the body is required to maintain the functional integrity of cells and the osmolality (concentration) of body water compartments. Sodium (salt) is the most important inorganic ion in the body. It regulates a variety of biological functions, including nerve conduction, blood pressure, muscle contraction, acid base balance in the body, etc. Excess sodium is usually excreted quite well in the urine, and elaborate mechanisms exist for conserving sodium when intake is restricted. If salt is lost, the body perceives this loss, stops urine output of salt, and initiates hormonal mechanisms to reabsorb salt and water. A sodium level lower than 135 milliequivalents per liter (a number used by clinicians to define pathology), whether or not the decrease in sodium is absolute or relative (dilutional), is diagnosed clinically as delusional hyponatremia. Common symptoms associated with fluid overload (dilutional hyponatremia) are confusion, headache, anxiety, restlessness, nausea, vomiting, apathy, fatigue, and weight gain.

We have known for some time that progesterone promotes salt loss because it antagonizes the salt-retaining hormone aldosterone. What is very important to understand related to this discussion is that where salt goes, so does water. When body water volume and/or concentration of solute changes in the vascular system (as in the example of sugar in the glass of water), whether an increase or a decrease, hormone-mediated mechanisms are activated to restore a "normal" state of water and electrolyte (sodium is the major electrolyte) balance. In the hierarchy of survival responses, maintenance and/or restoration of body water (circulating plasma volume) is top priority. What this means for premenstrual women is that when the ability to regulate (retain) sodium is temporarily impaired, as salt leaves the body, so does water. What results first is a decrease in circulating body-water volume, which triggers hormonal mechanisms to restore body fluids.

In the process of restoring body water, a transient dilution of the solute portion of the blood occurs. Sodium is the major solute that contributes to maintaining the osmotic balance of body fluids. Any increase in volume, transient or prolonged, dilutes the concentration of sodium, affecting the performance of all body cells.

During the premenstrual phase of the cycle, the body's response to restore water volume results in an overshoot of water retention, which is perceived by women as bloating, and which is measurable as weight gain. Premenstrual fluid retention is normal; premenstrual edema is not. An inappropriate response of the body to restore body water would result in edema, which is an excessive accumulation of fluid in the body. Excessive fluid may be sequestered in the bloodstream, or it may be evenly distributed throughout the body. Premenstrual edema is pathological and needs to be treated. A woman with premenstrual edema would have a measurable weight gain of more than 5 pounds over the short term (one to two days). Premenstrual edema would be accompanied by marked fatigue, inability to concentrate, marked irritability, marked mood swings, etc., mostly due to the dilution of salt in the body.

If a woman does not conceive, premenstrual changes subside; the corpus luteum regresses, hormone levels fall, menstruation begins, fluid is lost via copious and frequent urinations (the clinical term for the rapid loss of water in urine is "diuresis," physical and affective changes subside as osmotic (salt) balance in body cells is restored, and another cycle begins. However, if a woman conceives during the luteal phase of the cycle, hormone-mediated increases in body water are enhanced and maintained throughout the nine months of the pregnancy cycle. (More detail on the relationship between the menstrual and the pregnancy cycle is described in a 1982 publication, "Nausea and Vomiting of First Trimester Pregnancy" in C. M. Norris' *Concept Clarification in Nursing*. The physiological model explains how changes in water volume might be the cause of nausea during the first three months of pregnancy.)

WHY DO WOMEN MENSTRUATE?

Why women menstruate rather than resorb all of the materials found in menstrual discharge has been addressed by Profet (1993) in an intriguing hypothesis, e.g., that menstruation functions to protect a woman's uterus and the tubes that lead to the ovaries from pathological organisms. Profet argues that sperm are "vectors" of disease–during the act of sexual intercourse, bacteria from the male and female genitalia cling to sperm tails and are transported into a woman's body. The process of bleeding during menstruation exerts mechanical pressure on the uterus, forcing it to shed, which also delivers immune cells into the uterine cavity. The delivery of immune cells fights the invasion of pathogens, and thus, cleanses the uterus and protects the female against infection. If one views menstrual cycle function as essential for ensuring survival of the human species, that is, through preparation of the uterine lining for implantation, maturation of ovarian follicles, ovulation, and subsequent luteal phase changes, then premenstrual changes, while insufferable and painful for some women, can be viewed positively, not as a curse. According to Profet, menstrual bleeding is not a by-product of a failed pregnancy, a failed reproductive cycle. It is, instead, a functional mechanism. Profet's theory has been challenged by researchers who counter that menstruation, rather than ridding the uterus of bacteria, is more likely to be the time of greatest bacterial contamination because open areas are created by constriction and dilation of arterioles, with subsequent elimination of the necrotic (dead) tissue.

If Profet's theory causes your head to spin, a book by Judy Grahn, *Blood, Bread, and Roses: How Menstruation Created the World* (1993), might blow you away. Grahn explores menstruation rites and rituals in depth, concluding that blood is the center of human culture, and that menstrual blood is the center of all creativity on the planet. Grahn paints superb word pictures of bleeding and the origin of menstrual rites. For a multitude of people, she argues, menstrual blood was the primary life force (p. 6). Unlike the estrus of any other primates or other animals, Grahn argues: "Humans have a fundamental and unique tool of external-internal measurement in the synchronization of the menstrual cycle and the lunar cycle" (p. 7). " . . . Only the human cycle, at 29½ days, coincides with the cycle of the moon." The assumption here is that the cycles have been connected since the creation of the universe.

Lander (1988) theorizes that menstruation in humans is an evolutionary anomaly, that is, a new event on the evolutionary clock. As such, a woman's physiology has had little time to adapt to the change from estrus to menstruation. In other words, Lander thinks that modern-day woman's genes are the genes of a woman in the hunter/gatherer society who was always pregnant, and thus almost never menstruated. Presumably, a woman who never menstruated would never experience premenstrual tension, premenstrual syndrome or edema. Lander's hypothesis utilizes the Darwinian theory of natural selection. According to this theory, all sexually reproducing organisms are reservoirs of genetic and phenotypic variations (recall that the genotype is what is transcribed from the DNA; the phenotype is how it is expressed in humans, for example, blue eyes, black hair, etc.). For women the combination of two X chromosomes on fusion of egg and sperm determined genetic sex. The menstrual cycle, menstruation, and secondary sex characteristics associated with being "female" are the phenotypic expression of how the genes combined. What forces maintain genetic expression, create new ways of expression, or eliminate old ones within and among populations continues to be hotly debated among evolutionary biologists.

Theoretically, over time, Lander argues, circumstances that favor the obliteration of the genotype for menstruation (conceptualized by her and others as a genetic anomaly) will be obliterated. Would obliteration of menstruation obliterate the menstrual cycle as well? Or, according to the theory, would women continue to cycle as they now do–just not menstruating? This is an interesting biological question to ponder. Zeveloff and Conover (1991) have proposed that the concealment of ovulation has endowed primates with a reproductive advantage. Would the concealment of menstruation provide a similar advantage for women?

I appreciate Lander's feminist analyses of menstruation and her theorizing. I believe, however, that it is too similar to Aristotle's theorizing about women, which purported that women, because they menstruate, are imperfect and are in the process of development. Has Lander become trapped in her theorizing, using man as the standard for woman's evolution? Does the theory suggest that if women did not menstruate, they would be more like men?

Premenstrual changes and menstruation are normal processes. They are not evolutionary anomalies, nor signs of a disease; thus, I have developed no sophisticated theory for eliminating menstruation. The menstrual cycle is the phenotypic expression of woman's genetic heritage. Interpretation of menstrual cycle changes should not be made using either man or the PMS woman as the norm for reproductive biology. Each sex has a predetermined role to play in the grand scheme of species perpetuation. As such, the onset of changes throughout the menstrual cycle need to be celebrated, rather than derogated. A woman who experiences premenstrual changes needs to interpret these changes to mean that all is well in womb-world, that the ancestral genetic message has been decoded one more time, and that necessary physiological preparations have been made in the body should pregnancy ensue. This interpretation does not reduce women to the status of PMS sufferers or imperfect humans. Rather, it emphasizes the normalcy and necessity of such changes to ensure the capability to create life during each menstrual cycle.

In 1985, Linda Gannon speculated that even though interest in PMS had subsided and many PMS clinics had closed, the debate on whether or not to include a PMS-related diagnosis in the APA diagnostic and statistical manual was not closed. In February of 1993 I received a copy of a letter written by Mary Brown Parlee to Alice Dan, co-founder of the Society for Menstrual Cycle Research, regarding the newly proposed premenstrual diagnostic category. Excerpts from the letter follow:

> . . . the DSM-IV Task Force has recommended that PMS (a.k.a. late luteal phase dysphoric disorder) should be included

as a diagnostic category in the text of DSM-IV–as pre-menstrual dysphoric disorder, mood disorder not otherwise specified. In the DSM-III R it is listed in the appendix as a provisional diagnosis needing further research; moving it into the body of the manual itself will further consolidate PMS/LLPDD as an "official" mental illness.

. . . the scientific data are just not there to support this deci-sion. And there are cogent arguments against the proposed for-women-only "mental illness" based on social and political grounds. While nothing has changed (arguments or data) since the fight over including it in DSM-II R, there is good reason to think that more controversy at this stage can still affect DSM- IV.

In March of 1993, The Society for Menstrual Cycle Research (Board of Directors) forwarded a letter to Dr. J. T. English, President of the American Psychiatric Association, protesting ". . . the APA's deci-sion to include premenstrual dysphoric disorder (PMSDD) in the *Diagnostic and Statistical Manual of Mental Disorders.*" Arguments against including premenstrual dysphoric disorder in the DSM were the following:

- There is *no* sound empirical basis for such a category.
- It carries social and political dangers for women.
- There is no parallel category for men.

If women did not cycle and menstruate, would we be dealing with this issue? Who knows. Women would still become pregnant and birth babies; perhaps the focus of discrimination would simply shift from the menstrual cycle to the pregnancy cycle and the birth-ing process.

On May 22, 1993, the assembly of the American Psychiatric Association voted to accept the fourth version of the DSM. Included in the latest version of psychiatry's "bible" is a new class of depression based on hormonal changes in women: *premenstrual dysphoric disorder* (PMD). To meet the diagnosis, at least five of the following symptoms must be present and interfere with normal social activities and relationships: depression; anxiety; mood swings; anger; irritability; decreased interest in work, school, friends, hobbies; difficulty concentrating; lethargy; appetite changes; sleep disturbances; feeling overwhelmed or out of control; and physical symptoms associated with the menstrual cycle such as breast tenderness, headaches, weight gain, or bloating.

Clinical medicine and now some psychologists and other certified counselors are unrelenting in their efforts to cure menstruating women of being women.

SECTION III.
MENOPAUSE: THE CLOSURE
OF MENSTRUAL LIFE

Many women . . . the majority probably, suffer considerably during the transitional year or years of the menopause. Symptoms are of organic, physical and psychic character, but the psychic symptoms predominate.

There may be headache, capricious appetite, or complete loss of appetite, considerable loss of flesh, or on the contrary very sudden and rapid putting on of fat, great irritability, insomnia, profuse perspiration, hot flashes throughout the body, and particularly in the face, which make the face "blushing" and congested, are particularly frequent.

Then the woman's character may be completely changed. From gentle and submissive she may become pugnacious and quarrelsome. Jealousy without any grounds for it may be one of the disagreeable symptoms, making both the wife and the husband very unhappy. In some exceptional cases, a genuine neurosis or psychosis may develop.

It is my conviction, and I have had this conviction for many years, that many, if not most of the distressing symptoms of the menopause are due, not to the menopause itself, but to the wrong ideas about this period that have prevailed for so many centuries. (Robinson, 1917, pp. 285-286)

Wrong ideas indeed! Robinson would be astonished to read in the medical literature of the 1990s that menopause is viewed by medicine either as an estrogen-deficiency disease, or an endocrinopathy, rather than a normal process. This view has resulted in confusion and frustration for women who view menopause as a normal event in their growth and development. In Chapter 7, these two conflicting views of menopause are examined. I have also provided some background related to the events that led up to establishing menopause-as-disease ideology, which subsequently ushered in the era of steroid hormone replacement for women.

Several terms are currently used to describe the menopause experience: premenopause, perimenopause, artificial menopause, climacteric, menopause transition, and postmenopause. The terms, unfortunately, are used interchangeably by clinicians and researchers. The result has been ambiguity in definition about menopausal stages, and sometimes, confusion on the part of care providers regarding appropriate therapy. This ambiguity also makes it difficult to compare the findings of research studies. Because of this, I have devoted Chapter 6 to the problem of definition. Chapter 6 provides the framework for Chapters 8, 9, and 10, wherein I have included the voices of The Tremin Trust women who either have experienced or are experiencing and commenting on each menopausal stage. It is important to hear these women's voices. Through hearing and believing in the value of other women's stories and experiences, a much-needed and heretofore invisible perspective of menopause will emerge. Too often, women hear only the opinions of self-proclaimed experts.

Robinson also recognized that many changes were associated with the transition to menopause. Some, like hot flash and change in the bleeding pattern, are almost universal. Changes in vaginal tissue, skin tone, sexual drive and response, weight gain and/or redistribution of body weight, mood changes, increase in facial hair, prickly sensations on the skin, and thinning of head and body hair are fairly common. It is important to keep in mind that only a few of these changes are directly attributed to menopause. Most are related to the aging process in general. Menopause just happens to be one aging change that occurs around midlife. A change in the quality of bleeding, or the onset of hot flashes, for example, are menopausal changes, and may even herald entry into perimenopause. It is the onset of either one of these changes that motivates women to seek information and/or obtain the advice of care providers. In many instances they do both. These two common changes are discussed in Chapters 11 and 12, to include answers to most frequently asked questions on the topics and guidelines for coping.

Even though the most common changes associated with transition to menopause are quite normal, and in fact, should be expected, the dominant medical view of menopause continues to be one of women at risk for developing diseases and/or an endocrinopathy because of the loss of estrogen hormone. The two major diseases clinicians believe women are at risk of developing are osteoporosis (bone thinning) and coronary heart disease. As such, hormone treatment, which may be in the form of estrogen alone or estrogen in combination with a progestin or an androgen (male hormone), is the choice of treatment for these women.

Information on heart disease and osteoporosis is found in Chapters 15 and 18. In Chapter 14, I have included a detailed discussion of steroid hormones, and their mechanism of action. Risks associated with hormone use (to include the breast cancer controversy) are found in Chapter 16. Guidelines for decision making, i.e., "to be or not to be a hormone user," are presented in Chapter 17.

Chapter 6

Conflicting Views of Menopause

The view that menopause is a disease is dominant in medicine, where menopause has long been considered an estrogen deficiency disease, and more recently, described as an endocrinopathy. This view is a result of the scientific discourses and practices of the Western world, which have evolved a cultural stereotype of menopausal women as asexual, engulfed with hot flashes, and facing postmenopausal years with decaying bones and lipid-clogged arteries. The definition of menopause as disease, like menstruation, has its origins in patriarchal views and beliefs about women as defective and imperfect (as related to men), and/or machines that need to be fixed. This view of menopause has made invisible the concept of menopause as a normal biological event, i.e., the closure of menstrual life.

Menopause, clearly, is a biological event. It is, however, an event that is perceived privately in the context of a woman's physical and emotional health, culture, and social environment, and as you will read, it is an event that is not uniformly described or experienced. According to Madeleine Goodman (1991), a menopause researcher, the onus of proof that menopause is a disease requires more than a demonstration of declining estrogen levels. Rather, it requires proof of a causal relationship between hormone changes and clinical symptoms, and such proof is lacking. Without proof, the idea that menopause is a disease becomes an idea grounded in long-standing myths that have resulted in socially shared beliefs about women as inferior.

Opposing the menopause-as-disease ideology are feminist researchers and nonfeminist proponents of the women's self-care/health-care movement. These individuals argue that women are not diseased, defective, or disabled at menopause. They view menopause as a natural process, a normal growth and developmental event, one that women experience with a minimum of difficulty.

117

These opposing points of view have generated two ideologies, or theoretical camps, on the topic. Koeske's 1980 critique of menstrual cycle research conveys an important message even today for those who argue that menopause is normal, as well as those promoting the disease ideology.

CONFLICTING PARADIGMS: A PROBLEM OF REDUCTIONISM

Koeske separated menstrual cycle research into two ideologies: the "biological variable" approach and the "social or no-effect" approach. Koeske argued that the biological variable approach suffered from a profound and severe reductionistic bias, that is, it reduced the study of woman and her menstrual life to the study of ovary, uterus, and fluctuating hormones. Implicit in the reductionism is the "biology-is-destiny" ideology that equates menstruation with a disease to be treated. In Koeske's opinion, it was the biological reductionism that gave rise to the second ideology, the social or no-effect approach. Proponents of this approach believe that women are not different from men. The failure of the social or no-effect approach, argued Koeske, is that the "biology-is-destiny" and the "menopause-as-disease" assumptions of the biological camp are either totally denied or are replaced by sociocultural reasons for negative experiences during menstruation.

Extrapolating the tenets of Koeske's argument to menopause, one realizes that biomedical research about menopausal women has been based on a biological "deficit" model. The various physiological symptoms that appear at middle age are said to be associated with falling estrogen levels. Therefore, the psychological symptoms experienced during menopause, such as mood and affective changes, are related to an estrogen deficit. Using this model to design research, investigators primarily have studied clinical samples of women to understand and explain menopause; hence, Koeske argued, the conclusions and inferences related to menopause were drawn from a minority of ill women who sought either medical or psychiatric help. Koeske viewed this as the basic flaw in the biomedical model of research. A lack of concern for environmental events and social parameters that may affect the relationship between hormonal levels and menopausal changes was also identified. This latter point is made explicit in the voices of Tremin Trust women in perimenopause (Chapter 9), who not only are experiencing physiological change, but are also experiencing a variety of midlife changes which run the gamut from suicides of loved ones, job losses, drug abuse by children, caring for elderly parents, etc.

MENOPAUSE AS DISEASE: THE BIOMEDICAL MODEL

The biomedical deficit model has reduced menopausal women to a composite of biochemical and hormonal entities. This view is reductionistic and is in accord with the view of proper science, that is, complex entities, in order to be understood, need to be reduced to smaller, measurable, and quantifiable parts. This view of menopause, however, is new. According to Wilbush, menopause, the term as well as the symptoms coined from the label, first was used in France sometime after the French Revolution. At this time, the social stress to which women were subjected at menopause, and their complaints of various symptoms, were grouped together into a disease expression. Menopause, as a word, did not exist in the English literature until the last quarter of the nineteenth century, nor was the phrase "change of life" a significant theme in British or American literature until the twentieth century. In medical literature, commencing in the 1960s, menopausal women are described as hypogonadal, castrated, estrogen-depleted, or estrogen-deficient. Implicit in these words is that the totality of aging womanhood is reduced to the level of the gonads. At menopause, a woman is not considered wholly a woman without functional gonads, nor is she considered a man.

What then is a menopausal woman? The view taken by medical practitioners and biomedical researchers is that at menopause women become estrogen-deficient. And the argument that follows is that without estrogen replacement, diseases will develop. This definition is consistent with the menopause-as-disease concept. Menopause is the closure of menstrual life. It is a normal process. Yet, according to MacPherson, a powerful voice for feminism who is a nurse and researcher, no female function has been so degraded, dreaded, or made so unmentionable as this final phase of the female reproductive cycle (1981).

In 1963, menopause as loss and obsolescence was first sensationalized by Robert Wilson, writing with his wife, Thelma. In 1966 Wilson wrote his now infamous book, *Feminine Forever*, wherein he painted a most grim picture of menopause and menopausal women, making explicit the concept of menopause as disease, comparing woman's future (and, indeed, her destiny) without estrogen replacement as one of spending her life in a sort of living decay. The caricature of the menopausal woman as a castrate in a negative state, dependent, vapid, unfortunate, unseeing, and without vigor characterized the medical professional's view of a menopausal woman into the 1980s. The evolving ideology created by Wilson and followers was that menopause was a deficiency disease treatable only by physicians and only with estrogen.

Medicine has since tried to get Wilson "off of their backs," to retrench, to adamantly claim that menopause is not a disease. It is estrogen deficiency, not menopause, that *results in diseases,* osteoporosis and heart disease in particular. These estrogen-deficiency diseases are treatable only by physicians. The treatment of choice is estrogen hormones.

So powerful and convincing were Wilson's arguments in favor of estrogen replacement that in the 1970s estrogen hormone in the form of estrone (also known as E_1) was one of the top five prescriptions sold in the United States. Estimations of hormone use at this time suggested that one-third of women over age 50 were using it regularly. Estrogen at this time was promoted as a wonder drug. The benefits promised for menopausal women who used it would be to age more slowly, be sexually attractive, and avoid the psychological problems associated with menopause. Wilson also proclaimed that the hormone would protect against osteoporosis, heart disease, and cancers of the breast and uterus. Risks to health were minimized. More than 100,000 copies of *Feminine Forever* sold in seven months. Wilson presented a compelling picture of the horrors of women living postmenopausal years in bodies without estrogen–bodies that would ultimately betray women through crushing fractures; a dried, cracked, and bleeding vagina; clogged arteries; and unbearable hot flashes.

Consequences of the Menopause-as-Disease Model

In the mid-1970s, the myth that estrogen would forever keep women feminine and healthy was exposed when studies linked postmenopausal estrogen use to uterine cancer caused by a buildup of uterine endometrial cells and no menstruations. In 1984, an estimated 39,000 cases of endometrial carcinoma were reported, and 2,900 deaths from the disease were reported. Following the publicity concerning the estrogen/cancer connection, MacPherson noted that widespread treatment of menopausal women diminished and estrogen prescriptions decreased by 40 percent (1981). From 1975 to 1980, a concerted effort was made to rehabilitate estrogen therapy. When a progestin was added to the estrogen that women were taking in pill form, estrogen use was again said to be safe. The primary function of progesterone during a woman's menstrual cycle is to transform the rapidly proliferating uterine endometrium into a secretory organ. This transformation is necessary to prepare for pregnancy. In technical terms, according to Schenken and Pauerstein, progesterone antagonizes estrogen's powerful proliferative (or mitotic) cell-division effect on the uterus.

Commencing in the 1980s, estrogen replacement for a pre- or postmenopausal woman became "hormone replacement therapy," a combination of an estrogen and a progestin. The change from estrogen to hormone replacement therapy was quickly accepted by physicians, and recommended by the American College of Obstetrics and Gynecology. According to Barrett-Connor (1987), another drug regimen for use in healthy women became widely accepted with little critical study. Establishment of menopause as disease was completed when the link was made between estrogen deficiency and two diseases, osteoporosis (demineralization of bone) and heart disease. So eager was the crowd to join the parade that few bothered to consider that these links and endorsements were still questionable, and they formed erroneous, premature conclusions.

From Estrogen Deficiency to Endocrinopathy

In 1996, Wilson's estrogen forever/feminine forever myth has been partially dismantled insofar as estrogen has been identified as being very risky for a woman with a uterus. Nevertheless, treatment in the 1990s is grounded in Wilson's basic premise that menopause is somehow linked with disease. Fifteen years beyond the establishment of the causal link between uterine cancer and estrogen, the debate no longer is whether menopausal women should take estrogen; rather, the questions have become: For what disease prevention should estrogen be prescribed and what is the safest way to administer the hormone? The main difference between Wilson and modern-day clinicians is that menopause *per se* is not viewed as a disease to be treated; instead, treatment is thought to be necessary to prevent osteoporosis and coronary (heart) artery disease, which according to Utian (1990b), can occur as a result of a climacteric-related (which means menopausal in most instances) endocrinopathy.

Evidence to support the climacteric as an endocrinopathy was described by Utian. It is based upon the demonstration of four classical sequential steps: (1) a morphological change in the ovary, which is an endocrine gland; (2) an alteration in the endocrine milieu, that is, changes in the concentration of the sex hormones estrogen and progesterone; (3) changes in receptor target tissue, such as urogenital tissue (vagina, bladder) due to changes in hormone levels; and (4) the presentation to clinicians of women with complaints as a result of changes in endocrine glands, target tissues, and hormone levels.

Utian, a cofounder of the North American Menopause Society, believes that the nature of these four changes justifies some form of hormone replacement in appropriately selected women. What makes Utian's view of menopause important is that it comes from a trustworthy source. Wulf Utian is now the Executive Director of the North American Menopause Society, and a past President of the International Menopause Society. Like Frank, Utian defined the climacteric as endocrinopathy to represent only a subset of women in whom certain changes were viewed as outside the context of normality. Whether this definition will be appropriately applied or taken out of context remains to be seen. As mentioned in the preceding chapter, in 1931 R.T. Frank set about to identify and then appropriately treat a subset of menstruating women who suffered from severe premenstrual tension. According to Frank, many women experienced varying degrees of discomfort preceding the onset of menstruation. These discomforts, however, were viewed as normal. Only a small number of women were identified as having a grave systemic disorder needing treatment. These women were experiencing severe physiological stress as a result of undesired and/or abnormal tissue responses to fluctuating gonadal hormones.

Some clinicians associate menopause with disease. For example, in Chapter 12 the details on Gambrell's recommendation to perform the progestogen challenge examination on all postmenopausal women once a year, whether or not they are symptomatic, is discussed. Gambrell thinks that just being postmenopausal and asymptomatic may place women at risk for cancer of the endometrium. In other words, even if a woman does not bleed postmenopausally, this could be a sign that the uterine lining is building up to a dangerous precancerous level (Gambrell, 1992).

In summary, the definition of menopause as disease is embedded in patriarchal views and beliefs about women as defective, imperfect, or as Emily Martin suggests, machines to be fixed (1987). This view of menopause permeates society through the media, science, and medical practice.

MENOPAUSE AS NORMAL: THE SOCIAL OR NO-EFFECT MODEL

According to Koeske (1980), the behavioral sciences, or social or no-effect model, is also reductionistic; it reduces women to a set of roles and functions or a composite of reactions to society and the environment. Implicit in this model is the assumption that menopausal changes and the variations in these changes are interpreted either as social events or as cultural-symbolic events. The division of menopausal-associated changes into biologically and hormonally caused events, versus those that are socioculturally and/or environmentally caused, falls prey to the Western ideology of dualism. In other words, separating woman from biology and viewing her totally as a sociocultural being is as reductionistic as the approach taken by proponents of the biological deficit model. Let's examine these two models a little more closely.

An assumption associated with research involving this model is that women are no different from men. The implicit argument of much of the social or no-effect research is that there is no consistent relationship between biochemical or physiological changes and behavior. Specifically, regarding menopause, symptoms are viewed as a response to factors that repress women, leaving them powerless, such as sex-role conditioning, decreased status at this stage of life, and lack of alternative roles at midlife. For example, when the nest empties, loss of roles–particularly loss of the mother role–is considered a very important factor in menopausal depression. Proponents of the empty-nest concept believe that women who have invested most of their energy in motherhood may find the empty nest, not menopause, a depressing event. In the 1970s, Pauline Bart, a feminist sociologist, found that acute depression in the menopausal woman was associated with investment in the mother role and its loss, not with menopausal symptoms. There is good evidence that menopause does not result in higher depression rates for women.

The social or no-effect view appears to have been spearheaded by Marcha Flint, who argued that the "menopausal syndrome" found in American women is a reaction to the American societal abhorrence to old age and aging women (1975). Flint suggested that the reason Rajput Indian women she studied did not present with symptoms was due to heightened social prestige accorded menopausal women in that particular society. As they became menopausal, the women could remove their veils, sit with men, and participate in decisions related to village management, whereas prior to menopause they could not.

Flint's findings were interpreted by van Keep (in a review paper at the 1984 meeting of the International Menopause Society) as an "optical effect." That is, the impression of no symptomatology at menopause is an "illusion." Van Keep (1984) argued that findings related to women in different cultures must be interpreted in terms of the cultural context and the value assigned to critical life events. Yewoubdar Beyene's research on Mayan/Yucatan women and Greek women is a case in point. Like Flint, Beyene found menopause to be a liberating event for Mayan women, mostly because the culturally enforced taboos and rituals associated with menstruation were lifted at menopause. Unlike the situation for women in Western cultures, where menopause represents loss of youth and aging, for Mayan women menopause is not an end; rather, it represents a beginning.

Two problems are associated with the social or no-effect model. First, the negation and/or denial of the biological side of women results in an emphasis solely on sociocultural variables, rendering this model reductionistic to the same degree as the menopause-as-disease/biological deficit one. The exception is that here women are reduced to being reactive agents. Total adherence to a sociocultural explanation of menopause invalidates the fact that some physiological complaints are real. Feminist researchers who support the social or no-effect model may agree more than they disagree with a segment of the biomedical community who continue to believe that menopausal symptoms are largely in the minds of women, i.e., what they experience is all in their imagination. Clearly, much of what women experience at menopause is not in their minds! Physiological changes such as hot flashes and heavy bleeding are a natural response of body tissues to withdrawal or lowering of sex hormone levels, primarily estrogen. Women's bodies become quite used to estrogen; for some women (myself, for example) estrogen was present for 30 to 35 years. When it begins to fluctuate and decrease in concentration, a woman feels it. And when she feels changes and feels differently, she makes the transition from menstrual/reproductive life, the premenopause, to the perimenopause.

Perimenopausal women are very much involved in their world, solving problems, performing caregiving, supporting spouses, partners, and family members in crisis. They are not stagnant nor diseased, and they certainly are not rotting away physiologically. They are actively contributing to the whole of society as teachers, doctors, nurses, systems analysts, lawyers, students, engineers, truck drivers, mothers, wives, salespersons, accountants, secretaries, journalists, cooks, waitresses, mountain climbers, etc. And, yes, as they are interacting and reacting to what is happening in their lives, menopause is also happening. Midlife is a time of life when, in general, things become very complex. In Chapter 9, I have included the words of perimenopausal women who are experiencing the transition. It is important that we hear these voices, as all too often we hear only the opinions and definitions of what menopause is from self-proclaimed experts, who, until recently, have been proponents of either the menopause-as-disease concept, or the social or no-effect view.

Chapter 7

Menopause:
The Problems of Definition

If there is one thing clinicians and researchers agree upon, it is the ambiguity of terms and definitions used to describe the menopause experience. The continuing lack of clear definitions of menopausal terms, such as premenopause and postmenopause, makes it impossible to compare the findings of one research study with another. Women of various ages are grouped together as if they are homogenous, all having the same biopsychological status, when in fact, it is not known whether any two women of the same age have similar menopause experiences—or any other life experiences. Yet, definitionally, menopause, *the last menstrual bleed*, has been used as a dividing line, and women have been categorized as either premenopausal or postmenopausal, depending on whether or not they are menstruating. The assumption is that women *are* similar biologically and psychologically. The lack of precise definitions and the ambiguity with which terms are used has compromised the findings of much menopause research.

The most common error in menopause research is the ambiguity of the words used to define premenopause and perimenopause. This problem is at the root of other research problems, such as subject selection, data analysis, and interpretation/discussion of findings. These problems will be discussed in some detail in the sections on hormone use and heart disease, osteoporosis, and breast cancer.

The definition of menopause as a point in time, i.e., the last bleed, is useful to researchers, clinicians, and consumers; yet, nowhere is it clearly understood how one classifies women who have had their last menstrual bleed by virtue of a hysterectomy, that is, removal of the uterus with ovaries retained. These women, by definition, are menopausal; they have experienced their last menstrual bleed. Yet because they have retained their ovaries and thus the ability to continue to make ovarian estrogen (estradiol), they continue to cycle hormones monthly. How these women differ from those who experienced menopause naturally, or who have had menopause induced through surgery, radiation, or drugs, is unknown.

DEFINITIONS

For better or for worse, then, the following definitions, professionally derived, are offered in an attempt to provide more precision in menopause definition.

Menopause

The clinical definition of menopause is the cessation of menstruation, the last menstrual bleed. For naturally menopausal women, menopause is affirmed after one year has elapsed from the last menstrual bleed. Should a woman experience another bleed after one year of amenorrhea, her menopause would then be considered to be that time when she has her last menstrual bleed. Widespread use of steroid sex hormones, either for contraception or to "treat" menopause, and the implementation of aggressive treatment modalities (surgery, radiation, and chemotherapy) for some diseases, such as cancer, and other treatments, such as oophorectomy to prevent cancer, have necessitated expanding the definition of menopause to differentiate menopause as a natural occurrence from menopause that has been induced or affected by either surgery, hormone use, radiation, or chemotherapy. Whether menopause has been induced or occurs naturally, it is associated with a variety of changes.

Natural Menopause

Natural menopause is the final spontaneous menstrual bleed. It occurs on average at age 51.2. This definition applies to women who have retained their ovaries and who have never taken estrogen, whether in birth control pills or through estrogen replacement.

Hormonal Menopause

Hormonal menopause occurs in any woman who has ever been a sex hormone user. Hormone use includes use of any estrogens (such as estrone or estradiol) hormone-like estrogens (such as ethinyl estradiol or mestranol), and progestins (such as medroxy-progesterone acetate [MPA], norgesterol, and norethindrone).

Alan Treloar thought it was particularly important to introduce the latter definition because his analysis of data of menopausal women revealed that estrogen users experienced menopause at a later age: menopausal age for 294 Tremin Trust participants who had used estrogens was 52, versus 50 for those women who had never used estrogen.

Artificial Menopause

Artificial menopause is the induction of menopause by surgical removal of the uterus (hysterectomy), or removal of both ovaries and uterus (panhysterectomy, which is bilateral salpingectomy and oophorohysterectomy) by ablative chemotherapy (through drugs such as Tamoxifen) or by radiation. Women who experience an artificial menopause have had menopause induced precipitously. More women have menopause induced through surgery than through other means.

Menopausal Transition

Women and their care providers frequently have no overt indicators or index to use to monitor for subtle changes. Neither vaginal smears nor endometrial biopsies give any indication of the dynamics of entry into the transition. However, the closure of reproductive years is a dynamic process, a period of hormone fluctuations and change. As such, the static understanding of menopause as the last menstrual bleed needs to be differentiated from several other concepts.

The menopausal transition is a period of time marked by progressive changes in the pattern of menstrual bleeding, terminating at menopause. The pattern may be one of unusually long or short intervals between bleeds, and may be accompanied by bleeding that is very heavy, gushing, and with clots. Alan Treloar (1981) introduced the term menopausal transition, describing it as the period of time, premenopausally, when genital bleeding changes to either longer- or shorter-than-usual flow intervals. According to Treloar, change in genital bleeding was the crucial phenomenon characterizing the transition to menopause.

Definitions of other terms that are used as frequently as menopause also are not clear cut. The most frequently used terms are *perimenopause, climacteric, premenopause,* and *postmenopause.* I have defined the perimenopausal transition as an indefinite period of time that begins with the onset of the first hot flash and terminates when hot flashes disappear. This means that perimenopausal transition can begin many years prior to menopause and extend into the postmenopausal years. In contrast, The International Menopause Congress's definition of perimenopause is that period beginning immediately prior to menopause, when endocrinological, biological, and clinical features of approaching menopause commence and continue for at least the first year after menopause. This latter definition differs from the one I proposed in that empirical indicators are not provided to identify the onset of the perimenopausal phase, or the end of this stage. Neither definition designates specific biological or endocrinological indicators that may be used to characterize entry into or passage through perimenopause.

The issue of ambiguity of definition was addressed at the first International Congress on Menopause, convened in 1976 in Southern France. At that meeting, consensus in definition was accomplished with the cooperation of a panel of international authorities. Menopause was defined as the final menstrual period. Climacteric was differentiated from menopause as a phase in women's aging process that marks the transition from the reproductive to the nonreproductive state, which sometimes, but not necessarily always, is associated with symptomatology (van Keep, Greenblatt, and Albeaux-Fernet, 1976).

The ambiguity in definition also was addressed in the 1981 World Health Organization's (WHO) technical report, *Research on the Menopause.* A WHO scientific group conducting research on the menopause recommended the following stipulated definitions of menopause, perimenopause, postmenopause, and premenopause (pp. 8, 10):

Menopause: Permanent cessation of menstruation resulting from loss of ovarian, follicular activity.

Perimenopause (also referred to as the *climacteric*)*:* The period immediately prior to menopause when endocrinological, biological, and clinical features of approaching menopause commence, continuing for at least the first year after the menopause.

Postmenopause: A period dating from the menopause, although it cannot be determined until after 12 months of spontaneous amenorrhea.

Premenopause: The whole of the reproductive period prior to the menopause, not just the one or two years prior to menopause.

In 1996, the WHO group published Technical Report 886 on menopause, agreeing with the above definitions advanced in 1981 except for the term "climacteric." The term was dropped.

Comparison of findings of menopause studies is made difficult because of the lack of agreement among menopause researchers on how to classify women according to menopausal status. Nancy Woods suggested that the menopause period be divided into three distinct phases: premenopausal, menopausal, and postmenopausal. The premenopausal phase was defined as the phase during which nonpregnant women have had a menstrual period within three months. The menopausal phase was defined as the time period during which menstrual periods have stopped for at least 3 to 12 months. The postmenopausal phase was defined as a time period during which menstrual bleeding had stopped for one or more years. To increase precision in definition, Woods (1982) suggests subscripts be used to designate periods of time that extend beyond postmenopause.

HOW WOMEN VIEW AND DEFINE MENOPAUSE

In Chapters 8, 9, and 10, I include anecdotes written by women representative of the various stages of menopause. It is informative to know *how* women describe and define their experiences, and *what* they are experiencing. Views and attitudes among these women regarding menopause vary considerably. This is not too surprising, since premenopausal women in general do not experience menopausal changes, whereas perimenopausal women are in the transition and undergoing changes associated with the end of ovulation and lowered hormone levels.

In general, premenopausal women have no history and little information on menopause. Perimenopausal women are in the midst of the transition, and describe the full spectrum of changes possible. Postmenopausal women describe the experience from recall, and as such, what they recall and the intensity of the experience depends on whether they have been postmenopausal for a short or long time. The anecdotes of the women have not been edited except to remove material related to research record-keeping and/or identifying data. The age of these women ranges from 13 to 78 years, from very young postmenarcheal menstrual women to older women who have been postmenopausal for more than 20 years.

An examination of the material written by women in all menopausal stages suggests the following:

1. Menopause, in general, is viewed as a normal event.
2. Premenopausal women, on average, have little idea of what it means to be menopausal, except to be done with periods and to have no worries about pregnancy. The words of these women at times resonate the societal view of menopause as a negative experience. It is also an experience not yet identified with the self, similar to what Root (1992) observed with menstruating women as they described the menstrual bleed as an out-of-body experience. Menopause is described by young premenopausal women as "it," e.g., "When it comes, I hope it does not come too early," etc. However, as women move from the pre- to the perimenopause, the experience becomes more of an "in-body" rather than an "out-of-body" experience.
3. During the perimenopause, knowing what changes to expect does not make it easy to cope with the changes. The changes are annoying, stressful, and fatiguing, and interfere with activities of daily living. The anecdotes validate that hot flashes have never totally incapacitated or killed anyone. Yet the same women describe problems with fatigue and loss of energy, which sometimes were misdiagnosed or suggested to be depression, if hot flashes were frequent and/or heavy bleeding occurred over long periods of time, resulting in anemia. Some of these women con-

sulted a health care provider for treatment. Treatment options were either hormonal or surgical. Some women experienced painful intercourse, or no desire or diminished desire to participate in sexual activity, and treatment was necessary for these women to restore the quality of sexual relationships.

There was also confusion related to what changes are related to menopause and what is related to the aging process in general. The women report changes in body composition, wrinkles, decrease in height, increase in weight, onset of allergies, stiffness, joint and arthritic pain, as well as onset of and/or worsening of chronic conditions such as asthma, Ménière's disease (a problem with fluid in the ear, resulting in imbalance), and dry eye syndrome. Menopause may have a little to do with these conditions, but it is not the cause of them.

4. Postmenopausal women describe the experience as liberating and energizing. In retrospect, they insist it was not debilitating, unmanageable, or unnatural. It was just over!

Chapter 8

Premenopause:
A Time of Menstrual Stability

The term "premenopausal" includes the whole of the reproductive period prior to menopause, from menarche to menopause. Within the premenopause, then, is the perimenopause, a period of time closer to the menopause, which is identified by the onset of menopausal changes, e.g., hot flash or bleeding changes. The participants, whose voices are included in this chapter, have not experienced any menopausal changes. They are, for all practical purposes, menstruating women, experiencing the changes associated with normally fluctuating levels of hormones during the various menstrual cycle phases. They are not experiencing hot flashes or any other menopausal changes indicative of entry into the perimenopause. In essence, they have not yet begun the change process, although there is a strong possibility that the older women in this group (age 40 and older) are on the threshold of entering perimenopause.

VOICES OF YOUNG PREMENOPAUSAL WOMEN

Most of the young women (age 13 to 39) describe menopause as an event that is indeed very far off in the future. On average, they have not given menopause much thought unless their mothers were in the midst of the transition to menopause. As such, one source of information is their mothers, and as we would expect, this results in either positive or negative impressions. Some women plan to talk with their mothers at some time in the future, when "their time" comes, to obtain information. Generally, the young premenopausal women view menopause positively, and the majority look forward to the time when they will no longer have periods. A small sample of their comments follows:

I really have no fears about menopause, but knowing when it does come, a chapter of my life is over, and I am facing the unknown. The difference in my body is a scary thought.

It seems a long way off and a sign of getting past middle age.

I'm only 21 so it seems very far off. Right now it would seem nice to not menstruate and I'm looking forward to it. I imagine when it does happen I will feel a loss.

I'm not worried about it but I certainly don't look forward to it either. My mom is just starting to experience hot flashes, and I've read of lowered desire of sex—doesn't sound too fun!

Not looking forward to the process—fearful of becoming [a] "crotchety old maid."

I remember my mother being very unpredictable and irritable and I hope that somehow those days will be easier for me and my family.

I know nothing about menopause—it seems little information is available.

I have not given it much thought, which I guess means that I don't expect it to be difficult.

I can't wait. I hate periods. I also hope the transition goes smoothly.

Frankly I am looking forward to eliminating my period from my thoughts and concern.

I have mixed feelings, don't know what to expect.

I'm short (5'1"; weight 112 lbs.) and am concerned about whether to take hormones to prevent osteoporosis following menopause. My father, age 81, has osteoarthritis. It is confusing to me.

I don't expect to start a menopausal time for at least another twelve years, when I'm around 45 years old. When I do go through it I expect to be very emotional and get irritated very easily, but I hope that is something I can control.

I expect it to be a period of adjustment for my body—hopefully smooth—and I hope to not have to take any hormones.

Look forward to no periods. Hesitant/apprehensive of hot flashes/ mood changes, [and] unpredictable bleeding.

I hope it does not come too early, because of starting my family at age 32, and [I] would like to have several more children, possibly into my forties.

After a frank and open discussion with my mother about her menopause experience, I expect my experience will be a calm gradual change like hers, not the stereotypical "hysterical female."

[I'm] not really looking forward to menopause but not dreading it either. I view it as part of life.

[I hope menopause will] stabilize the physical/emotional patterns that dramatically change monthly due to my period. Because of my cramps, I'm looking forward to its end.

I haven't thought about it. I hope by the time that I [reach menopause], they take my uterus out and put me on hormones—that will hopefully eliminate the menopause experience.

A lot of people have gone through it, so I'm sure I'll be able to, too. From what I've heard, the symptoms are not as bad as publicized. I'm looking forward to no longer menstruating.

I look forward to not having my periods!

Don't really know, haven't really thought about it, only being 29.

I hope I don't hit menopause until my fifties. I enjoy my natural hormones now, especially estrogen. I will take hormones when I reach menopause. I have some concerns on how it will affect my sex drive and sexual relations.

It is part of life, haven't thought much about it.

It sounds like a real pain in the **!!

It would be a great relief not to have to cope with these inconveniences every month. I would feel very free. My family doesn't attain this state until age 60 years, so I still have a long wait.

I don't know enough about it.

Menopause is a natural process which is removed from me personally and from my age (21). I am aware of its psychological associations and potential problems, but I do not yet really contemplate this occurrence.

I am not exactly sure what happens.

I have a ways to go before I have to feel anything about it.

I think I'll be okay, at least I won't have to put up with my period, or have to worry about birth control. [I] am concerned about mood change things.

Will be a new phase in my life as a woman.

I have never considered the eventuality of menopause and therefore find myself without an opinion of any sort.

I haven't thought about it, since I'm only 19 years old. I really don't know that much about it either.

I expect to feel a little depressed that a certain period (pardon the pun) of my life is over. I don't expect physical pain of any kind.

VOICES OF OLDER PREMENOPAUSAL WOMEN

The ages of the "older" premenopausal women range from 40 to 55 years. Some women, particularly one 55-year-old woman, were old enough by virtue of age alone, to be either perimenopausal or postmenopausal, and as such, to be experiencing changes. Yet none were! These women, just as their younger cohorts, also expressed what a relief it will be to no longer have periods, although one woman ambivalently indicates that while she will be glad to no longer have periods, she is saddened by the loss of a friend (her monthly period). Menopause is described as a time of excitement, the next phase of life. Common changes associated with aging, such as weight gain, hair changes, skin changes (wrinkles), etc., appear to be concerns more than typical menopausal changes. And as one would expect, chronic diseases are more evident in this age group. Whether by virtue of age and/or being part of our mid-life study, these women are thinking about menopause more seriously than their younger cohorts. They observe friends and sisters experiencing perimenopausal changes, and they question whether or not they should be hormone users. They are ambivalent about what to do, and sometimes angry, because menopause has been brought into their conscious awareness. Others deny that anything negative associated with menopause will happen. These Tremin Trust women comprise the largest group of menstruating women in the research program (they were enrolled in the mid-1960s).

The anecdotes that follow are a random selection of responses to an open-ended question on a survey regarding thoughts, fears, joys, concerns, etc., about menopause, from a total sample of about 400 responses.

I get a yearly Pap smear, but I don't ask too many questions about menopause, as I just figure what happens, happens. If I felt I needed answers to a question, though, I would not hesitate to call my doctor.

My mom was over 50 when she went through menopause, so I don't expect to have to deal with it for another ten years or so.

I have pretty much assumed that it's a natural process, and I'll just adapt. However, things like this make me wonder if there's something I should be doing to prepare.

I really know nothing about menopause—[I] don't focus on its "arrival," [and I'm] not even sure when to expect this change. I'm assuming [it will occur] in my fifties, so it seems "too far away" to "worry" about.

Because I was asked to participate in this survey, I have thought more about midlife. At first, I was shocked to find out that I'm considered to be at "midlife"! In fact, I was upset. But, it has made me pay attention to my physical and emotional health, and to begin to prepare myself for upcoming changes.

I feel like my life is ruled by my menstrual cycle/condition. I look forward to feeling well more than two weeks a month, and to not having to explain/make excuses to my husband (who is not unreasonable or demanding; he's just interested, sympathetic, but ultimately [he] can't really relate). It really does ultimately make me feel unattractive, somehow impaired.

My older sister (one year older) began missing periods this year and went to our family doctor. I was surprised how little doctors know about menopause and what to do about it. She started taking Premarin, she was told to take it when needed. Another doctor suggested Estrace and Provera at the end of the cycle; she got the worst periods and cramps. Another woman suggested Premarin and Provera together, and she started and it has worked fine. It has really helped her moodiness, but she has zero sex drive. Someone else suggested vitamin E, but it didn't seem to help. It scares me when I really don't know what to do when mine begins.

I have chronic mastitis, and a surgeon I've seen for 20 years regarding fibro cystic disease and other problems advises me not to take hormones—unless I am too uncomfortable or there is a history of breast cancer in my family (there is not). I worry about the effects of [not taking] hormones on my bones—particularly—I plan to discuss his recommendation with my OB-GYN doctor. The surgeon's reason for suggesting [not taking] hormones is so my breasts would be "less active."

Mostly, I feel in the dark about the process and choices available to me. I don't trust most of the information because there are studies on all sides of the issues. I mostly worry about osteoporosis and heart disease risk. I have received conflicting advice about hormone replacement therapy. I am inclined to avoid any and all medications, including aspirin. I am inclined to look for holistic ways to treat my problems. I am at the beginning of new behavior—especially physical exercise, but don't see much pay off. I thought I would welcome signs of aging—as a natural course of events, a journey towards wisdom—but I don't like jowls and liver spots! I was always fond of my periods, part of being a women connected to the cycles of time and nature.

I had no experiences of menopause this year. Friends who are my age are having symptoms—I started menstruating [when I was] around 11 years old, so I thought that I would go through menopause earlier than 49.

My periods have always been fairly regular and predictable (too close together for my liking: 22 to 24 days), but no cramps or other problems ever. The only symptom I have is greater tiredness just the day before and during the first day or two. I also get severe headaches occasionally, but I'm not sure if they are hormone-related. Because menstruation has never been a problem, I am not anxious about menopause. My mother, who is now 87, never experienced any problems other than hot flashes—never saw a doctor nor took drugs or hormones—and took it in stride just as she has done everything else in her life. I expect that I will deal with it in the same way. I am overweight now, but I attribute that to changing jobs, family stresses and problems, and not menopause.

I plan on taking menopause in stride like everything else I do.

Sorry I'm late [returning her survey]—went white water rafting in May for eight days and have been walking lots of miles to train for a marathon—hope exercise helps the loss of estrogen because I'm getting lots of that lately—feel better than I did when I was younger, except for morning "aches and pains." Still *have all the PMS symptoms before/during periods for several days, so [I'm] still looking forward to no periods.*

Do women really worry about this stuff? Seems like a man must have started this study, since the choices given do not reflect the full spectrum of feelings a woman could have (i.e., they are heavily weighted toward the negative, not *the positive, like freedom, joy, increased sexuality, etc.)* Wake up. This is the nineties!!

I really don't give much thought to menopause since I don't seem to be experiencing any of the things associated with it. I'm extremely healthy and look younger than my 46 years. I'm sure that when menopause does set in, I'll become very much interested in the changes that will be affecting me.

Except for loss of estrogen, I will be glad to be done with monthly periods, cramps, headaches, and PMS.

I am hoping that if my outlook is positive I won't experience any emotional or physical problems.

OK about it. I feel the positives will be not having to be aware of menstruation schedule, procedures, etc. But, [I] would hope that I won't have mood swings, as I do now. Am aware that with menopause I may be more susceptible to heart/cholesterol problems (it runs in my family), so I'll need to be more careful of my eating/exercise habits.

Looking forward to no more periods; not looking forward to dry skin, saggy bags of age!

I do not anticipate any difficulty with menopause. [I] probably will not have hot flashes. I am not sure how I feel about estrogen therapy, but will probably avoid it if I can. [I] prefer to continue my exercise program to guard against osteoporosis.

I expect my skin to wrinkle—I've been having hot flashes so I guess I will have some problem with that.

Menopause is just part of life and I don't think it is any big deal.

I expect it to occur in the next five to eight years. My current feelings are to avoid replacement hormones because of the strong family history of breast cancer.

None. Expect to take hormones for antiosteoporosis, heart, and mood (doctor's advice).

Not concerned—very low priority compared to all of life's "opportunities."

Haven't thought much about it.

Can't wait!!!

It's just fine except for the hot flashes, and I can live with those pretty easily.

Little change from how things are now except the wrinkles will come faster.

Nothing major. [I] wonder when it will happen for sure, and what my health situation will be like—emotional and physical.

I don't expect it to be very difficult. There may be some times when unpleasant symptoms occur—but not extreme.

I won't miss the unpleasantness of monthly periods, but I am concerned about feeling depressed during the postmenopause. I feel sad at taking this step in aging.

Dread because it is another sign of aging. Relief because it no longer will be a bother.

Am looking forward to not having to bother with menstrual periods. But on the dark side, it signals that most of my life will be behind me. I see it as a natural milestone as I progress through life.

I keep thinking I will stop having my periods, but so far not so. I'm 55 years old. Maybe this year it will happen.

I expect to go through menopause naturally—no surgery, no therapy. I exercise regularly, as I always have. I do have to eat less, however. How unfair!

I look forward to the absence of periods and do not expect problems.

Part of the life cycle.

It can't come soon enough, except I dread the symptoms that accompany menopause.

Since I feel so well, I look forward to it. Do not have depressing thoughts of aging, etc., as I am thankful I have reached my present age in good health, and feel as good or better than in younger years, which have been filled with much caring for family.

Not worried. I feel women tend to blame all their aches and pains on menopause. If your life is full, you will have no time to worry about these minor problems.

I look forward to sexual intercourse without worry of pregnancy.

I'm not worried about it; I feel it's a normal process. My feeling is that it would be very nice to just cease, rather than [having to] mess around with a lot of irregular "periods" for a length of time.

It's a very normal part of living. I'm concerned about osteoporosis. My mother is very stooped at 76.

I don't anticipate any problems with it, though I may be surprised. I have no idea how my mother did with it since she never talked about it, or menstruation, at all. I'm looking forward to it now as an end to concern about getting pregnant, which I certainly don't want.

I don't anticipate any problems—anxious to be done with occasional PMS headaches.

I'm afraid of finding the process annoying—abnormal weight gain, periods of hot flashes, cramps more severe at times, hair growth on chin—yuk. Early menopause (I'm 44) means having concern about calcium level, too. Expectations? Not really sure, take it one day at a time.

Concern about osteoporosis and increased heart risk after menopause. Will welcome not having PMS anymore—curious about how I'll feel going through menopause.

I don't expect any significant physical problems. I'm surprised to discover that with every year older I get, I am more apprehensive about the emotional impact of menopause, because having children isn't an issue. Perhaps I'm concerned about whether menopause will have an effect on my sexuality.

I don't have any concerns about menopause at this stage of my life.

I'm worried about it when it comes to mind, but I feel as though it's a long time off—that it's for old people, and I'm far from old.

I've not given it much thought. I expect no major problems in association with menopause, but will deal with any as the occasion arises. It seems like just another natural step in my life.

I expect to have hot flashes and I expect to have mood swings once I become menopausal.

After talking with my mother (who has been a contributor for over 50 years) and reading about menopause, I don't think I'll be too unprepared. I'll be pleased to not worry about pregnancy. If I do as my mother did, I may still have ten years of regular periods, or possibly less if I begin to skip periods during this time at all. Any symptoms, if not severe, will be coped with so I'll know what changes really are going on naturally. Now that I've remarried, I tend to panic when I don't have a period, as I check the change in mucus discharge to watch for ovulation. With this in mind, I have mixed feelings but it can't be any worse than the last two years, which have been unusual due to financial stress.

I hope I'm okay. Also I wonder how it may affect my Ménière's disease. Now, just before and during and about a week after my period, my ear ringing and balance are worse. The ear doctor said it may be fluid retention. If I stop my periods, will this change? Otherwise I really don't know much about menopause. Some people get kinda weird and moody.

No problem. I'll take hormones only if absolutely necessary.

Not worried about it. Will be glad to not have to bother with periods any more.

I am nervous about menopause–think I may be in beginning stages–[I] worry about possibility of hysterectomy.

I spoke with my mother, who was one of your original participants, and she shared with me what she went through. She did not indicate any adverse problems, so I don't expect any. She did say her mother had fainting or black-out episodes, [which were] never really traced to menopause, but that was a long time ago. Also, [there was] some problem of spasms with her mother! If I experienced any overt reaction, I would seek out a specialist. In my area there are many competent people to help in a problem.

May have already experienced a hormonal imbalance–don't expect menopause to be in the near future. Am not anxious about menopause.

I'm not really worried about menopause, but I'd like to put it off as long as possible. I think the longer your natural hormones are at work, the better. My mother didn't seem to have any problems with menopause.

I accept it as a normal process, and do not have any strong feelings about it one way or another. Although it has occurred to me that not having monthly periods will be nice.

I have no physical fears–just emotional fears concerning loss of a "friend."

I hope and expect it to be mild, not unpleasant, tapering off with no need to medicate. I have spoken to friends [about it, and] I will be talking with my mother soon about her experience of menopause. She once told me it was "no big deal."

Actually I'm anxious! (as in "excited" and "impatient")

Looking forward to no more periods and cramps, but not looking forward to hormonal replacement–such as birth control pills for estrogen (a woman at work was put on the pill to retain femininity, per her doctor).

I look forward toward menopause—or at least the end of menstruation when I will no longer have a period! I don't worry about pregnancy—have had my tubes tied—but can't wait to be rid of the mess and bother!

I do not expect much change because I've always been so regular, had no problems. I think I may experience emotional changes, i.e., [I may be] more emotional than normal.

I dread the aging process and I hope I don't have mood changes.

I can hardly wait! I have fibroids, and am hoping they will reduce in size during menopause.

Chapter 9

Perimenopause:
A Time of Transition and Change

In the words of the women in premenopause, one does not find great concerns about menopause. Primarily, for these menstruating women, the expectation is that menopause will be an uneventful transition from reproductive life to the end of fertility. In the words of women in premenopause, one does not find great concern about menopause. Primarily, for these menstruating women, the expectation is that menopause will be an uneventful transition from reproductive life to the end of fertility. Perimenopausal women, however, paint a different word picture. These women describe both somatic (bodily) and mood changes, which are normal and predictable. Unlike the changes experienced during the premenstrual phase of the menstrual cycle, which are mostly due to fluctuating hormone levels, common perimenopausal changes are a result of lowered levels of hormones, and the response of tissues and organ systems to withdrawal of hormones.

The beginning of perimenopause is typically marked by the onset of hot flash or a change in bleeding pattern. The exact duration of time women spend in the perimenopause phase is unknown, and varies from woman to woman. Work done by Alan Treloar suggests that once the duration of menstrual interval begins to change, women can expect to be in the transition, on average, for about two years. No additional definitive research has been conducted in this area.

The key word in perimenopause is "transition." A woman does not become menopausal overnight; follicular depletion and atresia occurs over a woman's lifetime. Prior to menopause the ovaries become less and less responsive to stimulation from brain hormones. During this period of time, which can be four to five years long, if estrogen is not made by the ovarian follicle, a woman may experience hot flashes, change in mood, and/or changes in bleeding. It may be that one or the other ovary suddenly becomes responsive to high levels of follicle-stimulating brain hormones, particularly FSH, to promote ovulation. For some women (and the reason is unknown), after a period of symptom experience, symptoms may subside or vanish, and a woman may again be symptom-free for six months, or even a year. Eventually, however, time runs out. At a genetically predetermined time, the last egg is ovulated, and estrogen (estradiol) and progesterone hormone production from the ovary ceases. No matter how much the level of brain follicle-stimulating hormone increases, the follicles remain unresponsive, ovulation ceases, and menopause occurs. Documentation that menopause has occurred cannot be made until 12 months without a menstrual bleed have passed.

COMMON CHANGES
ASSOCIATED WITH THE TRANSITION

The most common perimenopausal changes are the following: hot flashes/flushes, heavy and/or irregular onset of vaginal bleeding, vaginal dryness, stress or urge incontinence, and mood swings. Other changes women reported include: joint pain, redistribution of body weight, skin pigmentation, growth of body and facial hair or baldness, sleep disturbances, sexuality changes, restless and jumpy legs, and formications (a feeling that something is crawling on your skin).

As women enter perimenopause, most do not let the changes they experience dominate their lives. Instead, for some women, menopause is more than hot flashes, heavy bleeding, and mood fluctuations. It is a time full of change, and a time for reflection, challenges, sadness, "empty" as well as "full" nests, and lifestyle and career changes. These views are reflected in the words of perimenopausal participants of The Tremin Trust who responded to a survey that asked them to discuss any questions, problems, joys, stresses, or good experiences related to menopause over a one-year period. Specifically, they were asked the following:

- What has bothered you? What has been stressful?
- What is on your mind?
- What has been helpful?

- What questions do you have, if any, about changing menstrual cycles?
- What questions do you have about hormones?

A 50-year-old woman reflected on menopause as a time of challenge, change, and choices:

> *Menopause has been pretty much as I'd expected. It has positives and negatives, as with menstruation! Hormone replacement treatment eliminated the hot flashes and joint aches. As I became a full-time doctoral student and our youngest child left for college, I was kept very busy ([I] have a 4.0 average). I have not felt depressed or encountered hormonally related mood swings. I have a loving, supportive husband and wonderful, productive, bright, and healthy young adult children. This is a happy, fulfilling time for me! I feel good about life, myself, and the future—at age 50!*

This woman clearly does not view menopause as the end of useful life. She returned to school as a full-time graduate student. She has great support from her family as she pursues a career in a doctoral program and she maintains an outstanding grade point average. She is on hormone replacement to help cope with the hot flashes and joint pain, which, undoubtedly, would have affected her sleep and concentration, as well as her ability to perform in school.

Another woman, age 49, entered menopause and medical school at the same time, validating Margaret Mead's view that life begins rather than ends at menopause, and there is a time of postmenopausal zest (PMZ). An important lesson this woman teaches us is that we can fulfill the role of mother first, and then, at midlife, pursue a lifelong professional goal.

> *I entered menopause and began medical school in the same year. I am extremely happy and blessed to have the rest of my life focused on the profession I thought I traded for my first choice of a happy marriage and six great kids. Now I have all I wished for. I just finished my first year and I still love it.*

Another woman reflects on the meaning of being a menstruating woman, and what menopause really means to her. She also raises a frequent, as well as important, question about the "genetics" of menopause, i.e., will/would her menopause experience be similar to her mother's or her grandmother's?

> *I have some sadness about periods ending, not because bleeding was such a joy, but that clock, that regularity, that reminder of my ability to conceive–all were good feelings for me. Menopause is an unknown. All the elders in my family are gone. I can't ask a mother or aunt or grandmother or sister what it was like for them or whether what I am experiencing is natural for our family. I think of the generations and genera- tions of women who experienced menopause without drugs and hoopla. I see strong, vibrant older women everywhere. As I sit here thinking, my concerns are more about aging than about menopause. I am not 50 yet; I haven't accomplished many of the goals I set out to accomplish (I have accomplished many, however). My hair texture has changed, my skin seems drier, [and] I've been overweight for some time and wonder if I'll ever get into a good health bracket. The muscles at my chin and neck are going. I have lines in my face, and my eyes have led me to bifocals. Others are wrapping up careers and I haven't started one. Is it too late?*

The answer to one question this woman has, "Is it too late to start a new career?" is "Of course not." The voices of the first two women validate this assumption. Many women are either returning to school at midlife or beginning school. The ranks of nontradi- tional students have grown exponentially over the past decade. Unlike during the 1970s when I entered graduate school at age 40, today women comprise the largest number of nontraditional stu- dents in colleges and universities. If we continue to draw upon theories of growth and development generated from the study of men, then, yes, we would say that midlife is not a time to start a career. Most men at midlife have reached the peak of their careers. Women, unlike men, were working in the home, raising families, and receiving no monetary reimbursement and little or no recogni- tion that what they did was important. A theory or theories of growth and development based upon the study of women would reassure this woman that she is not off schedule in realizing her manifest destiny related to a career. This woman also paints a positive image of older women. Yet, at the same time, she despairs over aging changes. She raises the genetics issue related to menopause, age, changes, and expectations. It is important to have information related to the female elders' experience of menopause and to gather information on how those genetically closest made the journey. For this women, unfortunately, that opportunity is no longer possible.

A 49-year-old woman wrote about the freedom and sense of relief that menopause and midlife will bring related to lifestyle changes that are anticipated when she and her husband are no longer responsible, financially, for children.

> *Generally, I have no problems with menopause, although occasionally I think I would prefer not to have the saggy skin and wrinkled looks that go with it. I do look forward to a lifestyle that being older and not having financial responsibility for children will bring. This is just a few years off. The change in sexual desire is of some concern, but my husband is also experiencing changes, so we just need to work harder at coordination and understanding.*

This woman also addresses concerns about her changes in skin tone, wrinkles, and the effects of aging. None of us can escape the expression of our genetic endowment as we age. We can get a pretty good idea of what it will be like, however, if we climb our family tree, look around, and observe how the elders in our family are aging. One of the most misunderstood aspects of menopause is that it does not cause aging *per se*. Menopause is embedded in the aging process, and because it happens at a time when other changes are occurring, it becomes a catch-all for a multitude of changes. This woman also expressed concern about a change in sexual desire. Although she did not state specifically that she had a "decreased" desire for sexual intimacy, the findings of a study done by me, Dr. Phyllis K. Mansfield, and Dr. Patricia B. Koch, indicate that women experience changes in sexual desire, sexual enjoyment with a partner, and ease in reaching orgasm. Nearly one-half of the 400 women we surveyed indicated that they had experienced a change in their sexual response. Changes in sexual desire appear to be related to physical changes in vaginal tissue—that is, dryness and pain during intercourse.

Menopause as a time of life change is viewed by a 50-year-old woman as a time of connectedness with nature, with other women, and with the next generation.

> *I feel I am experiencing normal life changes and patterns that connect me to nature [and to] other women. My great joy is my first grandchild, a girl, whose birth I witnessed. I feel I have real value to her and her folks, and that I really fit with the role now.*

This woman conceptualizes her life as just beginning to take on a new dimension of caring and nurturing–responsibility for the next generation. Her life energy will be directed toward grandmothering and feeling very valuable in performing that role.

A 49-year-old woman shares random thoughts about the value of being in a research program. Being a participant in The Tremin Trust research study has helped her to do self-evaluation related to menopause.

> *I am really happy to be participating in this study. It's helped me to look at myself, take stock of my health, emotionally and physically, and evaluate where I have been and where I'm headed. I feel especially satisfied to realize that I am not experiencing many of the "dreaded" problems as I grow older. In the past five years my periods have reduced in number and gained in intensity. The GYN I see has suggested aspirin for the clots I experience and that has helped. He's added yearly mammograms too. This research program is doing all women a great service. There is so much to be learned about all of us. I'm grateful you are doing it.*

This woman is experiencing one of the most common changes associated with perimenopause, change in the quality of the bleeding as well as in the duration of the bleed. Passing clots in menstrual blood can be very frightening for a woman. Aspirin is used as a preventive against heart attacks, and particularly as an anticoagulant (blood thinner). Its use as a clot preventer or thinner in premenopausal bleeding has not been supported through research. However, this women does feel that the situation has improved. What is important is that she is taking aspirin under the care of a physician.

The words of these perimenopausal women illustrate that, contrary to the negative stereotype of the menopausal woman portrayed in the medical and professional journal ads and in some popular magazines, the end of reproductive life, although filled with changes, is also a time for new beginnings, growth, reflection, and decision making. It is a time when women come face-to-face with important issues: What will I do with the rest of my life, and will I be able to do it as an older woman without hormones? For some women, experiencing menopause translates into confusion, frustration, and concern in response to the controversy fueled by experts on both sides of the hormone replacement issue, osteoporosis, and heart disease. For others it is no big deal! They are clear that menopause is normal. How a woman views menopause is relative to where she is in terms of gynecological, not chronological, age. For example, the older women in The Tremin Trust Research Program who were enrolled in the 1930s are now mostly in their seventies. These women undeniably proclaim that menopause was "no big deal." Most women made the transition without hormones or other additive therapies. Menopause was welcomed; it closed the door to the menstrual and pregnancy rooms; it brought newfound freedoms and the opportunity to explore new options.

Tremin Trust women enrolled in the 1960s (now in their late forties or early fifties) by and large resonate the voices of their predecessors in saying that menopause is no big deal. In their anecdotes that follow, however, they clearly reflect contemporary societal attitudes regarding menopause as disease and the devaluing of aged individuals, as they provide rather detailed descriptions of how complex their lives have become as they reach midlife and enter perimenopause. They communicate also that the issues and problems they face related to relationships, family crises, deaths (natural and by suicide), life-threatening and/or chronic illness, employment, etc., are very, very stressful. For some, midlife stressors, combined with normal aging changes, become confounded with menopause. As such, menopause sometimes gets an unfair share of the blame for what is occurring in women's lives, since what is happening is more clearly related to sociocultural factors. Some of The Tremin Trust women are able to distinguish a stressful life event from menopause. When both combine, however, as the following anecdotes suggest, the quality of life for women in the transition is affected.

VOICES OF PERIMENOPAUSAL WOMEN

In February 1988 I lost my husband of 19 years to suicide. Suicide grief is hard work and I attribute much of the bleeding irregularity, etc., to my grief. (Maybe to the initial shock of finding his body.) At any rate, I feel I am now in good health mentally, physically, emotionally, and spiritually.

In and out of work for past two years with the airlines–[I] can't get a good job. I find the stress of working full time–keeping house and family together and happy–very hard sometimes. I'm emotionally stable, but sometimes it gets overwhelming and I break down.

About question 10, you left out natural disasters. If you're interested in how stressful things have been for me this year, please add in a few more change units for a series of disastrous winter storms, just before and after Christmas. Howling winds, thousands of downed trees, my lineman husband working 18 hours at a stretch in awful conditions, power outages lasting many days and affecting my whole community, and frozen pipes causing havoc when the thaw came. Oh, yeah, and the dog developed a miserable skin condition. It was a very hard winter, made much harder by my nearby father's increasing mental health problems. It seems to me I'm getting steadier as the years go by, and if it's menopause, I'll take it, dry skin and all. Thank you for your continuing efforts to help us all understand how women work.

My new husband wants to start a family. However, I am almost 47 and already have a 24-year-old daughter who just married. I don't really want to; I want to keep my career and my energy.

I am in the middle of a personal crisis and can't sort out what problems may be stress related and what may be physical changes not related to stress. My lover of three years died. I took over the operation of his business (in addition to running my own). His business is complementary to mine so keeping it running made good sense for a number of reasons. I'm feeling overwhelmed by every-

thing. My energy level is low, I feel physically ill, and I think I'm depressed. I plan to see a doctor in the next two weeks for an evaluation of my physical status.

I have had gas pains in my intestines off and on for over a year. About a year or two ago, I had barium tests. I was told it was irritable bowel syndrome. It comes a lot and I can't get rid of it often. The only way I get rid of it is if I don't eat at all, and since I rarely can seem to do that, I seem to get this a lot. In April my mother died. When she got very sick, I got this problem real bad and can't seem to get rid of it. Otherwise I feel okay usually. One thing about my period I've noticed, if I eat lots of sweets, my PMS [symptoms] are way worse. If I eat well, my symptoms are far less exaggerated. I crave junk food but it makes me worse overall if I give in and eat much of it. Chocolate, especially, makes me worse, and I crave it the most.

The past few years have been quite difficult with four teens, three children graduating from high school, children becoming sexually active, etc. I have a very strong marriage relationship and very supportive friends. I maintain a very close relationship with my parents (aged 75 and 84). I talk with them, see them, do things for or with them one or two times per week. We also had a very close relationship with my father-in-law who was very ill for an extended period with cancer and died one-and-a-half years ago. We continue a good relationship with my mother-in-law. My two adoptive children have been a real challenge to parent, and I am looking forward to the next phase in our relationship.

My menopausal transition coincided with the loss (repossession) of investment real estate that I had built and was enmeshed with for five years. [It] also [coincided] with the full expression of anorexia/ bulimia in my college-age daughter, requiring hospitalization and intense therapy for suicide attempts. This caused me to feel a failure as a mother, hence my depression and therapy.

I've had a bad year and I'm not sure how much I can relate to maturity. I broke my leg and had several months of total disability—couldn't drive, etc. (A state I had never experienced on the slightest level). My 83-year-old mother was placed in a nursing home. I am over 2,000 miles from her and struggle with the helplessness.

Placing in black and white (writing about) how I am doing hopefully will help me take some positive action to regain some control.

I suspect many of my changes are related to recent pregnancy, which was complicated by pre-term labor and four weeks of bed rest resulting in a successful birth. My periods have been erratic since then (I bled for over a month postpartum) and have had a dysfunctional pattern the past two months. I don't know how much of this is related to aging and how much to pregnancy—it is interesting that after my first pregnancy my periods have been much heavier the first two days and longer. Unfortunately, this continues. If the dysfunctional bleeding continues another month, I plan to try Provera. I think the changes in sexual drive are 100 percent related to fatigue with a four-month-old baby not sleeping the night plus full-time work and night call—I don't believe these are hormone related—[I] don't feel it's likely I'm menopausal in the near future.

This has been a very difficult year and I haven't given menopause a great deal of thought. My daughter (18-1/2) has been diagnosed as having clinical depression. There has been a tremendous amount of stress associated with this as she has been hospitalized once and the crisis situation tripled. Through therapy (family and individual), things are slowly coming together. I have finally accepted my husband's death and am in the process of beginning a new relationship with all its attendant problems and questions, to say nothing of sexuality (which moms are not supposed to experience). Perhaps, after things settle down, I'll have time to wonder about the changes taking place. All of this time, I haven't spent much time pondering them.

Actually, I'm very happy not to have had my period lately, but the hot flashes replaced that! Also, I am depressed, but this could be caused by the fact that any money we have goes toward basic needs such as food, shelter, repairs, insurance, and college expenses for our daughter. Money for lighter moments in life does not exist. As a professional, I need to wear nice clothing, but I am "growing out of" my clothing, and there is no money for new clothes (weight gain). Probably, though, the worst is real anger toward situations and people I don't agree with. It is often just like PMS (which I have had with periods for some time now). This bothers me because I work with many people all day long and cannot allow myself to be so crabby!

For the most part my periods have stayed the same. I hoped the missed period in March was the beginning of menopause, but that was untrue. I have Parkinson's disease and on March 1, my medication dosage tripled. That may have caused the skipped period. I have hot flashes, but they seem to be associated with another drug I take for Parkinson's disease. Parkinson's makes me stiff which affects my sexual response. You can see, I'm not sure what is caused by the onset of menopause and what is the Parkinson's disease.

[I] did miss [my] period during the month of February—possibly due to having a family of three from South Africa living with us for approximately three months? Not too "normal" living situation here!

I am somewhat surprised I am still getting my period very regularly (no change at all). I mentally feel 50 is somewhat over the hill, but physically I don't feel that way. My husband is 53 but acts 65 or 70. I attributed my feelings of "downness" to his acting and behaving older than his age, but maybe it is that I am starting my changes??? My mother was 49 or 50 when she went through her changes and two of her sisters had babies in their early forties—so I suppose heredity is involved.

I seem to go through an enormous *number of tampons and have now added pantiliners for added protection. This is a mere annoyance, though. I have concerns about lack of energy, changes in muscle tone (i.e., breasts), but don't know how much both are related to a different job situation which prevents me from exercising as regularly as in the past. I don't seem to have the same PMS complaints of other women. There always seems to be another plausible reason for a sense of stress. Bloat, weight gain, and some lower abdominal discomfort are minimal. Being a teenager was* worse!

[Regarding what has been stressful]: foot surgery, breast mass surgery, cystoscopy; mother recovering from colon cancer; aunt (Mother's sister) in poor health; father lacks energy and [is] reclusive; moved into a new home and moved into a new classroom at work.

My mother is 80 and lives with us much of the year. Her health is poor—she is very frail. We are 135 miles from the doctor and hospi-

tal. There are no adequate alternate living arrangements for her. She's had a mild stroke (1990), [and was] hospitalized several months a year for a throat abscess–[she also] has gum disease and is very underweight. My husband had colon cancer with chemotherapy for six months after. My husband has had bypass surgery and carotid artery surgery. His cholesterol is high, and the medication he is on has not reduced it much. My problems have gotten ignored! I'm experiencing mildly abnormal Pap smears in the past year, and some unexplained bleeding in June. Will see the doctor today again.

I have experienced a number of changes in the past six months making it difficult to assess the symptoms resulting from physical changes. We moved to a new city after 24 years in one community, my husband took a new job (he previously traveled 50 percent of the time and now his is in town all the time), we built a new home, and my youngest child moved a long distance from us. All of these events have a positive and negative side and have all had an influence on my emotional state. It is reassuring to know that the mood swings I am experiencing are a normal part of this transition phase, and I appreciate this opportunity to think all this through. It's much easier to cope when one understands what is going on.

I have experienced some stress-related health problems, but my physician doesn't seem to think they are related to menopause. I am enrolled in a graduate school program and working part time, so she believes that is the source of my problems. Other than that, I feel very healthy.

This last year has been very stressful—one son has developed a serious chronic disease, [and I have a] difficult job situation, too much work. My answers are probably more related to my stress and energy level. My health is really fine.

During the past four years, we have experienced serious family and financial problems. I am currently in therapy for depression (major) and on medication. I often wonder if my depression is not due partially to the approach of menopause. My gynecologist thinks not but he is a real stickler for taking care of myself by exercise and cutting down on salt and alcohol–which I have done for years. I'm also anxious about menopause because I had a blood clot in my leg during my last pregnancy (19 years ago) and was told that I prob-

ably shouldn't take hormones. My doctor says I am not approaching menopause since I still menstruate. He said I could add ten years to the age my mother was when she went through it because my generation is going through it that much later. It seems strange to me that I have most of the other symptoms, i.e., vaginal dryness, emotional changes, decrease in sexual desire, irritability, no energy, etc.

I have a problem with a reoccurring cyst on the cervix, the root of which is up in the canal and would require more surgery than the simple removal of cyst. I've been seeing my gynecologist two times a year because of being on the hormone therapy. [My] last two Pap smears have been the level 2. The last one [was] a slight improvement over the first negative one. I am struggling emotionally with difficulties in a career change. I'm having difficulties finding the job I want and am also feeling like it's too late to start over. Intellectually I know that is not true, but I struggle with it emotionally.

Dealing with our two children causes me a little to a lot of stress. The girl is a teenager who experiences a hard time in school keeping her grades up [to a] C or better. On the other hand, she brings us a lot of joy with her experiences in music, etc. Our son is 22, living at home, works part time, and has a GED certificate and only recently has taken two classes at community college. He has a serious girlfriend and enjoys drinking out late. He causes us a lot of stress and will be soon asked to relocate if he refuses to pay us rent. He also can bring us a lot of joy. My husband is a workaholic, so is rarely at home when I am as I work weekends and two evenings. This causes stress in our sexual relationship.

MANAGING THE TRANSITION

Perhaps the best advice that can be given to women regarding the perimenopause is that it is a transition, and it will end. It is however a journey that still has few road maps to follow. I am indebted to Carol Ashton for sharing a 1992 document titled *Managing Organizational Transition* by Bridges and Associates, which is a workbook designed to be a resource for employees who found themselves or their organizations in transition. Six of the seven rules of transition management are applicable to transitions in general, and I have summarized them here as a resource for women in perimenopause.

The first rule suggests that you have to end before you begin. The authors indicate that this is the most important rule. One cannot develop a new identity or a new purpose until he or she lets go of the old one. Menopause is a midlife passage for women from reproduction/fertility into the mature years. No longer will a woman feel the changes that indicate the potential to create life; this phase of life is over, and the more quickly a woman can deal with this ending openly, the more quickly she gains closure of the past and plans for the future.

Rule two indicates that between ending and the new beginning, there is a hiatus. And indeed there is a hiatus in the perimenopause. As indicated, the precise temporal parameters have not been established. And the journey is difficult, the passage has not been totally mapped out. It is a "journey through the wilderness" or "a time in between trapezes." This is a time when one can lose heart easily. Therefore it is important to build temporary sources of support and control to get through. The changes that happen during the perimenopause are normal, but they are also chaotic, especially when they coincide with stressful life events.

According to rule three, the hiatus can be creative. Instead of viewing the transition as totally chaotic, step back and take stock. This can be a time to view every problem as an opportunity to abandon outmoded ways of solving problems and create more adaptive and effective ones. As The Tremin Trust participants have documented, it is never too late to do those things you have always wanted to do but have put on hold for one reason or another. At menopause, women still have one-third of their adult lives to live. The hiatus is the time to take stock of how that time will be spent.

Rule four is particularly relevant for the perimenopause. What is about to end is not just one particular situation. Instead, it is a whole chapter and stage of development for a women, and a new life is taking shape. The old way was fine for its time but that now belongs to a world which is gone. In Chapter 1, I indicated that at menopause, women no longer need to divert life energy into reproductive activities. Now energy can be redirected first into coping with the changes occurring during the transition, and then toward the goals set for the next stage.

The postmenopausal women in The Tremin Trust (Chapter 10) are living examples of rule five: transition as a source of renewal. The leap from one stage of development to another, similar to leaps in nature, releases energy. Renewal results when an individual goes through the transition successfully, not stopping for a rest somewhere. Perimenopausal women taking hormones to treat and stop the transition may obtain relief over the short term only to have to deal with the transition at a later date, which, at an older age, may be more energy-consuming than liberating. The message here is: "Don't stop the change process." The goal is to clarify and celebrate the reason for the transition and the new identity that will emerge.

The last rule discusses the concept of a "transition deficit." What this means is that some people are not given a chance to complete the transition cycle. They are hurried along, and what results is an individual who has unfinished business remaining. Some perimenopausal women are hurried along through hysterectomy to end heavy bleeding. Women can also experience a "transition plus" if they choose to postpone menopause through hormone replacement. Sure, symptoms may be relieved by taking hormones, and a woman may even have a hormone-induced bleed, almost (but not quite) like it was during menstrual years. However, a woman on hormones is not menstrual, is not reproductive, but she has delayed the transition. When hormones are stopped, the changes associated with the transition commence. Sooner or later, the price to pay for delaying may be high if coping skills and support systems are gone, and transition energy has been consumed in the process of delaying the journey to menopause.

My advice is the following: Pack your bags, remember the rules, and have a safe journey into postmenopause.

Chapter 10

Postmenopause: A New Beginning

The postmenopausal participants of The Tremin Trust Research Program are separated into two distinct age groups. Group one, as mentioned, was the first group enrolled in the research program in the 1930s. They experienced menopause either in the late 1950s or the early 1960s. The second group of women are younger; they enrolled in the research program in the 1960s. Both groups of women were students at the University of Minnesota, and on average were around 20 years of age when they enrolled in the program. As one would expect, there are similarities as well as differences between these two groups with respect to how they view menopause. A major difference is chronological age. Women in group one are mostly in their seventies, whereas the women enrolled in the 1960s are in their late forties or very early fifties.

The responses of both groups of women to the open-ended questions about menopause, in general, resonate with the voices of premenopausal women, that is, that menopause is no big deal. Some women in group two, however, reflect society's contemporary attitudes toward postmenopausal women, i.e., that menopause is a disease to be treated, and aging individuals are necessarily devalued, particularly women. Like perimenopausal women, they also describe in some detail how complex their lives have become at midlife, describing issues and problems they face related to stressful relationships, family crises, deaths (natural and by suicide), life-threatening and chronic illnesses, employment stresses, loss of a job, etc. Here, too, menopause gets an unfair share of blame for changes being experienced coincident with the onset of the aging process.

However, the overarching positive outcomes described by women in both groups is the relief they felt when periods ceased and they entered a new phase of life. The words of one woman say it all: "No more periods, cramps, flooding. . . . ." Hormone therapy also receives praise related to symptom relief. The older women were the estrogen users of the 1960s when Wilson's ideology of "estrogen forever, feminine forever" was in full swing. Now, because of the documented association between estrogen and cancer of the uterus, the younger women who are symptomatic and have a uterus are receiving hormone replacement therapy, a combination of estrogen and progesterone, to prevent the development of a precancerous condition. The menstrual bleed induced by the addition of a progestin is viewed by many women as a negative outcome of therapy.

Sex was said to be either better or worse by some women in both groups. Others expressed no desire at all to be sexually active. One woman voiced concern over the myths that have been perpetuated by other women regarding sex, i.e., "Sex is gone at menopause, hot flashes are in." Women in both groups complained of vaginal dryness. For the older women, the complaint was less intense and there was less of a concern about not being sexually active than for the younger women. The differences between the two groups related to sexual interest, arousal, and responsiveness may be due to age (that is, older women not having a partner), or, if partnered, it may be that they truly are not interested in sex. The younger women are more apt to be partnered or married and quite interested in sex.

VOICES OF OLDER POSTMENOPAUSAL WOMEN

The voices of older postmenopausal women undeniably proclaim that menopause was "no big deal." Many, but not all, made the transition to postmenopause without hormones or other additive therapies. In fact, they welcomed menopause; it closed the doors to the menstrual and pregnancy rooms; it brought newfound freedoms and energy, and the opportunity to explore life anew. Some examples of their view of postmenopause follow:

It was over before I realized it in 1968, when I was 54 years old; [it was] much easier than my menstrual history had been.

Had [a] hysterectomy at age 32.

Menopause [was] over long ago, except flashes.

The rapid aging process is sobering! but one doesn't have to worry about pregnancy. I looked forward to getting rid of my severe cramps.

No problem–discomfort. [I experienced] hot flushes after hysterectomy in 1971, but that cleared up in a year or two. I then stopped taking estrogen.

No problem–I just stopped. It was a time my father was very ill. He was my responsibility.

Had ovariectomy (bilateral) in 1949–had hot flushes relieved by hormones for two years–did not continue hormones long after.

I had no menopause symptoms, just a tapering off of menstrual flow.

I experienced "surgical menopause" and was very pleased to be through with menstruation, "cramps," "flooding," etc.

All over!

Was glad when it arrived 27 or so years ago.

Never went through it because of hysterectomy.

I never experienced a "hot flash." I had no problems related to menopause except that I gained weight during that period.

I had absolutely no problems–simple cessation of menstruation.

Always upbeat for me. Back when I taught a health class in 1936 to 1940, I loved a book by an English gynecologist, Life Begins at 40.

No problems since onset. I had no preconceived notions. Onset was accomplished by feeling faint and unsteady. But after a regimen of Premarin shots for a week, I was okay once again.

It was a nuisance (hot flashes) for two or three years, but eventually disappeared. [My doctor] prescribed hormones at the time (1960s) but urged minimum usage.

I think a positive attitude means a great deal during this time!

Menopause was tolerable and not too bad! Uncomfortable at times, but able to cope and continue to function well during that time.

It wasn't as bad as everybody said it was.

I've never taken any hormones, [because I] am allergic to all–[I] had no problem with menopause.

I experienced menopause so long ago I can't really remember much about it. It didn't bother me much. I feel fine.

I've enjoyed all postmenopause years! Gone forever, good to be better!

No problem–relief.

I do not have the energy I used to.

Mine occurred abruptly after a D & C 17 years ago. I had no more periods, spotting, etc. I felt no hot flashes except mild ones in the evening. I started the Premarin to try to [prevent] any osteoporosis in the future; any passing feelings of depression were due more to the empty-nest syndrome, as my three children had all married and left by then.

At 73, I am through with all discomforts, although I had an uneventful menopausal period.

It was no big deal.

Over and done with! However, the vaginal dryness I used to have is no longer evident. Maybe it's because of vitamins I take–maybe it's because of the almost daily use of our hot tub. Maybe–?

Experienced quite a lot of nervous tension, and mild depression (which I was able to control by forcing myself to sing). The last menstrual periods had very heavy flow which made for discomfort!

[I] Am 73 years old, [and] menstruation [was] always a problem. Not married but [I have] problems enough. So relief, I guess, is the word. [I had] lung surgery in 1956, menopause during 1961 to 1962.

I am now 71 years old. I had no problems with menopause. I never was bothered with hot flashes.

Prior to menopause in 1968, I felt confident that I'd experience no discomfort or mood swings–and I didn't. Menstrual flow just tapered off with no hot flashes, no intense emotions, no cramps, no weight gain.

Menopause—about 15 years ago—was easy for me. I took Premarin under doctor's orders for a few years.

Went through menopause with no problem—no medication—started hormones on recommendation of doctor following broken arm. Spotting and suspicious Pap smear caused doctor to induce bleeding. After two clear Pap smears it was discontinued. Thank God!

[I've had] no problems except hot flashes which began in 1969 and caused depression and great discomfort until I started to take hormones.

[It was] not troublesome except for long duration of hot flashes (not the individual flushes but the mere occurrence, into the 1970s). I discontinued estrogen years ago (i.e., 1962) because of a family occurrence of cancer of the endometrium (paternal aunt and two paternal cousins—not sisters) and because of a clinical impression that prolonged exposure of endometrium to endogenous or exogenous estrogen could lead to endometrial cancer.

Glad it's over. It wasn't nearly the ordeal that women have been led to believe. I should emphasize that I'm glad the reproductive and sexual phase of my life is over—not menopause itself.

At age 70, I still get hot flashes!

At first I was glad to be done with menstruation but then the vaginal dryness and hot spells (generally at night) bothered me and I finally asked to go back on estrogen therapy (I had once been taken off Premarin alone because a D & C showed up some possible precancerous cells). This time I was put on hormone replacement therapy and it's okay, although I'd rather not have to put up with the "periods."

[I have] the feeling of inadequacy as a sexual partner.

Menopause, for me, was much milder than I expected. Hot flashes were not severe, though I still experience them occasionally.

Perhaps menopause accounts for my reduced sexual desires, which is somewhat upsetting for our marriage.

At first I felt it might make me feel less feminine, but now that it is a fait accompli, how nice to be rid of all that bother!

I think all the books, lectures, TV shows about menopause are a great help. It was kept in the "closet" too long, and [there was] not much discussion about it. Male doctors not too understanding of this.

No special expectations when I started menopause—I was glad to end the periods. But my body "thermostat" has changed since before menopause. I'm warmer if it's warm and colder when it's cold (more so than other people). The "warmer" is more irritating to me; no flushes, though.

VOICES OF YOUNG POSTMENOPAUSAL WOMEN

The younger postmenopausal women expressed concerns related to lost fertility, regret at having only one child, loss of sexual desire, lack of information on menopause, disgust with myths, hot flashes, depression, freedom from cramps and bloody sheets, satisfaction with hormones, worries about going off the deep end, early onset of menopause, etc. These women enrolled in the program around age 20, in the 1960s, so most are still in the perimenopause. The words of a small sample of women who have become postmenopausal follows:

Sorry, I couldn't answer more questions, but it has been over five or six years since my last period, and since I have been on hormones for several years, I had no symptoms. It is wonderful not have a period anymore.

I never had menstrual cramps. Didn't have morning sickness when pregnant. Didn't expect—and haven't experienced—any problems with menopause. I have a vague regret that I didn't have more than one child, even though realistically this was never possible. Now that it's physically impossible, I think about it more.

Except for uncomfortable hot flushes and perhaps no sexual desire, I went through menopause fine. The [lack of] sexual desire may have started before menopause, and may not be entirely due to menopause but to other reasons. Today I am free of hot flashes—and feel very good except [for] no sexual desire, which I fear is not normal for a healthy woman like me.

Feel more depressed at times, more so than at other times.

[I feel] some sadness, as menopause means aging.

I had looked forward to not menstruating, and felt wonderful for about a year and a half after menopause. I do not feel as well on hormone replacement therapy (weight gain, unusual disturbances, feeling of sadness, and sometimes withdrawal building up).

I still have difficulty sleeping; [I am] anxious, and hot flashes [are] unpredictable.

I'm pleased I've had so few symptoms. While previously ambivalent, I now feel fine about being menopausal.

When it began I didn't really know what to expect, other than hot flashes. [I] was not well informed. I since have done some reading and discussing with friends and physicians so feel I know more.

I was looking forward to menopause. My family (three children) was complete. The thought of being free of periods and cramps is great. I had no idea I was going to have as much trouble as I've had. Also, menopause started much earlier for me than I had expected.

I have found menopause somewhat mystifying until I received your delightful booklet Menopause Me and You. *I was in the dark. Thank you so much for sending it. Prior to your book I found other women a source of myth—commonly shared—that sex was gone, and hot flashes were in! Often mentioned was some particular woman who went off the deep end! I wasn't experiencing these things, but I did have bladder problems and some hot flashes. My gynecologist specializes in fertility, not those of us on the other end of the continuum. I also have a vaginal crack (?), and he just said to buy some over-the-counter steroids. Never, until I read your book, did I know this was common. Thanks again for sending it.*

There is a great freedom in not having a monthly period, PMS, and sore, tender breasts. I don't like the dryness and itching in the vaginal area.

Glad to be finished with menstruation. Initially, I did not want to take hormones, but decided in favor when it was pointed out that they could help prevent osteoporosis. If I should acquire a sexual partner, my concern is that vaginal dryness would make intercourse painful, but I also know there are methods to combat that problem.

I'm just glad to be finished with the periods. I haven't been experiencing the wide emotional swings I did when I was menstruating.

[I] do not fear that change other than having concern about osteoporosis, which is in my family.

My hot flushes and cold chills were not as severe, and I expect they will gradually decrease.

I've had no problems at all, and have found menopause not difficult–nor did I expect it to be.

Increased interest in sexual intercourse. Happy adjustment to kids being grown happily and gone from home; vaginal dryness a problem at times. Don't like getting older–feel wise–younger people will vary in response to me (i.e., seeking out my ideas and observations and experience, or ignoring it!).

Menopause [is] much more tolerable now than it was about five years ago–probably due to hormone therapy.

It's wonderful! Helped cut down on PMS symptoms and no more bloody sheets!! Whoopee!

I felt a sense of loss at first; now [I] feel relieved it is over. Am enjoying life as much as ever.

I should have taken hormonal therapy early on after menopause. I do think the hormones have helped with the moods, and certainly with vaginal dryness. General sense of well-being improved with hormones.

Yes, it was very easy. It happened about four years ago–hot flashes only occurred when I was feeling stressed. I have never had so much energy; I love not menstruating.

Since it was surgically induced, once it was done I don't think about it. When it does come up, I realize it is a relief from the problems of having periods and PMS.

Since I have had a hysterectomy, I don't expect any changes other than possible vaginal dryness and hot flashes. I am exercising a lot more to help bone thinning, as well as many other benefits.

Since my hysterectomy (am now 48), I am wondering how I will know when I am experiencing menopause.

Chapter 11

Hot Flashes: When You're Hot, You're Hot!

It is the worst heat. I think I am going to smother. It's a horrible feeling. I feel hot, like a glowing furnace. But the heat is a different kind of heat than you get from running or mowing the lawn; it is very much internal and suffocating. When I have hot flashes, I break out in perspiration–on my feet, legs, in fact everywhere–to the point where sweat runs down my back and down the front. I always carry tissues, towels, handkerchiefs to wipe myself under my eyes, my forehead, anywhere I can wipe. Most of the time I look like I belong down south in the winter instead of in the north country. In below-zero weather, I can walk around with my coat open when I have a hot flash but when it is over I'm terribly cold because the sweat starts, and then I'm wet and shivering all over. When people see me this way they think I'm sick, and I'm not. I asked my doctor when the flashes would stop and he said that eventually they go away. When I asked when, he said he didn't know.

The above anecdote dramatically describes a hot flash, the most common bodily change associated with menopause. It identifies the question most frequently asked by menopausal women who experience hot flashes: "How long will they last?" Unfortunately for women, researchers do not yet know the answer to this question. The good news, however, based on work done with colleagues in my laboratory, is that even though women can expect to experience hot flashes for ten or more years, the frequency and the intensity of the experience decreases over time. The research findings also suggest that most women can expect to experience hot flashes through postmenopause, and that the experience will vary from woman to woman and over time in the same woman. I have experienced hot flashes for 15 years.

The variability in the hot flash experience is illustrated in excerpts from interviews with two women participants in my hot flash research. I have also included completed hot flash body diagrams that these women completed (see Figures 11.1 and 11.2). In the early 1980s, I developed the body diagrams as a research tool in order to map the origin and spread of the hot flash. This research tool emerged out of the interviews I conducted with women. During my interview with the third woman, I asked: "Describe your hot flash to me in your own words." I was astonished when the woman said: "Well, it starts in my cheek, goes down to my chest, and then it spreads to my arms and legs." I had not thought of the hot flash as having an origin and a spread, nor had any other researcher. When I

FIGURE 11.1. Hot Flash Pattern for Interviewee Number One

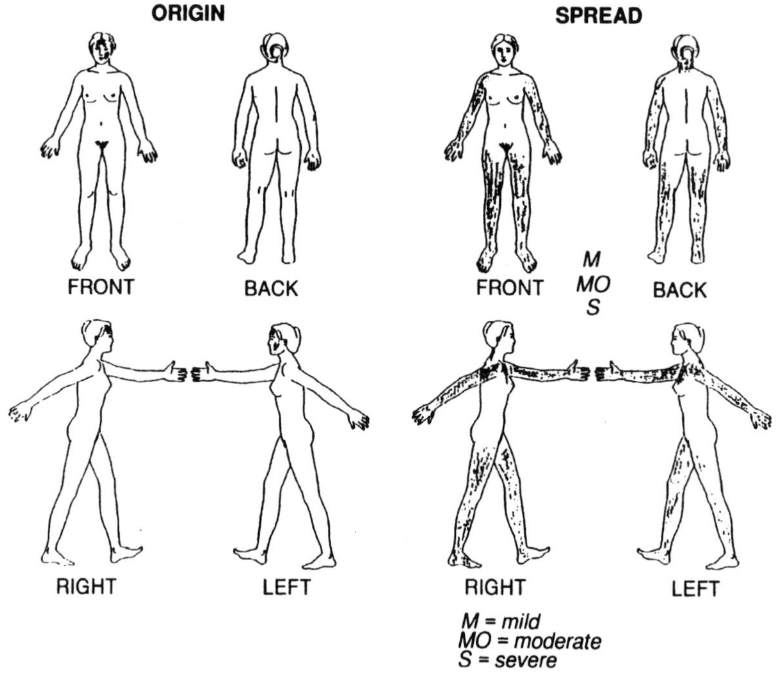

ORIGIN

FRONT   BACK

RIGHT   LEFT

SPREAD

M
FRONT   MO   BACK
S

RIGHT   LEFT

M = mild
MO = moderate
S = severe

incorporated a question on origin and spread into the interview guide, I discovered that no one hesitated to answer the question. The women knew where the hot flash started, and they knew its spread. In retrospect, now that I have experienced flashes as a postmenopausal woman for many years, I realize that if I had been experiencing hot flashes when I did these early interviews, the question about origin and spread more than likely would have originated out of my own personal experience.

To achieve more precision in locating the anatomical site of origin and spread of the hot flash, I asked all of the women to fill in body diagrams, which were hand-drawn sketches of naked women. Thus, the body diagrams were born and have proved to be an extremely useful research tool.

Dr. Brian du Toit, an anthropologist and a menopause researcher, has found the body diagram tool to be a useful nonverbal way to study hot flash in women in nonwesternized cultures. Du Toit (1989) used the diagrams in his research on menopause in South African Indian women.

Instructions on how to use the body diagrams as well as a hot flash diary I also developed are included in Section Four, Keeping Records and Keeping in Touch.

The first interview describes the hot flash experience of a 51-year-old woman who did not begin flashing until after her periods had stopped. Most of her hot flashes occurred at night. The origin was on the face, spreading into the lower extremities, out from her toes, and the back of her neck. This woman's hot flash origin and spread are shown in Figure 11-1.

This woman's hot flash was not debilitating. As such, her hot flash was categorized as mild, as it lasted for only a brief number of seconds and was of low intensity. Her description of her hot flash follows.

INTERVIEW NUMBER ONE

Please describe your hot flash, from start to finish, in your own words.

Well, it doesn't seem to come with any regularity. But most of them are at night, in the middle of the night. And maybe that's just

*because I'm so busy during the day, maybe I don't think about them.
I haven't quite figured that out. But since I knew—like I told you—that
I was going to do this, I did wake up one morning at 2 and I got
right back to sleep again, but I thought, "I'll see when these things
are happening." I never looked at the clock before. I just would
throw a foot out of the blanket. I have an electric blanket. Maybe it
doesn't even last for one minute, [but it] seems like an eternity in the
middle of the night. It probably isn't longer than half a minute and
then I go right back to sleep.*

You don't have any trouble getting back to sleep?

No, none.

Where does your hot flash start?

*In my face, my upper body. My face. . . . it just seems to be my
whole face where I really get hot. Not the top of the head or back of
the head, but now that we are talking about it, I'll have to think
about this more when I get another one.*

Once you feel the hot flash in your face, then what, does it stay
there?

*Well, it just kind of lightly, seems like it just goes out my toes, and
I don't really get hot. . . . Well, I guess I do, though. My husband
knows I'm doing this study so he felt me the other night and said,
"You're really hot." So it must kind of go down but not to any, you
know, where I'm going to lose my mind. And it leaves so suddenly
that it is not irritating.*

Have you ever awakened when you were in a hot flash?

*Well, it must be what wakes me up, I've decided, because I'm a
very sound sleeper, and I don't wake up. But it must wake me up
when it starts, I've decided. So, in other words, it's kind of simulta-
neous, that when the hot flash comes, I wake up and know it's there.
And, like I say, the last week or so I've been looking at the clock and
I've just remembered the times. I didn't time it at all. It just must
wake me when it happens. I'm thinking that must be what wakes me
up, because I'm not a light sleeper. I don't drink coffee, so I just
don't ever wake up.*

I see. You've always been a good sleeper. You put your head on
the pillow and go to sleep?

Yes.

Do you have any urgency to go to the bathroom when you wake up?

No. I just throw my foot out the blanket, or push that big husband of mine away from me because he seems so warm, and I'm warm, and then I go right back to sleep.

So, your hot flash is a facial experience, and you think that your whole face is the origin of the flash and that's the way you wake up at night. And, then, after awakening, you have this perception of heat which slowly leaves. It leaves to go to the rest of the body, and then out the toes. How about the fingers and hands?

No, that never seems to happen. And my toes never get really hot. In the back of my neck, now that I think of it, is where it gets hot, particularly if I have one during the day. I haven't had them during the day for some period of time, but the back of my neck gets really hot during the day.

Like on fire?

Yes, but not to the point where I'm going to lose my mind. I would notice that when I'm awake, that it's more the back of my neck and the front of my head. That might sound crazy, but that's the way I interpret it.

No, that is not crazy. Do you have any feeling around the breast area, or under the breasts, of intense heat or warmth?

No, just my head and the back of my neck. I'll have to be more aware of that. I think the reason I never noticed them during the day is because I seem so busy (they kid me in the office once in a while about being warm all the time). But, I tend to be warm rather than cold. You know, some females are always having two to three sweaters on, and I tend to be the other way.

You don't feel warmer now than you felt prior to the time when you stopped your periods?

No, no difference. I don't think so.

Do you dress any differently during the day than you did ten years ago in terms of selection of fibers, turtlenecks, etc? I see you have a turtleneck sweater on today even with a hot neck.

No, I never even think of that.

So, the way you cope with the flash, is to put your foot out, pull the covers down, move away from your husband?

Yeah. Maybe I'll release a . . . . I've got this electric blanket, and my husband doesn't like it (it's a dual control) so, he switches if off and I don't know when he does that. Maybe I also lift the sheet or cover away from my neck or something for a minute or so, but when I wake up in the morning I've got that blanket up there again. It's not that I must release my whole body outside the bed. I've never done that.

You were saying that some of the women you know have two or three sweaters on, and maybe these women go to bed with socks on and wear flannel nightgowns because they are cold. They refer to themselves as cold-blooded. Have you ever thought of yourself as cold-blooded?

No, once in a while my feet will be cold, and I will put my golf socks on when I first go to bed, but I just kick them off, leave them at the bottom of the bed, and in the morning I find them there. And I'm definitely not a flannel type.

If you had to classify your hot flash—mild, moderate, or severe—which would it be?

Moderate, I think. I must have had them before I really realized what they were. Suddenly, one day, I thought "My word, I am getting older; this must be what these things are."

Does your hot flash have an odor, color?

Oh, no. I never thought of it as a color.

Where do you think your hot flash comes from?

Well, there is something in the old bod that's changing. That's what we want to know, don't you?

Does your hot flash tell you anything?

Not a thing, except I am getting older.

Do you tell your hot flash anything?

I don't think so. I just think it's something that a female is going to cope with, and my attitude is that there is nothing we can really do about it. I don't tell it anything. I just know that it's going to be gone. It's not that uncomfortable.

Does the hot flash interfere with the activity that you were doing when it comes?

No, it comes, and I think it will be gone in a minute. I might just kind of kid about it once in a while. Gee, I'm getting hot, and I'll fan my neck. But, it's a joke. I remember the women my mother played bridge with years ago, there was a woman that was always fanning herself and I thought "That's strange." No, that's never occurred to me to do that.

Did you say that you have a hot flash every night?

No, but they kind of go in streaks, I think. Like I might have them maybe four or five nights, and then it might not hit for another three weeks. At one time I was trying to equate the hot flash with the period. "I am having this hot flash instead of having my period," I was thinking that to myself.

About your menstrual periods, you said that you stopped your menstrual periods, bang, just like that?

Right. And the last one I had (you know you never know it's the last one), the next one never came. So I guess I really am sorry I didn't keep a ledger or diary on that but I just never thought about it, because I thought another one would be coming. Well, then when it didn't come, you know, months go into years and I'm sure it had to be two years ago. But nothing before that. I am pretty sure I never had a hot flash until after my periods were gone.

What is the greatest number of hot flashes you've had in a 24-hour period?

Oh, I would say, three or four at the most.

Do you associate the hot flash with any particular function. Is there a trigger, other than sleep, that seems to bring the flash on?

No, I don't think so. I was trying to think maybe if anxiety did it. But, in this marvelous job I have—I do love it but I do hate it too— maybe something there, anxiety? I don't think that it does. I can't see anything that would trigger it. It is just there. It just comes.

Have you ever had a hot flash during sexual intercourse?

I don't think so.

What is the most discomforting aspect of the hot flash for you?

I suppose it is just being warm for a second. There is no discomfort other than the heat.

What is the heat like? Describe it, please.

Maybe it would be like if you had to, as a child, watch a fire. I'm thinking of a campfire or fireplace. We don't have a fireplace, but when you are close to the fire and maybe the wind fans it and the wind makes the fire come closer to you, in your face, just this feeling of sudden warmth. Like a fire, not in a fire, but close to the fire.

Do you want to be touched or talked to during a hot flash?

About touching, I would say to anyone, "Just leave me alone."

But talking, when it does happen, I would probably say I carry on a conversation.

INTERVIEW NUMBER TWO

This interview was conducted with a 56-year-old postmenopausal woman who had a hysterectomy and removal of one ovary and three-fourths of the other ovary at age 38. At age 40 she began estrogen replacement for relief of hot flashes because she was so uncomfortable. She stayed on estrogen for 15 years, stopping when her doctor advised her to stop because of the reports published about the link between estrogen use and cancer of the uterus. When she was on estrogen, she took it for three weeks, and then was off for one week. During the off week, she was so bothered with the flashes that she took the drug Bellergal, and she continues to take it. According to her, Bellergal did not stop the hot flashes but made them tolerable. This woman's hot flash origin was on her face and her feet, which then spread throughout the torso and the lower extremities (see Figure 11.2). Another hot flash origin for her was in the chest, over the sternum, between the breasts. This hot flash spread, however, remained in the upper body. This woman reported experiencing more cold flashes that hot flashes. Here is her interview.

Describe your hot flash to me, in your own words.

Well, at about 20 minutes to 9 almost every evening, I start getting quite warm. And I do not get flushed. I have different degrees of flashes. Sometimes they are very warm, where I will feel perspiring, but at other times they are just warm and I do not feel perspiring. But I also have an opposite; I also have cold flashes. Sometimes before the hot flash comes I'll have a cold flash, where I get quite cool. So, I dress in layers, so I'm either taking off or I'm putting on. They don't really last a very long time, except not too long ago, I had a hot flash that lasted for quite a while, and I don't remember if there was any specific reason for it or not. I have more cold flashes than I have hot flashes. I hope that the Bellergal is counteracting the cold flashes, if there is any relationship with the hot flashes.

Interesting. What is your cold flash like?

Well, I can get quite cool. Not shivering, but where I really feel cold. And I do have low blood pressure. So I don't know if there's a

FIGURE 11.2. Hot Flash Pattern for Interviewee Number Two

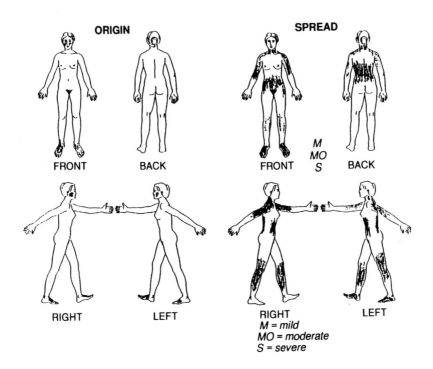

relationship with low blood pressure and cold flashes. But it almost seems like my hot flashes are preceded by a cold flash, but not all the time.

What is the heat like in your hot flash?

Well, It is not as intense as it used to be. And I just sort of feel very warm all over. If I'm in bed, I'm taking the covers off. A few minutes later I can be putting the covers back on because I'll get cool.

Where does your hot flash start?

I think it is in the upper part of my body. Or sometimes, I can get so hot with the covers on, with my legs covered up, that I have to get cool, so maybe they start down with my legs. I don't know. I really don't think I can give you an answer, but I feel the heat first in my head from the neck up, and then it goes into the rest of my body.

Do you tell your hot flash anything?

No.

Do you have an aura with your hot flash? Any other feelings other than a cold flash?

No, I don't think so. I could have had, but I can't think of anything right now.

Do your hot flashes occur every day?

I'm not so sure now, not even the evening one at 20 to 9, and they don't wake me up; they used to. When they do come, I usually have a glass of cold ice water at my bedside. I drink water, throw the covers off. For many years I only wore cotton nightgowns because nylon was too hot and sometimes I would have to get up and change that nightgown. But I don't have to do that now.

When you have a hot flash now, do you sweat?

Not on my face. I think I mostly perspire under my arms. But I can also have a sensation, it seems to me, of having a cold flash and a hot flash at the same time. Is that possible? I seem to remember there are times when I can be cold on the outside and like, well maybe it's that term cold sweat, maybe that's what I'm thinking of. But it seems to me that I've had occasions like that but I can't pinpoint it.

Do you to stop what you are doing when you have a hot flash?

No, I don't think so. I usually just take off my jacket. I dress in the layered look—I take my coat on and off. My husband says he never knows what I'm going to do—"you're either putting it on or taking it off," he said.

Does anything other than estrogen and Bellergal that gives you relief from the flash?

Nothing.

What is the most discomforting aspect of the hot flash?

Perspiring under my arms. I just hate that.

Have you ever had a hot flash during sexual intercourse?

Yes, several times.

Did you continue?

Yes, it bothered me to do so, but, you know, there are times when you just don't stop.

Do you think the activity had anything to do with it, a trigger?

Very possibly.

Do you want to be talked to when you have a hot flash?

That doesn't seem to bother me—in fact, it's better to have that to take your mind off of it.

Have you changed the way you dress?

No. I'm wearing a silk blouse today. The corduroy is cotton. I think the scarf is polyester, not silk. Polyester used to bother me at one time, but no more, and I wore a lot more cotton blouses a few years ago. Now, it is not a problem. At home I wear sweaters because I'm always cold. With slacks. I keep the thermostat at about 68. It's fine for downstairs and it's good for sleeping upstairs. But if I work at my desk—and I do have a lot of business I take care of—I have to have the heat pushed up if it's a cold day.

What does your hot flash mean to you?

I guess it means that I'm still functioning. I'm not dead; I'm there; I'm a living being. There are things worse than death. There's got to be something worse than hot flashes. If you didn't have hot flashes, particularly, at my age, it would probably mean that I wasn't around, so?????

COMMONLY ASKED QUESTIONS ABOUT HOT FLASHES

What Causes the Hot Flash?

No one knows what causes hot flashes. The first scientific study did not occur until 1975, when Dr. George Molnar, a physiologist, undertook the research in the hope of finding some relief for his wife who was experiencing severe discomfort from hot flashes. Prior to Molnar's research, the hot flash was either treated as simply another indication of female emotionalism, or as a disease to be treated with drugs such as estrogens and Bellergal, a drug used by the woman in interview number two. Bellergal is a combination of chemicals that will bring about balance in the autonomic nervous system. It has been used to treat hot flashes for years, based upon the assumption that the hot flash is a disorder of the autonomic nervous system. My own work on the hot flash suggests that most women cope with the hot flash without using drugs or hormones.

What Is a Hot Flash?

Even though we do not know what causes a hot flash, much work has been done to tell us what a hot flash is physiologically and endocrinologically. Technically, a hot flash is defined as "vasomotor instability." This is a fancy term for describing blood vessels that appear to dilate (open) and then constrict, to first dissipate and then conserve heat. The point to keep in mind is that this physiological activity appears to go on ignoring normal temperature control mechanisms. Research suggests that prior to a hot flash, peripheral blood vessels constrict, increasing internal body temperature, which is followed by vasodilation, an opening of blood vessels in order to cool down. Because body temperature has increased, another mechanism, sweating, is initiated in order to further cool the body through evaporation. The heat dissipation phase is the hot flash, and the cooling phase enhanced by the sweat is often described as a cold sweat; however, the woman in interview number two experienced a cold flash prior to her hot flash and no cold sweat.

Dr. Fredi Kronenberg at Columbia University has studied the thermoregulatory and cardiovascular changes that accompany a hot flash. These are described in a review article in Rogerio Lobo's 1994 edited text on menopause. According to Kronenberg (1990, 1994), the most typical physiological response that occurs with a hot flash is a sudden increase in heart rate, which is often sensed as palpitations (a rapid, throbbing, or fluttering of the heart). There is also an increase in peripheral blood flow (into the extremities–hands, arms, legs), which may be the cause of the flushing, the visible part of the flash, which is a change in skin color, ranging from pink to bright red. Following the flash, there is a sudden onset of sweating, particularly on the upper body. Kronenberg observed that it was the evaporation of sweat, a natural way of cooling the body, which resulted in a decrease in body temperature. Some women sweat and flush, some just flash and flush, and some women, for example, the woman in interview two, have cold flashes prior to a hot flash.

Consistent with the anecdote at the beginning of this chapter, a variety of sensations are associated with hot flashes, as well as varying intensities which may range from mild to severe. It is important for women to know that the hot flash is real; it is associated with an increase in body heat (from less than one-half degree to more than three degrees Centigrade) that radiates from within the body or from some part of the surface of the skin. It may affect only a portion of the body, as illustrated by the woman in interview number one, or it may spread uniformly over the whole body, as described by the woman in interview number two. The flash may last less than 30 seconds or more than 12 minutes. Also, as just mentioned, the flash may or may not be accompanied by a flush, which is a change in skin color.

How Prevalent Is the Hot Flash?

Results of research done in collaboration with Drs. Bernadine Feldman and Evangeline Gronseth, suggests that more than 88 percent of menopausal women will experience the hot flash (1985). It appears to be as universal as menopause itself. The high prevalence of hot flash found by our research strongly suggests that it is a normal part of the menopause transition. An event this prevalent cannot be abnormal or a symptom of a disease.

How Long Do the Hot Flashes Last?

I have already mentioned that the duration of the hot flash is unknown. I have had 30-year old women as well as 80-year old women report hot flashes. For 25 women followed over a three-year period, the average duration of the hot flash experience was between eight and nine years. These findings differ from those reported in texts and journals. Kronenberg suggests that most hot flash experiences last for six months to two years, but for some women (for example the older postmenopause Tremin Trust participants), the flash continues relentlessly for 10, 20, and even more years. Advising women that the duration of the hot flash may be no more than two or three years is the reason some care providers prescribe estrogens for women in order to "ride out the menopause," to treat the symptoms for two or three years, and then stop! There is no research-based data to support the assumption that taking hormones "prevents" menopause. *When hormone therapy is stopped, the hot flash returns, as do other symptoms.*

Are All Hot Flashes the Same?

No. I have discovered that there are three distinct hot flashes. Analyses of randomly selected self-report record cards kept by women over a two-week period suggests that women differ considerably in both the quantitative and qualitative aspects of the hot flash. Twenty women recorded 1,041 hot flashes over a two-week period, with an individual range of 2 to 247 over this same time period. The mean duration of the flashes (timed by the women themselves) was 3.31 minutes, with a range of 5 seconds to 60 minutes. Analysis of body diagrams showed unequivocally that the hot flashes were not restricted to one body area (as described in the literature). Instead, they had a distinct anatomical origin and spread that differed from woman to woman (refer to interviews one and two), and which may or may not affect the entire body. Finally, I found that the hot flashes varied in severity from mild to moderate to severe.

Mild hot flash is a warm feeling, lasting less than a minute to two minutes, sometimes barely noticeable (as for the woman in interview number one), with no interruption of activity, sometimes accompanied by dampness, sweating, and slight flushing. A mild hot flash may include sensations of tingling and rushing blood.

Moderate hot flash is a warm to extremely warm feeling, lasting from less than a minute to five minutes, often accompanied by sweat and sometimes by flushing. A moderate hot flash may include tingling, throbbing, rushing blood, light-headedness, chills, swelling of extremities, and a need to urinate; however, there is little interruption of normal activity.

Severe hot flash is an intense or extremely hot feeling, lasting from less than one minute to 12 minutes, usually accompanied by profuse sweating or flushing and extreme or unbearable discomfort that requires disruption of normal activity to seek relief. A severe hot flash may include a feeling of waves of heat, dizziness, chills, suffocation, inability to concentrate, and chest pains.

When Do Hot Flashes Begin?

They may begin many years prior to menopause and precede changes in menstruation. The woman in interview one said her hot flashes did not begin until her periods stopped. But, don't be concerned if you begin to feel warmer or experience night sweats in your late thirties or forties. Many women do. As menopause nears, the hot flash experience may become more intense and frequent, occurring night and day.

Is There a Time of Day When Hot Flashes Are Most Frequent?

Yes! Though some women's experience may differ, my research shows that hot flashes most frequently occur between the hours of 6 and 8 a.m., followed by a cooling-down period during the day. Frequency of hot flash increases during evening hours, that is between 6 and 10 p.m., followed by another cooling-down until approximately 6 a.m. However, don't be alarmed if hot flashes occur only at night or only during the day. For some women this is the pattern. The woman in interview number one had hot flashes only at night. I still experience flashes during the day and night, although the night-time experience has diminished greatly. My own hot flash experience is predictable. I will inevitably have a mild hot flash following ingestion of hot coffee (with or without caffeine), wine, or food, or due to emotional stress, but, interestingly, when I am physically ill, I do not have any hot flashes.

Is There a Seasonal Variance for Hot Flashes?

Some women report experiencing more frequent hot flashes during the summer than winter. But there has been no systematic study of the effect of the seasons on hot flashes.

Are Hot Flash Frequencies and Patterns the Same for Women Who Have Menopause Induced?

Yes, if you have had your ovaries and uterus removed, or have had menopause induced by radiation or drugs (such as Tamoxifen, which is an antiestrogen used to treat breast cancer), you can expect hot flashes to occur. In the case of surgery, you can expect hot flashes to occur almost immediately after surgery. In the case of radiation or drugs, the time of onset of hot flash will depend upon the dose administered to ovarian tissue, as in the case of radiation, or, as with Tamoxifen, menopausal symptoms may not appear for a week or two. Tamoxifen acts initially as an estrogen agonist, in other words, it mimics the action of estrogen. In time, the agonistic effect diminishes and it becomes antagonistic to the receptors in the ovary, and no estrogen is made.

Does Hot Flash Frequency Change Over Time?

Thankfully, yes. In the women I studied over three years, frequency decreased for both natural and induced menopausal women. This is encouraging information, as it indicates that the hot flash diminishes naturally and, if women can "ride it out," they settle into a new biological rhythm consistent with decreased levels of estrogen hormone.

Does Hot Flash Intensity and Duration Change Over Time?

Yes! The Tremin Trust women and I are living testimonials to that. It has been my choice not to take estrogen or hormone replacement. As such, I have not altered the closure process in any way with hormone or drug use. My hot flash frequency, intensity, and duration have decreased considerably. Most women report a lessening of hot flash intensity, and that it seems to be of shorter duration. Laboratory measurements of the hot flash have validated women's self-report (perception) that the intensity and duration of hot flashes decrease over time. For example, analyses of hot flash frequency data across a three-year period for 25 women I followed (based on analysis of self-report records over a two-week period for three years) showed a decrease from 1,802 to 1,127. When another group of women had their hot flash measured in the laboratory over a three-year period (a four-hour measurement once each year), a decrease from 73 to 39 hot flashes was observed.

We found also that as hot flash frequency decreased, so did hot flash intensity. The "climax" of the hot flash, that is high frequency associated with moderate to severe intensity of long duration, appears to cluster around the time of menopause.

We do not know with any certainty how long hot flashes will last. For all we know, we may take them to the grave with us, albeit with greatly diminished frequency, intensity, and duration. My mother, who recently died at age 89, commented from time to time that she was having a hot flash. Until we get the answer to the question of how long hot flashes last, I can suggest some methods for coping that were developed based on my research.

ANN'S ADVICE: COPING WITH THE HOT FLASH

The following are 13 suggestions regarding how to cope with hot flashes:

1. *Don't worry.* The hot flash is not a disease. It is a normal and natural part of the menopausal experience. It may occur while you are still menstruating and your periods are regular. Worrying about it may increase hot flash incidents.

2. *Know thyself.* Keep a record or a diary of your hot flash. Time it. Identify where it starts on your body and where it spreads. Try to identify your trigger(s), then devise ways of avoidance. Others who have kept such records say they are better able to manage their hot flashes. They report that the more you know about yourself, the better you'll feel about the whole experience. A few women report that daily record-keeping forced them to pay more attention to their hot flashes, made them dwell on it more, and made them miserable. Try it and see how it works for you. I have included the hot flash diary and body diagrams in Section Four.

3. *Dress in the layered look.* Many women cope with the heat sensation by taking off a layer or layers of clothing and then putting them back on as cooling commences. Others have found that certain fabrics are hot flash triggers: polyesters, for example, are avoided, while cottons are preferred.

4. *Avoid hot areas.* They trigger hot flashes for many women. I have found that even a subtle source of external heat, such as the heat generated from a computer terminal, can trigger a hot flash. Keep your thermostat low, about 65°F or lower if possible. If you can't control the heat, dress in layers and keep a fan handy, one you can hold in your hand as well as one you can plug into an electrical socket.

5. *Avoid highly seasoned, spicy foods, coffee, tea, and alcohol.* These are common triggers for hot flashes. Try to find your specific trigger, but don't worry if you can't identify one. For some women a particular time of day is the trigger (like the woman in interview two who had a hot flash at 8:40 every night). Time of day suggests that internally triggered hot flashes are related to a resetting of biological rhythms. I predictably have a hot flash after my morning coffee, after a glass of wine, and particularly after food containing jalapeño peppers. I guess some things in life have to become a trade-off. The flashes are not so bad that I will give up everything that is pleasurable as well as palatable.

6. *Avoid getting excited.* Keep cool (no pun intended). Emotional stress is a trigger for some women. It is a trigger for me. If I have lost a document, or if I am in a horrendous time-crunch to get a job done, you can bet that I will have flashes. If I am having an unpleasant conversation, I will inevitably experience a hot flash. If I am frustrated, I will flash, etc.

7. *Try to stop the hot flash in its tracks.* One woman stops flashes by imagining herself doing something very pleasurable. Another imagines herself walking in snow without shoes, forcing herself to shiver, or anything to fool her body into being cool instead of hot. Other women cope quite well by seeking a cooling device, a fan, by showering, or by applying cold cloths or ice cubes to certain body parts, such as the back of the neck or the cheek.

8. *Do not take tranquilizers or mood elevators.* Psychotropic drugs are worthless against the hot flash.

9. *Stop smoking.* Smoking is associated with an early age onset of menopause. The earlier you begin menopause, perhaps the longer you will experience hot flashes. Also, most smokers tend to have more lean tissue than body fat, which means that there is lessened ability to make estrogens in fatty tissue.

10. *Consider vitamin therapy, but only after consulting a nurse, physician, or nutritionist.* Many women appear to relieve debilitating hot flashes with 400 to 500 I.U. of vitamin E and protein powder; yet others with 500 mg of vitamin C per day. For most women who use vitamins, research indicates that the hot flash is only relieved, not eliminated, and the relief is short term. No research-

based information on how much vitamin E to take, for how long, and whom it might benefit is available. My best advice for additional information on vitamins, nonhormonal options, and other nonconventional remedies is Dr. Sadja Greenwood's book, *Menopause Naturally*, 4th Edition, 1996, Volcano Press.

11. *Consider hormone treatment only after you have considered all of the risks as well as the benefits, over the short term and the long term.* Taking hormones will alleviate and maybe even eliminate the hot flash. Taking hormones may also increase the risk of developing serious side effects that can result in a chronic disease.

12. *Be informed.* There are risks associated with vitamin and over-the-counter replacement substitutes. We have many studies to consult that identify the side effects associated with hormone use. We do not have any systematically designed studies on the nonconventional remedies, such as vitamin replacement and herbal remedies. So, obtain as much information as possible on health food replacements as well as on hormones.

13. *Discuss your hot flashes with other women.* One great resource for women that is frequently overlooked is other women. Don't be a closet flasher. Most women are destined to experience hot flashes. The more you talk about it with other women, the more natural the process will seem. The hot flash is a part of menopause. We will cope more successfully if we aren't ashamed of it.

I believe that the hot flash is telling us something important about our bodies. I don't know what that message is. But, I'm not giving up. So, until we have more data, buy fans, keep records, dress in layers, stop smoking, consider taking vitamin E, cut down on alcohol consumption, increase dietary sources of estrogens, and consider hormone treatment as one of many options.

Chapter 12

What a Bloody Mess!
Changes in Bleeding Pattern

Two significant events which occur in the lives of all women are menarche and menopause, the onset and closure of menstrual life. Between menarche and menopause, on average every 23 to 38 days, for an estimated 35 or more years, a woman's body prepares for the implantation of a conceptus in the uterus. If implantation does not occur, the uterine endometrium is shed over a period of four to seven days via a process familiar to all women: menstruation. This process is described in Section II.

Reproductive endocrinologists agree that the menstrual cycle is not simply switched on at menarche and switched off at menopause; hormonal and bodily changes precede the first menstruation and follow the last. During the period of hormonal change, the onset of menstrual bleeds becomes unpredictable, and the quality of the bleeding can change quite markedly. It is estimated that about 88 percent of women experience irregular bleeding patterns as they experience menopause.

Several Tremin Trust participants describe their menstrual bleeding changes. The first woman, age 50, describes a common change associated with the transition—irregularity and unpredictability of onset of the menstrual bleed.

This year, I have begun to actually look forward to my periods ending! (Which is much different from last year, as I recall.) The irregularity is getting to me. I used to be like clockwork. Now I never really know when a period is coming. I find I think about it more. It will be nice not to have to deal with it. Enough else is going on in my life.

A 51-year-old woman describes her concerns regarding the change in the quality of the menstrual bleeding:

> *I have asked my doctor several times about the dark, muddy-looking discharge that I have up to four days before my period and occasionally between. She doesn't seem to know why it happens. At times it concerns me even though I have no other signs of a problem.*

Another woman, also age 51, describes a different situation. Her most recent bleeds are very heavy. She also experienced a change in the duration of the menstrual interval:

> *I don't particularly have any questions. I would just like to finish with monthly periods. I don't have the rhythm I did for years. Sometimes they are closer together, and sometimes further apart. I have experienced a couple of very heavy periods, one in February and another in May of this year.*

A 50-year-old woman also describes unpredictability in her bleeding, and the consequences of heavy bleeding. At the same time, she realizes that the closure process, which she describes as "complete cessation," has another meaning as well:

> *The unpredictability of my menstrual period is bothersome. I never know when to expect it, or how long it will last. Also, heavy bleeding at times has ruined some of my clothing. Nevertheless, I have mixed feelings about complete cessation. I think I will feel older then—as if I'm passing into the last phase of my life—it is a melancholy feeling for me.*

A 55-year-old woman believes she has been in the menopausal transition for about three years. While age 55 is at the upper end of chronological age to bring closure to the process, being five years beyond the average age of menopause (age 50 to 51) does not mean that her closure is abnormal. There is wide variability regarding age at menopause. Some women stop bleeding in their late 30s. These women are described as experiencing premature menopause, which is menopause prior to age 40. How many women experience premature menopause is unknown. The few studies done, however, estimate that the risk in the general population ranges from 3 percent to 9 percent. I have been unable to find research-based estimates on the probability of experiencing menopause in the middle and late fifties. In the anecdote that follows, this woman describes the changes associated with the transition and asks important questions related to bleeding and the fate of uterine fibroids:

> *My periods have been in this transitional-type stage for about three years now. For approximately one and one-half years I experienced hot flashes; they have disappeared completely in this past year. I do have a fibroid, which the doctor says is about the size of a five-month pregnancy, and would like to remove surgically. And a friend who is a nurse thinks my heavy flow is probably due to the fibroid. Does my flow seem unusually heavy for a woman in transition? Can you offer me any opinions about how long I might be in transition, and how likely it is that the fibroid will shrink or disappear when I stop menstruating?*

Uterine fibroids are benign tumors, masses of muscle tissue that start as a single smooth cell, which become enclosed by fibrous connective tissue. They are also rich in blood vessels. Fibroids can grow on the inside surface of the uterus, on the outer surface, or within the uterine wall. Often, they are symptomless, but just as often they can cause spotting between menstrual bleeds, and bleeding so heavy that anemia may result. Fibroids are estimated to occur in at least 30 percent of women, and of these, 20 to 25 percent of the time, the fibroid is in a submucous location, which means that it can bleed with "ferocity" during a menstruation.

Little data are available to clinicians or women about the qualitative or quantitative aspects of menstrual flow. A heavy menstrual flow is defined *clinically* as more than 80 milliliters of blood loss per menstrual period (one fluid ounce equals 29.53 ml, so what we are talking about here is a little less than three ounces of blood). Heavy bleeding is referred to as *menorrhagia*. However, the definition of heavy bleeding as blood loss of more than 80 ml is only useful in a research laboratory. In order to quantify the volume of blood loss, menstrual products would have to be collected, blood extracted from the products, and then the hemoglobin concentration of the blood fraction would have to be measured. The process is very time consuming and expensive, and appropriately belongs in a research laboratory.

Until recently, no reliable and valid rating scale was available for women to rate the quality of menstrual bleeding. Not having a scale to estimate menstrual blood loss resulted in a lack of information on how menstrual bleeding changes from menarche to menopause. This has important implications for perimenopausal women who report to their care providers that they are experiencing "heavy bleeding," and the heavy bleeding is interpreted as a sign of pathology, i.e., a condition that needs to be treated.

As discussed in the chapters on menstruation, the work of Vollman, and Treloar and colleagues, informs us that regularity in onset of menstrual bleeding is not common in the first few years following menarche. The interval between postmenarcheal bleeds can range from 10 to 60 days. As women move into young adulthood, between ages 20 and 39, a regular pattern of bleeding ensues, in large part due to maturation of the reproductive system, and which, according to Vollman (1977), is characterized by a preponderance of ovulatory cycles.

Recall that during prime reproductive years, the duration between menstrual cycle intervals shows a characteristic length and variability that remain stable until the transition to menopause. Most women become very familiar with their menstrual cycle pattern, time of onset, and typical quality of bleeding, so that even minor changes are noticed.

Don Gambrell, a physician, and the creator of the "progestogen challenge test," notes that the most frequent problem encountered by physicians who treat female patients in general, and peri- and postmenopausal women in particular, is a complaint of change in the vaginal bleeding pattern. Any change in bleeding is a concern to physicians because it is thought to be a precursor of a serious condition, such as cancer. Potential causes of abnormal bleeding, according to Gambrell (1992), can range from hormonal disturbances, polyps, fibroids, and even pre-malignant or malignant lesions of the cervix or uterus. As described in the chapters on menstruation, breakthrough bleeding may result from oral contraceptive use, as well as progestogen contraceptive regimens, and irregular bleeding is associated with hormone replacement therapy and IUDs.

When taking a patient's history, Gambrell recommends that clinicians carefully concentrate on the characteristics of the bleeding, the duration and frequency of flow, as well as any previous episodes of abnormal bleeding. Each peri- and postmenopausal woman who is diagnosed with abnormal bleeding should undergo a thorough evaluation. Thorough means Papanicolaou smear (Pap smear), biopsy of cervical lesions, bimanual examination to detect uterine enlargement or masses, and cervical and uterine curettage (scraping of a cavity).

In the absence of normative guidelines to assess the bleeding, perimenopausal women, in particular, are at risk for both physical and emotional disruption as the pattern of bleeding changes. As suggested in the perimenopausal women's anecdotes, in psychological terms, loss of predictability of a previously predictable event is translated into a sense of loss of control of an important bodily function. This sense of loss of control becomes a source of anxiety in that the change in pattern is perceived as a sign of "illness," and becomes a vitally important emotional health issue for women. Findings from research done with Dr. Phyllis Mansfield strongly suggest that anxiety, confusion, and psychological distress can be directly related to women's lack of understanding of what constitutes normal perimenopausal menstrual cycle changes. This lack of information has adversely affected women's health through emotional strain and worry, and the performance of unnecessary procedures such as hysterectomy.

The number of women in the perimenopause is increasing rapidly. Approximately one-third of all women in the United States are age 50 or older. By the year 2000, it is estimated that 719 million women over age 45 will inhabit this planet (Kronenberg, 1990). Many women have no idea what changes may occur in their menstrual cycles as they become perimenopausal. Some women might expect to have altered bleeding patterns when going through the change, but they do not understand—nor should they be expected to understand—what kind of change in bleeding pattern is an indication of a serious problem. According to Wulf Utian, documentation of physical and emotional changes that occur during menopause will have a significant impact upon the emotional and physical well-being of increasing numbers of aging women. Dr. Mansfield and I concur with Utian. We believe that being able to accurately assess the volume of menstrual blood loss is very important, and needs study now. Not having information on bleeding patterns is one reason why the hysterectomy rate in U.S. women has increased. Only a small number of laboratory-based studies have been done on menstrual bleeding. And, except possibly for in-house research done by the feminine care product companies (the results of which are kept secret), no published data are available documenting how the quality of menstrual bleeding changes over time as women enter perimenopause.

An Australian researcher, Ian Fraser, believes that most clinicians are unaware of the extent of errors in a woman's perception of volume of menstrual discharge when they report this complaint to their care providers. In the 1960s, self-report of excessive menstrual blood loss by women was a symptom that was commonly treated by hysterectomy. Fraser reported that large numbers of hysterectomies were being done in the 1980s on Australian women who reported heavy bleeding, even though the complaint could not be subjectively or objectively confirmed.

In 1990, Dr. Mansfield (now Professor of Women's Studies, Pennsylvania State University) and I began a series of studies on menstrual bleeding. We are indebted to Pennsylvania State University and Friends of The Tremin Trust, University of Utah, for funding the first study, wherein we collected data on the quality of bleeding using a self-report scale that had been created by Drs. Mansfield and Jorgensen. The tool, now known as the Mansfield/Voda/Jorgensen Bleeding Scale (MVJBS), is a six-point scale women use to rate the quality of bleeding from spotting to very heavy bleeding. The scale is found in Chapter 19.

Dr. Mansfield and I are also grateful to Tambrands, Inc. (Palmer, MA) for funding a second study on menstrual bleeding. The goal of this study was to measure the volume of menstrual discharge on a small sampling of pre- and perimenopausal women, ages 35 to 55, across three menstrual bleeds, in order to validate the MVJBS. Dr. Kimber Richter, former Medical Director and Vice President, Medical/Regulatory Affairs for Tambrands, realized that normative guidelines on how the pattern of bleeding changes in perimenopausal women needed to be established.

STUDY ONE

Between March and May of 1990, we mailed a total of 845 surveys to two groups of women. One group consisted of pre- and perimenopausal participants of The Tremin Trust. The second group were former college classmates of Dr. Mansfield. Using the MVJBS and the clotting scale, we asked these women to rate the quality of menstrual bleeding and clotting they experienced during their most recent menstrual bleed. Five hundred and five women returned the surveys, which accounted for a good return rate of 60.5 percent. When we compared the data obtained from women who reported that they were menstruating regularly with those who said they were irregular, we found the following: (1) the estimations of heaviest menstruations for both groups, on average, were reported for Day Two; (2) the average menstruation rating, based on the 6-point scale, for the regularly menstruating group was 3.8; for the irregularly bleeding group, the mean rating was 3.9 (not much difference); (3) by Day Six, approximately 50 percent of all women had stopped bleeding; only a small percentage continued to bleed until Day Twelve.

For the women who reported passing clots, we found that the highest mean clot rating was reported for Day Two; by Day Six, more than half of the women had stopped clotting, and only a small number of the irregularly menstruating participants continued to clot until they ceased menstruating on Day Twelve. However, for women in the 46 to 47 and 48 to 49 age groups, clotting continued until flow ceased. Details on this study are reported in the *Proceedings of the 9th Conference of the Society for Menstrual Cycle Research*, Seattle, WA, 1991.

STUDY TWO

In Study Two, our goal was to evaluate the validity of the six-point bleeding scale. In a measurement sense, we needed to know how accurate the scale was when women used it to estimate the volume of menstrual discharge. In other words, was the scale sensitive enough for women to rate differences in the volume of discharge? To establish scale validity is no small task. The work would have been easier had an established, valid bleeding scale been available. We could have had the women use both scales, and then compared the findings of our scale with that of the established scale. Unfortunately, no valid scales existed; we had to start from scratch, trying to decide how we could proceed to accurately measure the volume of menstrual discharge. We decided to weigh used menstrual products (tampons and napkins). We hypothesized that when a woman rated her bleeding as a "1" (which is the low end of the scale), the weight of the product would also be low. We reasoned that at the end of the study we would be able to statistically evaluate whether there was agreement between what a woman rated her bleed (what she perceived in terms of quality and volume), and what was weighed. Weight of the used products, then, was the objective criterion we used in order to validate the rating scale. To carry out this study, it was necessary to collect all used menstrual products over three menstrual bleeds from 40 consenting pre- and perimenopausal Tremin Trust participants. We asked the women to place each used napkin and tampon into a plastic bag with a "zip"-type closure, and to rate the quality of the bleeding using the bleeding scale, which was printed on a label pasted directly on the bag. We were pleased that 31 women completed the study.

What did we find from this study? We did not validate the scale in the purest measurement sense. However, we did find a statistically significant association between the weight of 1,508 used products and 1,508 ratings. Even considering statistical significance, on close examination of the data, we were not satisfied with the amount of disagreement observed between the ratings made by some women and product weights. Specifically, if a woman rated her bleeding as "low," we expected that the product weight measured would be low rather than high. And conversely, if a woman rated her bleeding as "high," we expected her napkin or tampon to weigh in the high range. We did not obtain this kind of correlation among all women. We were puzzled, as some high raters had low weight measurements, and low raters had high weight measurements. We decided to ask the women what factors influenced how they rated their bleeding. Following an informal poststudy conference with eight study participants, we realized that a variety of factors influence how a woman rates her bleeding. For example, if a woman lost a lot of menstrual discharge into the toilet, or on her body and/or clothes (which was described in one woman's anecdotes), or if many products were changed per day, or the color was bright red versus brown, or the odor was offensive, or cramps, gushing, oozing, or passing of clots were present, the rating may be high even though the volume of discharge weighed was low.

The findings of Study Two generally agree with the findings of Study One: Day Two was the heaviest day of bleeding for the 31 women. One particular difference in day of heaviest bleeding was due to one woman who was a *very* heavy bleeder who dropped out of the study after Cycle 1. We discovered also that there were differences in the duration of bleeding among women between cycles. In Cycle 1, the longest duration of bleeding was 9 days, whereas in Cycles 2 and 3, two women menstruated for 13 and 17 days, respectively. Interestingly, by Day Five in all three cycles, 96 percent (29 out of 31) of the women had stopped bleeding. Bleeding beyond Day Five was accounted for by the same two women, who were categorized as "long, but not necessarily heavy, bleeders."

Another interesting finding that emerged when we calculated the total volume of menstrual discharge for each woman was that the highest volume during one cycle was 553 grams, measured on a participant who was a very heavy bleeder and who dropped out of the study after Cycle 1. No other woman in the study during the three cycles eliminated as great a volume of menstrual discharge during one bleed.

We were curious to find out who else might be a heavy bleeder. Using a formula derived by Fraser (1985), we calculated the percent of total discharge that was estimated to be blood (minus fluid and other materials in the discharge) for each woman. When we did this, we found that five women had lost more than 500 grams of menstrual discharge over three cycles, and were categorized as heavy bleeders, or to use a clinical term, were menorrhagic. According to Fraser, the percent of blood in the total volume of menstrual discharge in women who have high and moderate losses is around 48 percent, or about half blood and half discharge. These five women, thus, had lost substantial amounts of blood. Remember that a heavy menstrual flow is defined as one which exceeds 80 ml of blood loss. Fraser also calculated the proportion of discharge that is blood in women with low volume discharge to be about 27 percent, or about one-fourth blood. A rule of thumb that can be applied is that for women who have a high volume of discharge, one can estimate that about one-half of the discharge is blood, whereas for a low volume, about one-fourth is blood.

Eight of the 31 women who completed the study were categorized as moderate bleeders, and 18 were light bleeders. The total volume of menstrual discharge measured on each woman for all three cycles is shown in Table 12.1. The letter T in the table next to an identification number indicates that a woman had a tubal ligation for contraception. Reports in the literature about the effects that a tubal ligation may have on bleeding are controversial. Whether a tubal ligation affects the pattern of bleeding is unknown, although one study suggests that women with tubal ligations may have an earlier onset and a bloodier transition to menopause. Three of the five heavy bleeders had tubal ligations; however, as shown in Table 12.1, eight light bleeders also had tubal ligations. We will be monitoring these light bleeders to find out whether they will be heavy bleeders as they progress to and through perimenopause.

INDIVIDUAL PATTERNS OF BLEEDING

When we examined the data on how each woman rated each product, and then compared the rating with the weight of the product, we observed considerable variability among women in bleeding patterns, as well as variability in patterns of bleeding for each woman from cycle to cycle. Bleeding data on these 31 women will be published soon.

The bleeding pattern data Dr. Mansfield and I have described are only a beginning. More study is needed to describe how the pattern of bleeding changes during perimenopause in order to dispel myths and assumptions that now guide clinical practice. Such myths indicate that any change in the pattern of bleeding, whether of long duration or heavy bleeding, is abnormal and/or dysfunctional,

TABLE 12.1. Total Menstrual Discharge, Heavy to Light Bleeders, Across Three Menstrual Cycles

Heavy (> 500g)		Moderate (250 to 499g)		Light (< 250g)	
ID	Grams	ID	Grams	ID	Grams
7465	990.28	11122	423.93	7570	238.38
13139 T	696.91	10279	419.22	11114 T	227.76
7640	635.71	10016 T	386.26	10230	224.31
11089 L,T	565.87	9117	330.78	11109	215.50
10062 *,T	552.94	11455	310.14	10219	199.54
		11470 T	292.54	12017	199.52
		7759 T	289.89	9120	197.72
		12099	252.46	9106 T	192.83
				20022 T	189.67
				12122	174.25
				7617 T	154.78
				13142 T	150.52
				11159 **Hx,T	146.27
				13323 T	134.55
				11343	121.74
				13153 L,T	102.65
				9102 **	67.36
				7628	2.68

* 1 cycle, ** 2 cycles, T = Tubal Ligation, L = Long Bleed, Hx = Hysterectomy

requiring treatment. Only one participant was placed on hormones to regulate her bleeding. Whether her bleeding needed to be regulated is unknown. In other words, menopause may have been imminent for this woman, and the change in bleeding she experienced may have been a normal variation in menstrual pattern as she moved toward closure of menstrual life. All 31 women expressed different patterns of menstruation across the three cycles.

The prevalent clinical view of reports of change in bleeding is that it is evidence of a problem that needs to be fixed. "Fixed" means treated with hormones to restore a regular ("normal") premenopausal menstrual pattern, or removal of the source of the bleeding problem by surgically removing the uterus. Reynolds, a nurse, writing on midlife health concerns, cited studies indicating that women generally have four or five years of abnormal bleeding prior to menopause (1995). She indicates that this can be remedied; low-dose oral contraceptives can be prescribed to restore menstrual regularity. Of course, menstrual regularity is the *last* thing a perimenopausal woman's body needs. The body is sending a message that it is preparing for closure.

Several Tremin Trust women described their experiences with medical interventions to regulate bleeding:

> *I (probably as a result of tracking my bleeding more carefully) went to a gynecologist in November because my periods were long and drawn out, and sometimes heavy. I tried progestin in December and January, which did result in shorter periods, but I had many unpleasant side effects. Now I'm taking a nonsteroidal anti-inflammatory drug that is supposed to help lessen bleeding and control cramping. It seems to have helped.*

> *I'm really not particularly concerned about menopause. I'll be delighted not to menstruate any more, as I find my heavy periods to be a great nuisance since I can't use tampons easily. I'll start taking hormones when my gynecologist thinks I should start.*

> *I had a physical in April, and no sooner [was it] done [that I] had massive bleeding in May. The doctor seems to think that I'm producing estrogen and not progesterone, and that I need to get this bleeding regulated like it was before. I'll be going on hormone therapy soon.*

On May 8th I started taking Ortho-Novum 1/35 because I wanted to hold off my period because we were going on vacation for eight days. On May 18th I took my last pill. On May 22 I thought my period had started, but all I did was spot for three days. Who knows what is going on right now? Maybe taking those pills messed me up, or maybe my period could have been like that anyway (but I doubt it). There have got to be other options when it comes to hormones so I don't have a period monthly after menopause. I haven't discussed this concern with anyone just yet because I don't need them yet.

I have much more discomfort associated with my periods now than ever before. I get very painful cramps with the heavy bleeding, which at times have been so bad I couldn't sleep. I also have lots of migraines, which are related to my periods. I look forward to getting rid of them. Getting older has meant some health problems for me, particularly diarrhea, which becomes worse around the time of my period. My doctor wants to put me on hormones to get me regular again. What do you think?

The discomfort mentioned by these women—the spotting; the unpredictability of the bleeding; the recommendation and belief that hormones can regulate the bleed, eliminate menstrual pain, and migraine headaches—are all important issues. No research-based data have been found to support the widespread clinical use of hormones to regulate the menstrual cycle. Instead, hormone use may complicate an already poorly understood situation, stopping the transition and trapping the woman in premenopause. Long-term hormone use may necessitate the need to perform an even more risky and invasive procedure, hysterectomy.

ANN'S TRANSITION

My own transition to menopause was similar to that described in the anecdotes of many of The Tremin Trust women. It was a time of unpredictability, many migraine headaches (which are now gone), menstrual pain, and even flu-like symptoms before and during my period (which I now believe were probably pre–toxic shock due to the fact that I spotted for days, and perhaps was careless regarding the length of time I used one tampon). I had a diagnosis of fibroids, but not the size of a five-month pregnancy as described by one of the women in our studies. And, I was fortunate to have had a very conservative physician, who took a "wait and see" attitude about the fibroids. That attitude paid off. Since my last bleed, I have not menstruated, and every indication from frequent physical examinations is that the fibroids have regressed.

In Chapter 1, I discussed the reason I began keeping a record of my menstrual bleeds. In Table 12.2, I have included three years of my own bleeding data, years 1975 (premenopausal), 1980, and 1981 (perimenopausal). In 1975, at age 45, my menstrual bleeding pattern was regular. The number of days between bleeds ranged from a minimum of 20 to a maximum of 44. The bleeding interval averaged five to six days. In 1975 I had no episodes of heavy bleeding. Regularity in my pattern of menstrual and bleeding interval, duration, and quality did not change until 1979, when, at age 49, I began experiencing severe migraines during menstruations, and episodic heavy bleeding.

In March of 1980, at age 50, my menstrual interval began to lengthen, and in May I began to bleed heavily during each menstruation, and passed clots. I also observed that I spotted before and after the heavy flow. I experienced miserable headaches, and at times, severe nosebleeds associated with my menstrual bleed. (Strange, I thought, to be bleeding from two places simultaneously!) Even though my menstrual-cycle interval changed, the bleeding interval, for the most part, remained fairly constant. I experienced only one long period of bleeding–12 days in August 1981–which was two months prior to the time that I would experience my very last bleed. My menstrual and bleeding interval data are shown in Table 12.2, as well as how the 1980 and 1981 data appear when recorded on The Tremin Trust Menstrual Calendar Card (Figures 12.1 and 12.2).* Like many women in The Tremin Trust, I know the date of my menopause because I kept this record.

---

*Instructions on how to record menstruations using The Tremin Trust Menstrual Calendar Card and the MVJBS are found in Sections IV, Keeping Records and Keeping in Touch.

TABLE 12.2. Duration of Menstrual and Bleeding Intervals During Premeno-pause and Perimenopausal Transition for Ann Voda

DATES OF MENSTRUAL INTERVAL	NUMBER OF DAYS IN INTERVAL	NUMBER OF DAYS IN BLEEDING INTERVAL
1975 1/20 - 2/17	28	
2/17 - 3/18	29	
3/18 - 4/12	25	
4/12 - 5/6	24	
5/6 - 6/19	44	
6/19 - 7/9	20	
7/9 - 8/2	24	
8/2 - 8/29	27	
8/29 - 9/23	25	
9/23 - 10/16	23	
10/16 - 11/13	28	
11/13 - 12/8	25	
1980 1/13 - 2/6	24	5
2/6 - 3/6	29	7
3/6 - 4/8	33	6
4/8 - 5/11	33	3
5/11 - 6/18	38	4
6/18 - 7/6	18	5
7/6 - 8/23	48	5
8/23 - 12/11	110	5
1981 2/11 - 1/19	39	6
1/19 - 3/24	64	5
3/24 - 4/27	35	7
4/27 - 6/20	55	5
6/20 - 8/19	51	7
8/19 - 10/2	55	12
10/2 - 10/6		5
10/6 - Infinity		

FIGURE 12.1. 1980 Menstrual Bleeding Data (Voda)

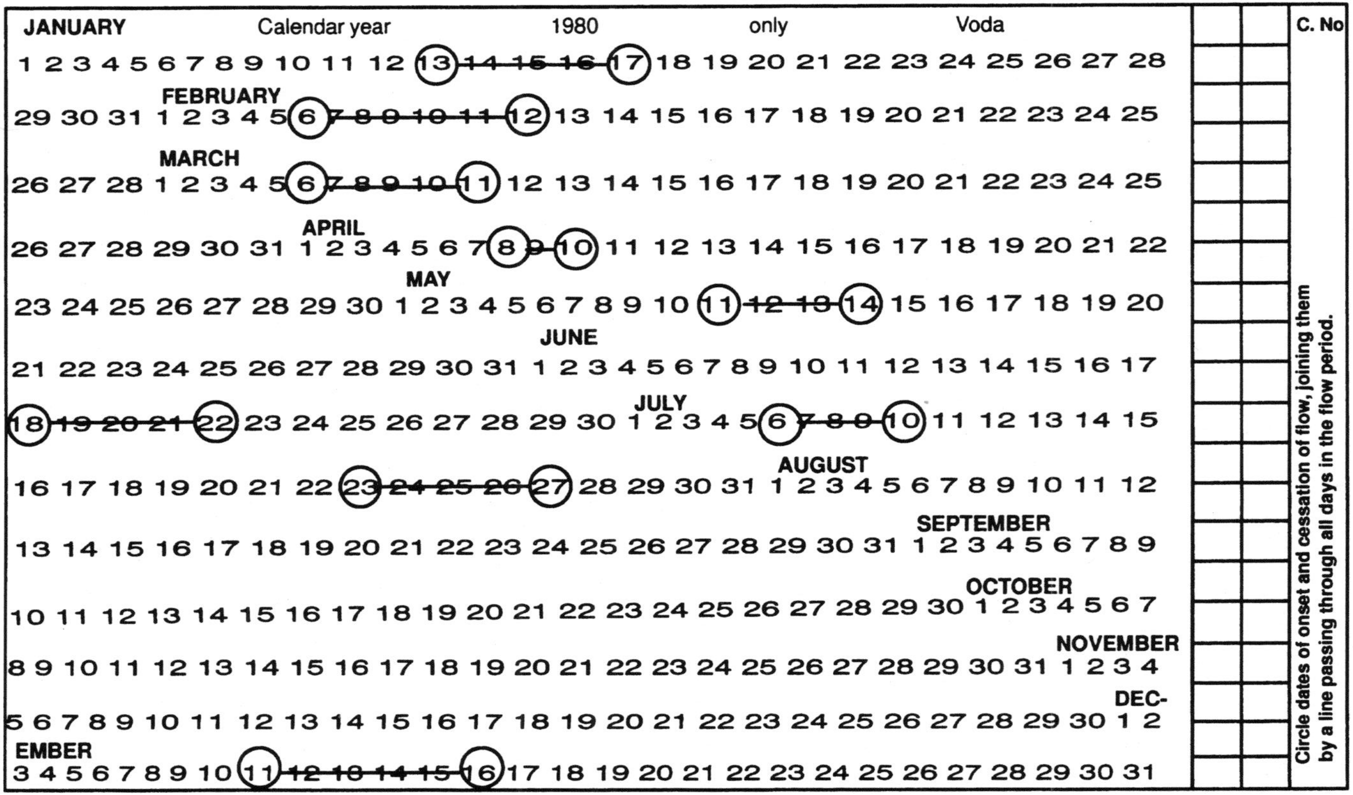

FIGURE 12.2. 1981 Menstrual Bleeding Data (Voda)

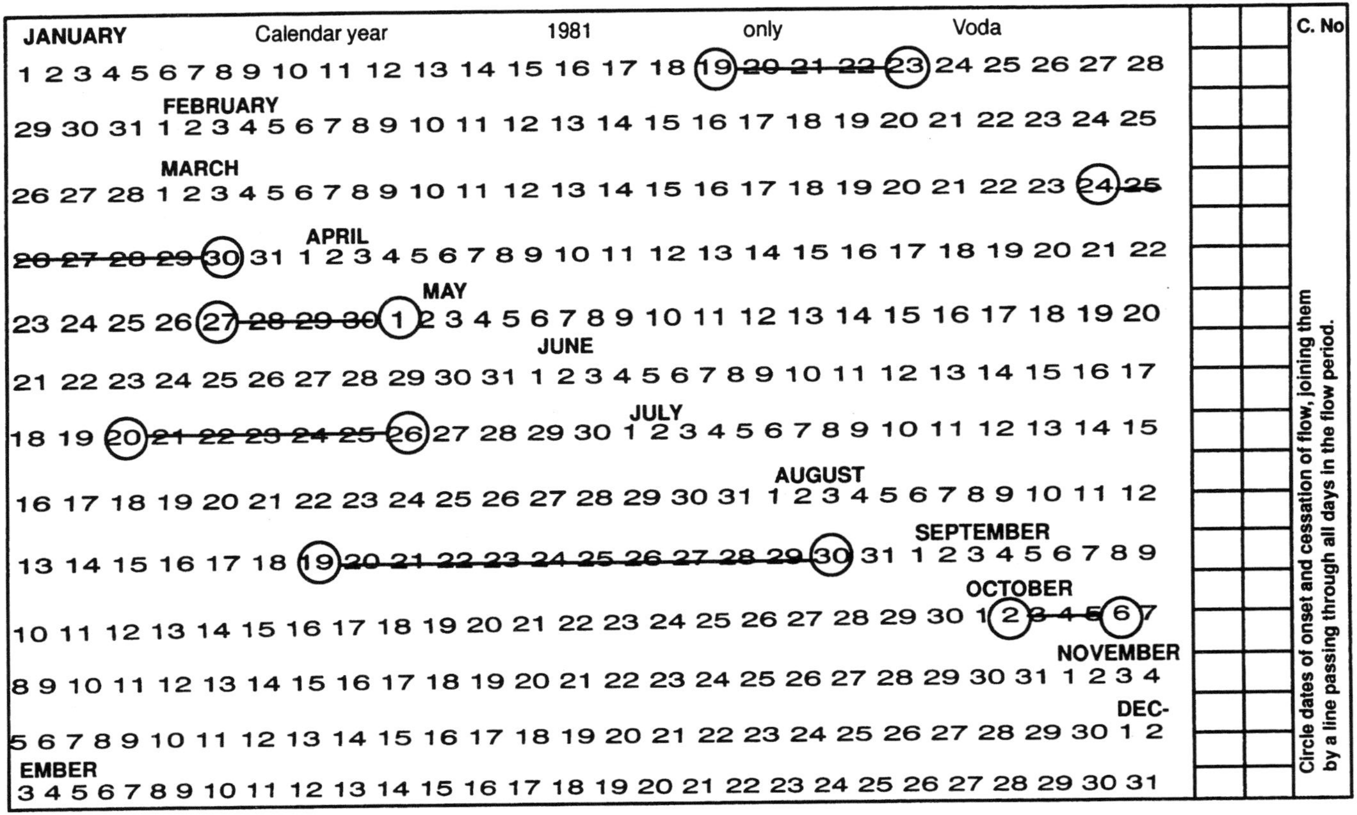

207

TREATMENTS AVAILABLE TO REGULATE BLEEDING

Some clinicians believe that almost every woman at some time in her life will have an episode of abnormal uterine bleeding which will require treatment. Abnormal uterine bleeding may be an indication that the uterine endometrium has built up excessively; in other words, hyperplasia has developed. If a woman's endometrium is hyperplastic, there is a concern that it may also be neoplastic, which means that conditions may be right for cancer to develop. Whether one or both of these pathological situations exist in all cases of a change in bleeding reported by women is unknown. In any event, once a woman receives a diagnosis of dysfunctional bleeding, clinicians have available to them a variety of medical options to treat menorrhagia (excessive menstrual bleeding), which may or may not be due to fibroids. The treatments that may be suggested to a woman are: surgery, which means hysterectomy (removal of the uterus); endometrial ablation, which is burning or cauterization of the uterine lining; antifibrinolytic agents (drugs to promote clotting); prostaglandin synthetase inhibitors (drugs to control the blood vasculature, constriction, and dilatation); oral contraceptives (birth control pills); and replacement of synthetic and artificial hormones, such as equine estrogens, progestogens, and androgens.

Each treatment is associated with risks. Well-defined risks are associated with any surgery, and hysterectomy is no exception. Endometrial ablation is a fairly new procedure, and little data are available about either short- or long-term side effects. Regarding hysterectomy and ablation, the goal of treatment is to eliminate the source of the bleeding. Hysterectomy removes the entire uterus; endometrial ablation removes the lining of the uterus that is hormone-sensitive. The remaining methods, hormonal and nonhormonal, are based upon hypotheses that have been advanced regarding mechanisms that regulate menstruation.

Dilatation and Curettage

The conventional treatment for regulating abnormal bleeding is dilatation and curettage (D&C), which is often followed by some form of hormonal therapy. In women under age 35, a D&C may be effective in reducing heavy bleeding for several years, but inevitably, the bleeding problems resume. Perimenopausal women are often encouraged to have a hysterectomy rather that a D&C to cure the problem. A D&C is considered minor surgery. It involves first dilating (widening) the opening of the cervix in order to permit the introduction of a larger instrument, such as the curette, a sharp metal instrument which is used to scrape away the lining of the uterus. Even though a D&C can be performed on an outpatient or short-stay surgery basis, it is not without risk. Too aggressive scraping can cause uterine perforation, adhesions, and scar tissue buildup. Curettage can also be performed using a suction device, or a small pump to vacuum the uterine lining. This procedure is called "aspiration curettage," and according to Dr. Vicki Hufnagel, it can be performed with a minimum of discomfort in a doctor's office. It is also much less risky than the scraping done with a sharp metal instrument. Hufnagel cautions women to never sign a consent form to undergo a D&C that also gives permission to perform a hysterectomy. She advises having the D&C performed, getting tissue sample (histological) results from the pathologist, and only then agreeing to surgery if the diagnosis is cancer. Hufnagel also recommends that women send slides of the tissue samples off to a different pathologist to obtain a second opinion *before* agreeing to have the surgery (1988). Any surgery is anxiety producing and is risky. It takes time to prepare for such an event, both emotionally and physically. A woman's life can change drastically following hysterectomy. It is not as "simple" a procedure as it is made out to be. As I will discuss later, the aftereffects from the procedure may affect a woman's sexual response, possibly inducing a premature menopause. *Always get a second opinion, and do not agree to have a hysterectomy in conjunction with a D&C.*

Endometrial Ablation via Rollerball or Yag Laser Ablation

This procedure involves the destruction or cautery (burning) removal of the lining of the uterus. A laser light is used in the uterus, cauterizing and destroying the tissue lining the inside of the uterus. The procedure requires long training on the part of the physician. When compared with hysterectomy, which requires hospitalization, the ablation procedure is performed on a less expensive, outpatient basis. Not enough procedures have been done to assess whether or not the complications that may occur will be fewer than those associated with other procedures. One physician, Dr. Duane Townsend (1990), who has pioneered the technique, predicts that in the future endometrial ablation will become a standard procedure, and many women will choose the cautery method to cease menstruation, if for no other reason than to bring an end to the "nuisance" of menstrual flow. There is no doubt in my mind that women do view the change in bleeding as a nuisance, a bother, and a mess, and look forward to getting rid of it. However, I am not convinced that many women will opt to have their uterine lining burned to stop menstrual bleeding.

The roller ball technique has been utilized for many years to treat other conditions, such as prostate problems. It is fairly new in the treatment of menorrhagia. The method is said to be effective in 95 percent of the cases followed to date. However, the long-term impact of endometrial coagulation is unknown, particularly the risk of cancer. According to Townsend et al. (1990), questions regarding safety will be determined with long-term follow-up of women who have had the procedure. The DES experience taught us that it sometimes takes decades for sequelae to develop. So, it is too soon to comment on the safety of the procedure over the long term. Prior to using either the rollerball or cautery techniques, menstrual cycle physiology and uterine function has to be modified. First, a drug, Lupron, must be taken. Lupron is a long-acting gonadotrophin-releasing hormone analog (which means that it mimics the releasing hormones in the brain that stimulate the pituitary gland). After Lupron is injected, there is a brief period of stimulation of the pituitary gonadotrophic hormones, LH and FSH. This means that at first Lupron acts as an agonist, causing pituitary cells to *secrete* LH and FSH. This stimulatory, or agonistic, action is followed up with the desired antagonistic action of Lupron, which is *suppression* of LH and FSH synthesis.

Lupron effectively prevents the pituitary gland from stimulating the ovaries to make estrogen and to promote ovulation. This results in an almost immediate, albeit temporary, menopause. The menopausal effect of Lupron lasts about one month. According to drug company literature, the effect of Lupron is reversible when treatment is discontinued.

Following Lupron administration, the uterus is cauterized. Then the treatment protocol is to give the woman an injection of Depo Provera, a long-acting progestogen, in order to minimize postcautery bleeding and uterine discharge. As with any procedure that carries risks, always get a second opinion.

Hysterectomy

Hysterectomy is the surgical removal of the uterus. It is an invasive procedure with a high risk of complications. The hospital stay time for the procedure ranges from two to four days. Recovery time can take from four to six weeks. According to Nora Coffey, President of the Hysterectomy Educational Resources Foundation, the impact the surgery has on a woman's life has not been broadly disclosed, nor has the effect that it has on family and friends been studied (1993). Many men and women have been socialized to believe that men are strong and women are weak. A woman's weakness is said to derive from the reproductive organs (the theory of the defective woman). Consequently, women are concerned that the ovaries and the uterus are superfluous—excess baggage. At midlife, and particularly perimenopausally, as the pattern of bleeding changes (whether or not it is associated with fibroids), women, more often than not, are encouraged to have a hysterectomy to end bleeding; they are told they will function better if they eliminate that monthly nuisance. In other words, according to Coffey, "if women had been made right to begin with, they would not have been born with these useless, bleeding, and potentially dangerous sex organs." She is concerned that some gynecologists have set out to right this "mistake of nature" (p. 3).

Hysterectomy generates about $4 billion a year for gynecological surgeons. This is not a small amount of money. But, according to Coffey (1993), Hufnagel with Golant (1988), and Cutler (1988), there may be more to this picture than greed and money. Why does any doctor become a gynecologist? Until the last two decades, there was no counterpart to gynecology for men, i.e., a department of andrology. This is strange, since it is far easier to examine a man's reproductive organs. Traditionally, men did not see a doctor every year to find out if there were problems with their reproductive organs (although I think they should, and there is a movement toward this goal in order to detect prostate cancer in the early stages). However, the bottom line here with respect to menstrual bleeding is that it is women, not men, who menstruate, and at midlife it is women who experience heavy, gushing bleeding, sometimes with the passing of clots. It is easy to rationalize having a hysterectomy when one uses man (who does not menstruate) or, for that matter, premenopausal woman, who bleeds with predictability and regularity, as the standard. Understanding how the female uterus functions will provide information necessary to understanding why hysterectomy causes women so many problems. I am indebted to Nora Coffey for the material that follows, which was published in a 1993 *HERS* newsletters. The article is summarized as follows.

The uterus is not free-floating in the pelvis. It is attached to four broad bands of ligaments that attach to the sacrum in the lower back. It is also attached to a major blood supply and a large bundle of nerves. When the ligaments attached to the uterus are severed, they are then hanging at one end, and tied in bundles, no longer attached to anything at the other end. Those are the supporting ligaments for the entire pelvic structure. When those ligaments are severed, it permits the pelvis to broaden and widen. It is not an old wives' tale that women become broader across the pelvis and backside following hysterectomy. It is a reality.

When blood vessels to the uterus are severed, much of the sensation to the vagina, clitoris, and nipples may be lost. If you were to examine a diagram of the pelvic nerves, they would look like a bundle of spaghetti, attached to the uterus in several places, and branching out to different parts of the body, including many different parts of the spine. The impulses that travel along these nerve pathways provide sensation and feeling in various parts of the body. When those nerves are severed, sensation is lost.

If the uterus and cervix are removed, they are excised by cutting all around the cervix. If they are removed through the vagina, the top of the vagina is sutured shut, and sutured to one of the hanging ligaments. The result is that the vagina becomes like a closed pocket. There is a loss of elasticity and a scar at the top of the vagina. Many women report that they are unable to have intercourse at all following hysterectomy because the vagina was made too short or too narrow. Other women find intercourse painful because of scar tissue. In addition, everything in the abdomen and pelvis drifts down into the area previously occupied by the uterus, displacing remaining organs. When women report they are having problems posthysterectomy, or are no longer having sexual feelings, they often are told that these problems are "in their heads."

The moral of this story is the following: *The successful problem-free hysterectomy is related to the level of skill and experience of the surgeon.*

Finally, hysterectomy is not a simple procedure. It will eliminate the bleeding problem, but at the same time, it increases the risk of developing chronic conditions and may profoundly alter sexual arousal and responsiveness. Whether or not to have a hysterectomy is not a decision that should be made based upon one physician's opinion, nor should the decision be made based upon a woman's self-report of heavy bleeding. There is an unacceptably high incidence of mortality with hysterectomy; 1 in 2,000 will die. Because there is no simple way to estimate or measure blood loss, one researcher, Dr. Steve Smith (1991) of Cambridge University, believes that about one-half of the patients who attend gynecological clinics complaining of heavy bleeding do not, in fact, have heavy bleeding; these women are being treated for a disorder that does not exist. Smith does not belittle the patients, for whom the bleeding probably is quite unacceptable, whether light or heavy. Instead, he stresses how important it is for clinicians to be able to make the diagnosis of abnormal or dysfunctional bleeding correctly. Smith hopes that drugs to reduce blood loss will be found soon, since drugs are, in most instances, a less risky form of medical treatment than surgery or ablation. For more in-depth information on hysterectomy, or myomectomy, see Hufnagel with Golant (1988), Cutler (1988), and Coffey (1993).

Drugs

Prostaglandin Inhibitors

The use of these agents, which are local hormones released in the lining of the uterus, is based upon a hypothesis that the initiation of menstruation arises from the constriction of the arterioles. Once bleeding begins, control is obtained by the process of vasoconstriction and subsequent dilation of the vessel. The use of prostaglandin inhibitors, then, is targeted at controlling the local vasculature, the uterine blood vessels. An example of one drug that is used to control blood vessels is Flurbiprofen, a potent prostaglandin synthetase inhibitor, which has been shown to be effective in the treatment of primary dysmenorrhea, as well as menorrhagia. Side effects associated with the drug are fatigue, stomach pains, and nausea.

Antifibrinolytic Agents

The use of these agents is based upon the finding of a highly significant increase in fibrinolytic activity in the clots of women who were evaluated as having menorrhagia, menstruation which contained more than 80 ml of *blood* per day (not just discharge). The site of action of antifibrinolytic agents is local, within the uterus. They block the enzymatic conversion of substances that promote clotting of the blood, transforming fibrinogen into fibrin. When fibrin is formed, it is deposited as fine interlacing filaments, in which are entangled red and white blood cells and platelets. An example of an antifibrinolytic drug is Tranexamic acid. Side effects are associated with it, such as nausea, dizziness, numbness, restless legs, headache, and sometimes difficulty in swallowing.

Oral Contraceptives

These estrogen- and progestogen-like agents are used to shut down the body's (endogenous) synthesis of estrogen and progesterone. They have more of a central rather than a local site of action. The central mechanism of action is exerted at the level of the central nervous system (the hypothalamus and pituitary), to suppress the synthesis and release of the gonadotrophins, FSH and LH. Without FSH and LH, follicles on the ovary do not develop. Hence, no estrogen or progesterone is made within the body. Since the oral contraceptives are taken in low dosages, they do stimulate reproductive target tissue, but at a much lower level than that achieved when a woman produces her own hormones, so the local site of action of these agents is the uterine lining. Uterine buildup is kept to a minimum, and bleeding is minimal.

Progestogens

Any progestogen or progestin, such as Depo Provera (medroxy-progesterone acetate), when administered at recommended dosages, inhibits the secretion of gonadotrophins, LH and FSH, which, in turn, prevent follicular maturity and ovulation. Without ovulation, as indicated above, endometrial thinning occurs, and subsequently amenorrhea (absence of menses). Side effects associated with progestogen use are as follows: an increased risk for osteoporosis (bone thinning), breast cancer, heart disease, and thromboembolic disorders. Progestogens must not be administered to women unless the cause of the abnormal bleeding is diagnosed.

Progestogen Challenge Test

Aside from the problem of heavy bleeding in the perimenopause, Gambrell (1992, p. 29) recommends the progestogen challenge test be administered to all peri- or postmenopausal women who have their uterus intact, in order to detect whether a precancerous condition exists. The women Gambrell recommends be screened may or may not be women in perimenopause who are bleeding heavily. Rather, they may be menstruating regularly, may be women who are being evaluated for estrogen replacement therapy, or may be estrogen-treated patients who are not currently taking a progestin with the estrogen. Gambrell recommends screening asymptomatic postmenopausal women as well. Screening of asymptomatic women is based upon well-documented knowledge that many women produce sufficient endogenous estrogen (estrone) in the fatty tissue of their bodies. These women are asymptomatic during the postmenopause. These women, more often than not, are obese, and are able to offset some of the changes associated with a state of "true estrogen deficiency," such as osteoporosis, because they are making considerable quantities of estrogen in their bodies. Gambrell hypothesizes that within this group of obese and/or nonobese asymptomatic women are women who are in the greatest need of cyclic progestogen therapy to shed an estrogen-stimulated buildup of the endometrium. Recall that during the menstrual cycle during premenopausal reproductive years, it is progesterone that transforms the uterine endometrium from one that is in a phase of rapid cell division to one that is hospitable for implantation of the developing organism. Progesterone does all of this by antagonizing the proliferative or hyperplastic effects of estrogen. During the perimenopause, little or no progesterone is produced in a woman's body to antagonize estrogen. During postmenopause, no progesterone is available. Thus, Gambrell concluded that the test is needed to determine whether or not women have built up the endometrium, which could predispose them to cancer.

The progestogen challenge test challenges the uterus to eliminate any cellular buildup. If there has been a buildup of the uterine endometrium, after stopping the progestogen, a woman should experience withdrawal bleeding. If there is no bleeding, it is assumed that no excessive buildup was present.

The test is performed by administering a 13-day course of either Depo Provera, 10 milligrams, or norethindrone or norethindrone acetate, 2.5 to 5 milligrams. If withdrawal bleeding occurs, then the progestogen should be continued for 13 days each month (or each menstrual cycle), for as long as withdrawal bleeding continues. Gambrell believes that the test should be repeated annually in asymptomatic postmenopausal women who do not bleed following the test. Side effects are associated with the test. Taking the progestogens for the 13-day period causes cramping, headaches, bloating, weight gain, and in some women, PMS-like symptoms.

Myomectomy

Traditionally, the only option to hysterectomy to control bleeding due to fibroid tumors was a surgical procedure called "myomectomy," which is the removal of a fibroid tumor. Myomectomy does not remove tumors that grow within the wall of the uterus, ligaments, or abdominal cavity, or any that are difficult to reach. Hufnagel with Golant (1988) say that conventional myomectomy is not routinely offered to women because multiple incisions are made on the surface of the uterus at every tumor site. Bleeding and complications such as weakening of the structural integrity of the uterus can result. Hufnagel provides detailed information on fibroids and alternatives to hysterectomy in her book *No More Hysterectomies* (1988), which was written with Golant.

ANN'S ADVICE REGARDING CHANGES IN BLEEDING

Until more information is available on how the bleeding pattern changes during premenopause, here are a few suggestions on how to cope with this very common change.

1. *Know thyself.* Just as with hot flashes, keep a record of the onset and stop of menstruations using the menstrual card to track the menstrual interval. Rate the quality of menstrual bleeds using the 6-point scale.

2. *Don't worry* unless *bleeding is very heavy over a long period of time, and periods are close together* (that is, less than two weeks apart). A change in the bleeding pattern premenopausally is normal. However, heavy bleeding over a long duration is not! If bleeding is heavy over two menstruations, and periods are close together, do not hesitate! *Seek out a care provider* and take along your bleeding record card. Do not wait, as anemia may develop. Anemia is a serious condition. It causes fatigue, and it makes the heart work very hard in order to circulate the red blood cells that carry the oxygen needed by all cells in the body. No tissue in the body can function without oxygen. If the number of red blood cells is decreased, there is less oxygen available to meet the energy demands placed upon the body, even basal needs.

3. *Be prepared for the unexpected.* As The Tremin Trust participants have discussed, what is most frustrating is to have bleeding begin without any warning. So, carry a good supply of napkins or tampons of various absorbencies, and keep a good supply in a desk or locker if employed outside of the home. Phyllis Mansfield and I discovered that the 32 pre- and perimenopausal women we studied used 46 products of different absorbencies.

4. *Do not wear a tampon for more than a few hours.* If a menstrual bleed is characterized by spotting or is light or very light, or bleeds have become unpredictable in onset, and appear to happen without any warning, *do not* wear a tampon for long periods of time! This could increase the risk of developing toxic shock syndrome or urinary tract infections.

5. *Eat a well-balanced diet, particularly foods high in iron.* If bleeding heavily and passing clots, consult with a nutritionist regarding iron supplementation. The body has a minimal capacity for storing some iron, but with prolonged bleeding from any cause, the storage source is quickly depleted. A normal hemoglobin value for menstruating women is around 13 to 14 grams per deciliter. A care provider will probably measure hemoglobin as well as the percent of the blood in the total circulating volume of fluid. This latter measurement is referred to as the hematocrit. If the hematocrit is low, less than 40 milliliters per deciliter, this will indicate that red cell mass is lower than it should be.

6. *If menstrual blood soils clothing or bed linens, consider this tip: pour hydrogen peroxide on the bloody spots.* The oxidizing action of the solution will/should lift the blood right out.

7. *Consider drug, hormone, surgical or ablation therapy only after a valid diagnosis of abnormal or dysfunctional bleeding has been made.* Read as much as possible from the list of readings compiled by the North American Menopause Society. Make a list of questions to ask of a care provider. Expect that questions will be answered in a respectful manner. Realize that every treatment carries some kind of risk. Don't submit to treatment and then ask questions. The mechanism of menstruation is only now being understood at the cell molecular level. Treatment with drugs is based upon "hypotheses" related to bleeding and coagulation mechanisms. Treatment with hormones is based upon knowledge of how estrogen and progesterone function during the menstrual cycle in prime reproductive years, not what they do in a uterus that has been genetically preprogrammed for closure. A hysterectomy stops the bleeding by removing the uterus. Endometrial ablation eliminates the lining of the uterus; it destroys a portion of the uterus, but does not remove it. *Always* get a second opinion related to the results of any test performed–especially when surgery has been recommended based on a test.

8. *Appreciate that we do not have the information we need to say with any confidence that the change in perimenopausal bleed-*

ing will last for a certain length of time and then stop. We do not have data on how the bleeding pattern changes, nor how long the bleeding will be irregular, heavy, and unpredictable. And, we do not know whether the bleeding pattern or the duration of the bleeding will be prolonged with drug or hormone use. This lack of information may be related to our cultural heritage, long-standing superstitions, and beliefs about menstruating women as polluted and impure. When Phyllis Mansfield and I were asked to explain our menstrual bleeding study, when we said we were collecting and weighing used feminine care products, people said, "You're doing *what*? How gross!"

9. *Debunk the theory of the defective woman.* Menstruation, PMS, and menopause may be out of the closet, figuratively speaking, but in reality, little has changed. The theory of the defective woman is alive and well. Menstrual blood is still thought of as unclean and impure. Women shed this "polluted" blood periodically in a process called menstruation. At menopause, when reproductive life has ended and menstruation becomes unpredictable and out of control, a woman's uterus is described as a useless, diseased organ. Cut it, scrape it, prime it, burn it, purge it, drug it. By all means, get that uterus under control. Implicit in controlling the uterus is controlling the woman.

    It is fascinating to realize how "uterus-intensive" gynecological practice is as a medical specialty. It is akin to an obsession. Until recently, most gynecology practitioners have been male, individuals who have never experienced pregnancy, menstrual cramps, or the shedding of menstrual blood.

10. *Appreciate the importance of the uterus to the quality of post-menopausal life.* Even though the uterus may appear to be out of control as the perimenopause commences, it usually is not. Menstruation and reproductive life were genetically preprogrammed for closure. The onset of certain changes, such as the change in the menstrual and bleeding interval, are part and parcel of the normal process of closure.

Chapter 13

Estrogen Deficiency

Ever since my entry into the field of women's health, I have been concerned about the medicalization and hormonal treatment of menstruating and menopausal women. On one hand, when women have sex hormones circulating during menstrual/reproductive years, it is the hormones that are responsible for premenstrual syndrome, or in the worst case scenario, they are the cause of luteal dysphoric disease. On the other hand, at menopause, when hormones are mostly absent, women are diagnosed as "estrogen-deficient," and at risk of disease if the lost hormones are not replaced. Women are *not*, let me repeat, *not* estrogen-deficient at menopause unless they are diseased, or have been made estrogen-deficient through drugs, radiation (X ray), or surgery.

The most frequently asked question I hear from menopausal women centers on the issue of hormone replacement, that is, to be or not to be a hormone user. The answer to this question necessitates a full understanding of the risks and benefits associated with the hormones being replaced. What do these agents do in the body once they are administered? What tissues, other than reproductive tissues, do they affect? How and why do they cause cancer? Do they reduce heart disease, heart attack, and stroke? What are the major benefits of taking hormones? And what are the major risks, i.e., what are the trade-offs, to prevent heart disease? Does one increase the risk of breast cancer through hormone use?

Many women have been exposed to estrogen- and progesterone-containing drugs during their adult lives. Steroid hormones were used and are used today as a contraceptive, and commencing in the 1960s, estrogen was used widely by pre- and postmenopausal women. Once the undesirable side effects associated with estrogen use were known, women and some care providers became very skeptical that benefits outweighed the risks associated with use.

Women who are experiencing menopause naturally are concerned about the risks associated with hormone use, and need information that is supported through research. Unfortunately, as we found out related to the estrogen/uterine cancer connection, years can elapse before enough information is available on all the risks associated with these agents. A 52-year-old woman shared this concern and others about hormone replacement:

> *Most of my current questioning centers around hormones and hormone replacement therapy. Is there good information supported by solid research? Should all menopausal women be on a hormone replacement program? What are all the indications for hormone replacement? What if symptoms are not dramatic? Is prevention of symptoms a good reason for hormone replacement?*

To answer her questions, there is good information about the cancer risk to the uterus when estrogen is taken, and there is good information to support that women with a diagnosis of osteoporosis will benefit from estrogen replacement. There is no research-based data, at least not yet, to support that all menopausal women should be on hormone replacement. Recall Gambrell's words that some women continue to make sufficient estrogen pre- and postmenopausally, and are asymptomatic. If symptoms are not dramatic, this is not an indication to take hormones, nor is age or menopausal status an automatic sign that hormone replacement is indicated or even warranted.

Whether or not a woman will be a hormone user needs to be the woman's decision, based upon all the facts available at the time she is searching for information. Advice from a care provider is but one source of information that can be considered, not the *only* source.

A 49-year-old woman uses her mother as a reference point to voice concerns about hormones:

> *What concerns me the most about menopause is hormone therapy. There is so much disagreement on whether it is good for you or not. My mom started on hormones after menopause, and her next Pap test was abnormal. So, she stopped. But they*

do say that estrogen protects against heart attacks and bone loss, so it's hard to know what to do.

Yes, it is hard to know what to do. We know that hormones are potent initiators of metabolism, which includes the synthesis of growth factors, some of which may initiate or promote cancer. With the lack of needed information on all metabolic processes that might be affected, it is frustrating not knowing whether taking a hormone may increase the risk of developing a disease that has not been identified. I will discuss the postulated heart disease and osteoporosis benefit later.

Two women expressed a fear of cancer with hormone use. The first said the following:

My mother died of cancer. She took hormones. I am afraid to take hormones. I'm bothered by the irregularity and uncertainty of it all. I'm concerned about whether or not I should take hormones upon the onset of menopause, since there is a history of breast cancer in my family.

Yes, a history of cancer is an important risk factor to weigh when considering hormone use, since there is no clear-cut evidence that hormones do not cause breast cancer, and we know that breast tissue is hormone-responsive tissue.

The second woman pondered the fear of cancer along with the benefit that might be obtained related to heart disease and osteoporosis:

I have mixed feelings about pursuing hormonal treatment, as I understand there's a tendency toward cervical cancer with medication. Yet, my paternal medical history [puts me] at risk for heart disease, and my mother appears to have osteoporosis, both of which would be improved with medications.

This woman tries to put the pieces together in order to make a decision about whether or not to be a hormone user. She definitely is at risk for developing uterine, and perhaps cervical, changes with estrogen use. She is at risk for breast cancer with estrogen and progesterone use. Her bones will benefit with hormone use, which will at least prevent further demineralization.

Another woman wrote the following:

> *I am concerned about the unknowns associated with pro-*
> *gesterone therapy. I wish I could find a physician who would*
> *take an interest in PMS and my experiences. I am worried*
> *about the changes menopause will bring and what kind of*
> *therapy will be appropriate for me.*

This woman must take progesterone *with estrogen* if she has a uterus. Progesterone replacement therapy is the new kid on the hormone block; there is much we need to learn about the long-term effects of progestogens on bones, the heart, breasts, and many other tissues in the body that have receptors for steroid hormones. The woman has raised an excellent question regarding PMS and progesterone use. If Katharina Dalton's theory has credibility, that is, that PMS is due to progesterone deficiency, then this woman should see a lessening of PMS-like symptoms as she takes estrogen and progesterone. Unfortunately, we have no data on PMS-suffering women concerning estrogen replacement, or the effects of combined hormone therapy.

Another woman is on hormone replacement therapy, the patch, and progestogen for hot flashes. She, too, is "very concerned about the possible side effects, increased possibility of tumors, cardiovascular disease, etc." Two women, both age 50, express concerns about the logic of taking hormones and the lack of guidelines for asymptomatic women:

> *I question what the big deal is. It is part of the normal aging*
> *process, not a disaster. [I'm] just curious to see how it will*
> *play out for me. My physician (OB/GYN) has suggested hor-*
> *mones at the proper time, but my thought is not to use them*
> *unless I can be convinced that mother nature doesn't know*
> *how to run my body!*

> *My only serious concern is use of hormone therapy, its*
> *necessity, the dangers, and the lack of clear guidelines for*
> *women without significant symptoms.*

These women are questioning the logic of taking hormones to treat a normal process, particularly if there are no symptoms and symptoms result when the hormones are taken. For example, of clinical concern is the knowledge that progestogens produce side effects, some of which are described as nuisances, e.g., abdominal bloating, migraines, and even some PMS-like symptoms. An important metabolic side effect associated with progestogen use, however, is that it could decrease the concentration of the good lipoproteins in the blood, the high density lipoproteins, and increase the triglycerides, both of which are declared risk factors in men for increasing rather than decreasing heart disease in women who must replace progestogen with estrogen. The use of progestogens was deemed useless by Schenken and Pauerstein in 1989, if such treatment eliminates the protection against heart disease obtained with estrogen. Since the results of the Postmenopausal Estrogen/Progesterone Intervention (PEPI) trial have been published, the concern regarding the negative effect of progestogen on the lipid profile has been encouraging. More detail on estrogen and heart disease is found in Chapter 15.

What, then, are the major risks associated with hormone use? The answer to this question is ambiguous. If a woman with a uterus takes estrogen over a long period of time (10 to 15 years), she is at increased risk for developing cancer of the uterus. Fully understanding how estrogen may cause cancer, and how it causes other undesirable side effects in a woman's body requires a basic understanding of how the sex hormones function in the human body.

Few women understand all they should about how sex hormones function. Nor do they understand basic biological processes well enough to understand the risk-benefit picture painted for them about hormones.

And why should they? They are not trained in biology or biochemistry. In fact, many care providers are not knowledgeable either. The changes that occur in a woman's body perimenopausally are as normal as the changes she experienced with hormone fluctuations during the menstrual cycle. These changes are biologically determined: they have a specific and important purpose in the grand scheme of the survival of the human species. I have tried to paint as clear a picture as possible, indicating that the menstrual cycle is a life within a life. And I have repeated several times (and I have meant to be repetitive) that when the genetically predetermined time comes, closure of the menstrual and reproductive cycles must occur. All women, some with a little ambivalence, look forward to the end of menstruation; it is a liberating experience. To use the words of some women: "Whoopee, freedom! No more bloody sheets, no more tampons and napkins, no more cramps, no more pain, no more mood swings." Hormone replacement at menopause for a woman with a uterus means blood, tampons and napkins, cramps, bloat, pain, breakthrough bleeding, etc.

Hormone replacement is based upon the biological deficit model (Chapter 6), which purports that women are estrogen-deficient at menopause. But women are not estrogen-deficient unless they are made estrogen-deficient when their healthy ovaries are removed during a hysterectomy, or destroyed with drugs or X rays.

EXTRAGONADAL SYNTHESIS OF ESTROGEN

Within a woman's body there are well-developed endocrine mechanisms that function to provide a continuing source of estrogen pre- and postmenopausally. And, according to the research that has been done, the process becomes more efficient as women get older. This process, first described in the early 1970s by Grodin, Siiteri, and MacDonald, is called *extragonadal synthesis of estrone*. In more technical terms, the process is described as peripheral conversion of one steroid, androstenedione, which is an androgen, into another steroid (an estrogen), estrone. The conversion process occurs in fatty tissue. In the menarche chapter, I discussed the role fat plays in maturation and puberty, maintenance of the normal menstrual cycle functions, and steroid hormone synthesis. I also described what can happen to pre- or postmenopausal women who have either too little or too much fat for their height and weight—obese women are at high risk for cancer of the uterus because of the endocrine function of their fatty tissue. These women have an enhanced ability to convert the androgen precursor hormone in their fatty tissue into estrone.

Estrone is a weaker estrogen than estradiol, but it can bind with the estrogen receptor (which you will read about shortly). If there is a good concentration of estrone available to interact with the receptor, in the absence of progesterone, endometrial hyperplasia (growth of cells) results. Hyperplasia is a risk factor for neoplasia, cancer. Fortunately, most women, as they enter menopause, are neither obese or cachectic (too thin). They enter menopause with adequate body fat, and in fact, most women will increase body fat as they begin the transition and become postmenopausal. This body composition change is a concern to women, but it need not be. Perhaps the weight gain that most of us experience is nature's way of ensuring that we have a way to make estrogen in our bodies. A menopausal woman may not continue to cycle or make estradiol and progesterone, but she does have a continuing ability to make estrone, a weaker estrogen. The variability in the menopause experience among women is probably related, in part, to the variability in how estrone is synthesized; the fatter the woman, the greater the possibility of estrogen synthesis and the fewer symptoms she will have.

ESTROGEN DEFICIENCY AND HORMONE REPLACEMENT

It is encouraging to know that more menopause clinicians/researchers than in the past believe that most postmenopausal women will not experience serious illness or disease as a result of not receiving supplemental or additive treatment. These physicians believe that estrogen is appropriate for some women with disease and those who have had menopause induced prematurely by surgery, chemotherapy, or radiation. These physicians also believe that all women will experience some decline in estrogen levels during prime reproductive years. Fortunately for many women, the transition to and through menopause is gradual, and they do not experience a state of absolute estrogen deficiency unless they have been *made* estrogen-deficient.

CASTRATION-INDUCED ESTROGEN DEFICIENCY

Removal of a woman's ovaries is castration. Destruction of a woman's ovaries, particularly the follicles, through drugs (chemotherapy) or radiation is castration. A few of my feminist colleagues object to the use of the word castration when referring to women, suggesting that it is a term for surgical removal of a male's testicles. Actually, the medical term for surgical removal of the testicles is orchiectomy. Removal of the ovaries is oophorectomy. The term castration implies an inability to produce hormones from human gonads whether due to disease, medical procedures, and/or treatments, regardless of the biological sex of the individual. The most common form of castration in premenopausal women is through surgical removal of the ovaries (oophorectomy). Recall from Chapter 2 how Robert Wilson, in his 1960s articles and his book *Feminine Forever*, described menopausal women as "estrogen-deficient," "castrates," and "hypogonadal," with nothing to look forward to (without hormones) except a life of living decay.

Casting aside the degrading pontifications of Wilson, castration, no matter how it is accomplished, poses serious metabolic consequences for women and men. Castrated, young, premenopausal women have little choice for a healthy quality of life unless they replace the estrogen that has been prematurely eliminated from their bodies. These women are no longer able to synthesize estradiol, androgens, or other weaker estrogens such as estrone from the ovary. Estrone production, via extragonadal synthesis (androstenedione to estrone mechanism described previously, in fat tissue), is also diminished. Women who are castrated absolutely require hormone replacement.

HYSTERECTOMY- AND OOPHORECTOMY-INDUCED ESTROGEN DEFICIENCY

Until recently, hysterectomy was one of the most common surgeries in the United States. A woman who agreed to a hysterectomy was also at risk of being castrated, even if no ovarian disease was present.

Pinn reported in 1993 that the number of hysterectomies performed in the United States has increased over the years, peaking in 1975 at 725,000, and declining slightly in the 1980s to stabilize at about 575,000 per year. Most hysterectomies (on average about 1,500 per day in the United States) are performed to correct either a misdiagnosed condition, e.g., dysfunctional bleeding, a benign condition such as uterine fibroids, or endometriosis. Only 5 percent of the hysterectomies are performed to treat cancer of the uterus.

The median age of a hysterectomized woman is 40.9 years, with the greatest number of surgeries being performed on women between the ages of 30 and 49. In 1984, estimates indicated that between 20 and 30 percent of all hysterectomies performed were combined with oophorectomy. I do not know whether the rate has increased or decreased related to combined hysterectomy and oophorectomy. However, there is no reason to believe that it will, as there continues to be the belief that removal of a woman's ovaries, even though healthy, during hysterectomy on women age 40 and older, protects against ovarian cancer.

Oophorectomy does eliminate the risk of developing ovarian cancer. The American Cancer Society estimated that 26,700 new cases of ovarian cancer would occur in 1996, and 14,700 women would die from the disease (Parker et al., 1996). No research-based data are available to substantiate that the rate of ovarian cancer in women increases if ovaries have been retained when a hysterectomy is performed. The data available are appallingly unreliable. In 1990 Utian reported that rates of ovarian cancer in women who had their ovaries retained during surgery were estimated to range from 1 in 500 to 1 in 5,000. These data are inadequate to support the need for ovary removal, particularly since oophorectomy precipitously induces menopause, and an almost 100-percent guarantee that a state of estrogen deficiency will result. For surgically induced estrogen deficiency, somatic and affective changes occur immediately. Unlike women going through menopause naturally, these women have no time to adapt to changes in hormone levels. For older premenopausal women who have menopause induced surgically, the changes may have started prior to surgery. The response of these women to a precipitous reduction in estrogen levels may be less intense. In the final analysis, it matters not how old one is when menopause is induced: Castration is castration.

Several Tremin Trust women describe their castration experiences in the following anecdotes. The first woman underwent hysterectomy and oophorectomy related to fibroids, which were causing severe bleeding problems. She was also diagnosed with ovarian cysts. She describes the sudden onset of symptoms, as well as concerns she has about hormone use.

I have been going through a surgical menopause since last August. My uterus and ovaries were removed because I was having severe bleeding problems caused by fibroids and cysts on the ovaries and tubes. I am 47, and did not have any menopausal symptoms before surgery. My body was not ready for this. The most annoying symptom has been some very profuse night sweating. I went to my internist for a hypertension problem, and he told me to keep [my blood pressure] down myself, and was cautious about Premarin. I told him I was taking garlic, which will lower blood pressure and reduce hot flashes. He thought that was a good idea, as garlic is also protection for the heart. He wouldn't prescribe anything, although a very small dosage of Premarin is relatively harmless. My concern with temporary use of estrogens such as Premarin is that it should not be taken for more than a year, and after that time, I still may not be at a normal menopausal age, and the symptoms may return.

The woman obviously is being cared for by a very conservative physician. Most internists are more hesitant than gynecologists about estrogen prescription. The reason may be that internists and other nongynecological specialists are less familiar with the hormone literature, or they are more conservative in general, preferring diet and exercise prior to any therapeutic drug prescription. This woman's problem is really a catch-22. She is experiencing hot flashes and wants relief. However, her blood pressure is elevated; thus, estrogen may be risky for her as it can further raise her blood pressure. And, she thinks that a very small dosage of "Premarin is relatively harmless." Her concern also is that hormone use should be temporary, and that she may still have symptoms, since she will still not be at a normal menopausal age.

The response to the menopausal age question, and the fact that she may still have symptoms, is "Yes, that is true." Age of menopause is about 51 years, and research has shown that when hormones are discontinued, whether over the short or long term, symptoms do return. Taking hormones over the short term is not without risk. Still unknown is the risk associated with breast cancer in hormone users, and for this woman in particular, the risk of increasing her blood pressure. Perhaps the greatest risk faced by this woman, and all women over the short term, is the risk of increasing or exacerbating osteoporosis. Research documents that upon withdrawal of estrogen, bone mineral concentrations decrease at a rapid rate.

The following anecdote was written by a woman who experienced a chemical castration due to anticancer drugs.

A year ago I had radical mastectomy. I underwent chemotherapy for one year. Approximately one month after I started my therapy, I started my menopause. I have had hot and cold flashes ever since. They come about every hour during the day, and about three or four times during the night. Do you have any information that will help me?

There is not much information that will help this woman. She is unable to take estrogen, probably (but I am not sure) because her breast cancer was diagnosed as estrogen-receptor-positive. What this means is that the tumor was found to be estrogen-dependent; that is, it would grow in the presence of estrogen. The onset of hot and cold flashes for this woman was almost inevitable. The information I shared with her was on vitamin E intake, which suggested that women who could not take estrogen start with 400 International Units (IUs) of vitamin E daily, and increase the dose in consultation with a care provider. She also needs to keep a detailed hot flash diary in order to determine which events are triggering her hot flash, such as caffeine intake, a hot environment, etc., and then use this information to control some of the aspects of her life that may be controllable.

The next woman describes her experience 18 years postsurgical castration.

I had my ovaries removed many years ago. I took Premarin for 18 years, and had been off that two years last fall with only mild symptoms of hot flashes. Last August it was discovered that I had endometrial cancer, and I had a hysterectomy. Since that surgery, I have had steaming hot flashes at least every hour, followed by chills. I have asked several doctors why I'm having these now. They are mystified. Do you have an explanation?

Yes, I do have an explanation. I will always remember hearing Don Gambrell state at a conference that he is always concerned about pre- or postmenopausal women who say they have no symptoms. The woman in the preceding ancedote had been off estrogen for two years, was asymptomatic, and then developed endometrial cancer. Unfortunately, I do not have the chart data on this woman, which would enable me to state with any certainty that she was either obese or overweight. If she were, that could be the answer as to why she developed endometrial cancer–she was making a lot of the weaker estrogen, estrone, in her fatty tissues. However, that does not matter; if a woman makes enough estrone, she will be asymptomatic, but she is also at risk of endometrial cancer, since estrone can stimulate uterine cells to increase in number. As long as estrone is being made, the uterine endometrium will be stimulated. Also this woman might not have had both ovaries removed many years ago. She could have been making enough estrogen from one ovary, or a part of any ovary that was retained, which would minimize symptoms. All of this is speculative, however.

For whatever reason, this woman had some uterine cells that were predisposed to transform into cancer cells. When her uterus was removed, as Hufnagel with Golant (1988) and Coffey (1993) suggest, the blood supply to the ovary may have been affected. The result was hot flashes. Many women, when asked whether their ovaries were retained following hysterectomy, do not know. A pretty good clue as to whether or not they did have their ovaries removed is a prescription for estrogen replacement immediately following surgery. The following anecdote by a 42-year-old woman is living testimonial to this. She denies that her femininity will be compromised in any way because her uterus was removed. And she voices what many women say following hysterectomy: They are glad it is over–no more bleeding and pain–and they feel great.

> *I returned home from the hospital yesterday after a complete hysterectomy. I have no emotional hang-ups about being less of a woman. I know many women who have had the procedure, and they say they feel 100 percent better. I am 42 years old, and my doctor has immediately put me on estrogens; he says it does not cause cancer but can accelerate it if it*

is there. Would it be better not to take it at all, and to get menopause over all at once?

Yes, estrogen can stimulate a cancer if there are precancerous cells in the uterus. For this woman, at age 42, whether or not to take estrogen is a dilemma. As mentioned, the risk of initiating breast cancer is a possibility with estrogen use. Also, because of her age, 42, this woman is at risk of developing osteoporosis, or at least enhancing the demineralization process at an earlier age than would occur in a woman who did not have surgery. So, she must make a decision: If she takes estrogen to prevent osteoporosis, she will protect her bones but she may increase her risk of developing breast cancer. Truly a catch-22!

Chapter 14

Steroid Hormones and Cell Regulation

In the menstrual cycle chapters, I explained how the key menstrual cycle hormones were regulated; how the gonadotrophins, FSH and LH, are synthesized in the pituitary gland; and how these hormones function to regulate the production of estrogen and progesterone in the ovary. I emphasized how carefully regulated and controlled the process was. As one cycle ends, another has already begun. When estrogen hormone is increased to a certain level, FSH is suppressed, LH increases, and ovulation occurs. After ovulation, estrogen and progesterone synthesis increases. If a pregnancy does not result, progesterone and estrogen concentrations fall, FSH rises, and the process starts all over again. What is important to understand is that the hormones circulate and fluctuate to regulate each other and the menstrual cycle, rising and falling at fairly precise intervals. The menstrual cycle, as a life within a life, is a "system" under a great deal of control. This kind of regulation is absent when women take hormones or hormone-like drugs in pill, patch, or implant form, since these agents are not under any endogenous regulatory control.

In order for a woman to make an informed decision about whether or not to be a hormone user, she must first understand, at least at a conceptual level, the regulatory mechanisms that are operational during the menstrual cycle, and how the sex steroids, estrogen and progesterone, do what they do in the cells of the target tissues and other tissues and organs in the female body. To fully understand what hormones do, and how they do it, requires taking a journey into the center of the cell.

The following material is summarized from articles published in *The Menstrual Cycle, Volume 2* and *Menopause: A Midlife Passage.*

In general, hormones are part of the body's regulatory system, the wireless counterpart of the nervous system. Hormones function according to a basic physiological law of supply and demand. Very simply, when the stimulus to conserve, pump, or utilize water, sodium, calcium, phosphorous, or glucose is received, the demand is met partially by feedback relationships between these substances with the gland that secretes a specific regulatory hormone. In other situations, such as thyroid or cortisol secretion, or in the regulation of reproductive physiology, there is a dynamic state of hormone balance based on the principle of negative feedback.

The following concepts are important in understanding how hormones work in the body, and how they regulate metabolism. First, hormones are metabolic regulators. They do not initiate any action; rather, they increase, decrease, or inhibit basal metabolic processes. The ability to just maintain, or more specifically, to function at a basal level, is present in all cells. When a demand is placed upon an individual and there is a need to increase metabolism (for example, during the luteal phase of the menstrual cycle, there is a need to make receptors for progesterone), the hormones are made and secreted—some directly into the circulation—and eventually they bind with receptors on cell membranes or inside of the cell.

Second, the concentration of free hormone in the blood is very low. In the case of the sex hormones, estrogen and progesterone, circulating blood concentrations are extremely low; for example, in picogram (10^{-12} gram) amounts for estrogen, and nanogram (10^{-9} gram) concentrations for progesterone hormone. Hormones are degraded continuously; synthesis is a complex relationship of free hormone, degradative capacity, and feedback demand for its regulatory function.

Third, hormones are classified mainly as peptides, proteins, amines, prostaglandins, or steroids. At the cellular level they differ in mechanism of action, depending upon their classification and chemical makeup.

Fourth, hormones regulate metabolism indirectly via a process called *receptor-mediated signal transduction*. Now that is a mouthful! What it means is that all hormones regulate cell metabolism by binding with receptors. Protein, peptide, and amine hormones regulate cell metabolism by interacting with receptors on cell membranes. The cell membrane is a bilayer of lipid which contains a variety of proteins. It is the proteins in the bilayer that function as the receptors. Once the hormone binds with a receptor, a signal to initiate intracellular events is transmitted into the inside of the cell. Steroid hormones function by a different model. Because they are lipids, they are able to diffuse freely through the cell membrane lipid bilayer. Once inside a cell, particularly a target cell such as breast, uterus, or ovary, the hormones (for example, estrogen and progesterone) bind with a receptor. This binding functions mainly as a method of transportation for the final destination of all steroid hormones, which is within the nucleus. By a process referred to as *translocation*, the steroid hormone, still attached to its receptor, moves through the nuclear membrane to bind with a receptor on the DNA. Let's explore steroid hormones more closely.

STEROID HORMONES

The most important steroid hormones are the sex steroids, progesterone and estrogen (estradiol during menstruating years); the adrenal steroids, cortisol and aldosterone; the androgenic hormone testosterone; and vitamin D. All steroids perform different functions in the body. To understand the many side effects associated with taking steroids, a few additional concepts specific to these hormones need to be understood.

First, all steroids are structurally similar. All have the basic 4-ring structure of cholesterol as common building material. The different functions of steroids are attributable to the way in which side groups are attached to the 4-ring molecule.

Second, steroids bind first with intracellular (referred to as *cytosolic*) receptors. In uterine and breast cells, the process of binding creates a new compound, a hormone-receptor complex. This complex then translocates into the nucleus, where it binds to certain proteins on DNA, namely, the chromatin material, or the genome. In fact, in recent scientific publications, the mechanism of action for the most part is now referred to as the *genomic* action of steroids. In plain words, the final mechanism of action, the site of binding to initiate action, is the genetic material of target cells.

Third, after binding with DNA, steroids stimulate the synthesis of proteins that increase or decrease metabolism, enzyme synthesis, synthesis of receptors for hormones, growth factors, and so on. As an example, during the follicular phase of the menstrual cycle, the genetic message transcribed via estrogen hormone binding onto uterine cell DNA is to promote growth of the uterine lining, also referred to as *cell proliferation.* Following ovulation, during the luteal phase of the cycle, progesterone binding with DNA initiates synthesis of a protein, an enzyme that stops cell division and changes the structure and function of the uterine cells.

Fourth, the sex steroids are present in the blood in very, very low concentrations. The unbound, or free, concentration of estrogen is in picogram amounts (one-trillionth of a gram), whereas progesterone circulates in nanogram concentrations, which is one-billionth of a gram. In contrast, the concentration of artificial hormones found in oral contraceptives is in microgram quantities, which is one-millionth of a gram, concentrations greater than the amount of progesterone or estrogen that normally circulates in the blood during menstrual years. Thirty-five micrograms of ethinyl estradiol, an artificial estrogen found in some birth control pills, is a much larger concentration of estrogen than the naturally synthesized concentration of estradiol found in the blood. The daily dose of the most commonly prescribed estrogen for menopausal women, Premarin, is prescribed in milligram quantities, which, theoretically, is considerably greater than the concentration of natural estrogens. However, estrone is weaker than estradiol regarding binding with the cell receptor, so the increase in concentration is a moot point. What matters is how much hormone is available to the cells, and for how long, after the pill has been swallowed and passes through the liver, which is the first place metabolism occurs. The most common form of progesterone replacement in menopausal women is medroxyprogesterone acetate (MPA), or Depo Provera. This hormone is prescribed in 10 milligram doses, which is also greater than the concentration of progesterone normally measured in the blood. Less is known about progesterone's metabolism and side effects than estrogen.

In Table 14.1, information is provided on metric weights, ranging from one gram to picograms quantities.

TABLE 14.1. Metric Weights

WEIGHT
1 gram = 1/30th of an ounce
1 milligram = 1/1000 gram
1 microgram = 1 millionth of a gram
1 nanogram = 1 billionth of a gram
1 picogram = 1 trillionth of a gram

SIDE EFFECTS OF STEROIDS

The side effects associated with sex steroid use, whether for contraception or treatment at menopause, are a result of three factors: (1) the dosages of hormones prescribed, (2) the affinity these hormones have for binding with steroid receptors, and (3) the rate of metabolism. Regarding dosage, the dose of hormones prescribed for women is greater than those measured in the blood. As such, the dose is said to be *pharmacological* rather than physiological. With respect to receptor binding, even though the affinity for estrogen to bind with its receptor is very high, it can also bind with receptors for other steroids, such as receptors for cortisol, the anti-inflammatory and/or stress hormone, or aldosterone, the salt-retaining hormone in the body. Concerning the rate of metabolism, if artificial estrogens and progestogens are taken orally, they must make an obligatory first pass through the liver, the most metabolically active organ in the body. In the liver, some hormones are metabolized. Here, they can also bind with receptors for other steroids, albeit in a weaker way than would occur if the hormone was specific for a particular receptor in breast or uterine tissue. In other words, the sex hormones are able to bind with the DNA in certain liver cells. This binding can initiate certain metabolic processes (for example, changes in fat and lipid metabolism), and in some instances, alterations in the blood-clotting mechanism. Side effects occur because the hormone can "turn on" cells other than reproductive target tissue cells. They are able to do this because they are present in the body in pharmacological concentrations.

The steroids found in oral contraceptives provide an example of the binding capability.

The most common estrogen-like steroids used in the birth control pill are either ethinyl, estradiol, or mestranol. Unlike the natural hormone estradiol, these two substances, while resembling estrogen, are not the same substances synthesized in the body. They are, by definition, drugs. Both compounds have a chemical group (ethinyl) attached to the carbon-17 position of the four-membered cholesterol skeleton. In addition to the ethinyl group, mestranol has a methyl ether attached to the third carbon position. These modifications of the natural hormone are necessary in order to prevent metabolic inactivation of natural steroids in the liver. Examples of the natural and artificial hormones are shown in Figures 14.1 and 14.2.

FIGURE 14.1. Structure of 17 Beta-Estradiol (Endogenously Synthesized Hormone) Compared with Two Estrogen-Like Drugs, Ethinyl Estradiol and Mestranol

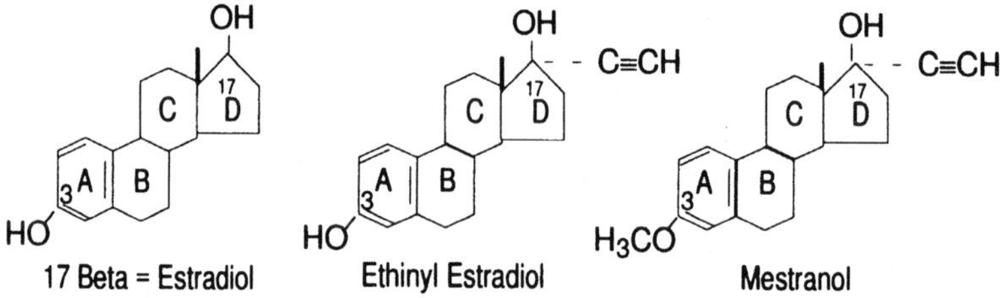

FIGURE 14.2. Structure of Progesterone (Endogenously Synthesized Hormone) Compared with Two Progesterone-Like Drugs, Norethindrone and Testosterone

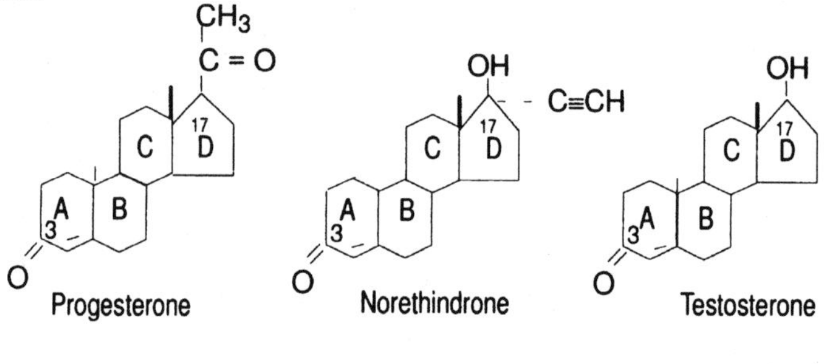

When these drugs are absorbed into the gastrointestinal tract, the liver, as mentioned, is the first organ that is affected. In technical terms, clinicians and researchers refer to pill ingestion and absorption as presenting the liver with a *bolus* of artificial steroid. By definition, a bolus means a large concentration of the steroid-like drug. In the liver, the bolus of drug increases the probability that binding with other steroid receptors, such as cortisol receptors, will occur. In the scientific literature, this process is referred to as agonism, the ability to turn on the cell. When the steroid binds with a receptor that has a high affinity for cortisol, it may initiate the synthesis of proteins that promote a process called *gluconeogenesis* (which means to make glucose from protein). If a lot of this kind of synthesis occurs via the agonistic action of estrogens or progestogens in HRT, a woman may develop what is called a prediabetic condition, which is an increase in blood sugar above normal levels. In women who have a history of clotting disorders, binding with other steroid receptors in the liver may result in an increase in the synthesis of certain liver enzymes that promote blood coagulation. These women could increase their risk of having a stroke or heart attack.

The side effects associated with steroid use are found in patient package inserts that accompany steroid prescriptions. All of these side effects are related to the ability of sex steroids or steroid-like drugs to bind with any steroid receptor, thus mimicking the action of other steroids and tricking the receptor. Sometimes, however, as in the case of aldosterone (the salt-retaining hormone that I studied related to premenstrual tension) binding produces an antagonistic effect that blocks a hormone's action. In Chapter 1, I discussed the concept of antagonism in relation to my study on premenstrual tension. I postulated that it was progesterone's antagonistic effect on the aldosterone receptor that resulted in initiating the events promoting premenstrual water retention.

Another example of antagonism is found in the use of the drug Tamoxifen, an antiestrogen, used to treat women who have breast cancer. In women who have had estrogen receptors detected in breast tumor tissue, Tamoxifen blocks the effect of estrogen at the receptor. By doing this, it is thought to block estrogen-induced production of tumor-promoting growth factors. Tamoxifen is a rather unusual drug. It is by definition a dual agonist/antagonist. By this is meant that it *blocks* the action of estrogen in some tissues (the breast and ovary), but *acts like* an estrogen in other tissue; for example, in bone it acts like estrogen to prevent the bone loss that occurs at menopause.

HORMONES MOST FREQUENTLY PRESCRIBED AT MENOPAUSE

Estrogens

Oral Conjugated Estrogens

Premarin. The most common form of estrogen used is in tablet form. The most frequently prescribed estrogen is Premarin, which is a registered trademark of Wyeth-Ayerst Laboratories, Inc. According to Wyeth-Ayerst ads, "Premarin . . . contains a mixture of estrogens obtained exclusively from natural sources, occurring as the sodium salts of water-soluble estrogen sulfates blended to represent the average composition of material derived from pregnant mares' urine. It contains estrone, equilin, and 17 alpha dihydroequilenin as salts of their sulfate esters." Recall that during reproductive years, women have three estrogens circulating naturally in their bodies. Estradiol is the major estrogen. It is the sex steroid that binds with the most affinity with the estrogen receptor. Estradiol is metabolically converted to estrone, which, by definition, is a weaker estrogen. However, estrone does bind with the estrogen receptor, albeit with a lesser affinity. It is the ability to bind with the receptor and to initiate estrogen-mediated metabolic events that results in relief of symptoms, as well as affording protection against osteoporosis.

Tablets are available in 0.3, 0.625, 0.9, 1.25, and 2.5 milligram strengths of conjugated estrogens. These dosages are color-coded for easy recognition: 0.3 is green, 0.625 is maroon, 0.9 is white, 1.25 is yellow, and 2.5 is purple. The usual dose for treating and/or preventing osteoporosis is 0.625 milligrams daily for 25 days.

For symptom relief, the dosage varies depending on the symptom being treated. For example, for hot flash relief, a care provider may prescribe 1.25 milligrams daily, while for atrophic vaginitis, the dose may range from 0.3 to 1.25 milligrams daily. Generally, however, the lowest dose that will control symptoms should be chosen. Of course, for a woman who has a uterus, any estrogen must be administered cyclically and with a progestogen, which also is taken for 25 days. On day 12 or 13 (a putative midcycle) it is combined with a progestogen until the twenty-fifth day. Then, both hormones are withdrawn for five days. For a woman who does not have a uterus, the estrogen is prescribed without a progestogen.

Estrace. Estrace is the registered trademark of Mead Johnson Laboratories, a Bristol-Myers Company. Estrace oral tablets contain 1 or 2 milligrams of micronized estradiol. Micronized, by definition, means pulverized into particles only a small micra in size (micra is the plural of micro). These tablets are also color-coded: the 1 milligram tablets are lavender and scored (can be easily broken in two), the 2 milligram tablets are turquoise blue-green. Similar to Premarin administration, Estrace dosages are administered cyclically, and the lowest dose that will control symptoms should be chosen.

Patches

Estraderm. Estraderm is the registered trademark of the CIBA Pharmaceutical Company, a division of CIBA-GEIGY Pharmaceutical Company. The Estraderm system releases small amounts of estradiol through the skin in a continuous way. The estradiol in Estraderm is contained in a patch that is applied to the skin. When on the skin, the Estraderm system releases estradiol, which flows from the patch through the skin and into the blood. Each Estraderm system is individually sealed in a protective pouch. Two systems are available to provide transdermal (through the skin) delivery of estradiol: a 0.05 milligram or a 0.1 milligram patch. Treatment of menopausal symptoms is usually initiated with the 0.05 milligram patch, and as in the case of Premarin and Estrace, the dosage should be adjusted in order to control the symptoms. It is recommended that the Estraderm patch be changed twice weekly. As with the other estrogen treatments, for a woman who has an intact uterus, the CIBA ad indicates that Estraderm may be given cyclically. Currently, there is controversy surrounding the use of the patch, and whether or not a progestogen should also be combined with this method of hormone replacement.

Estrogen and Androgen

Estratest. Estratest is the registered trademark of Solvay Pharmaceuticals. Each dark green capsule-shaped, sugar-coated tablet contains 1.25 milligrams of esterified estrogens and 2.5 milligrams of methyltestosterone. According to information in the 1991 Solvay ads, the esterified estrogen is a mixture of the sodium salts of the sulfate esters of the estrogenic substances, principally estrone, that are of the type excreted by pregnant mares. Esterified Estrogens contain not less than 75 percent and not more than 85 percent of sodium estrone sulfate, and not less than 6 percent nor more than 15 percent of sodium equilin sulfate. Methyltestosterone is an androgen, a synthetic derivative of testosterone. Estratest is recommended for use in women who have severe vasomotor symptoms (hot flash) not relieved by estrogen alone. Estratest is administered cyclically for short-term use only. The lowest dose that controls symptoms should be chosen, and it is recommended that the medication be discontinued as soon as possible.

Progestogens

Depo Provera

The most commonly prescribed progestogen is medroxyprogesterone acetate (MPA), better know as Depo Provera, a synthetic progestin. MPA is manufactured by the Upjohn Company, under the registered trademark Provera. Provera tablets are available in 2.5 milligram, scored, orange tablets; 5 milligram, hexagonal,white tablets; and 10 milligram, round, white, scored tablets. The chemical structure of MPA closely resembles the chemical structure of natural progesterone, but it is not progesterone; it is a progestin. Progestins, by definition, are a large group of synthetic drugs that have a progesterone-like effect on the uterus, breast, and other body tissues. Provera is administered to menopausal women to transform the uterine endometrium (from one that has been proliferating) into a secretory organ. A 10 milligram dose is recommended for transforming an endometrium that has been primed with either endogenous or exogenous sources of estrogens. Provera is administered for a 10-day period, commencing on the sixteenth day of cyclic therapy, to ensure that cellular proliferation has been stopped.

In 1978, Depo Provera was approved for use in 89 countries, but not in the United States, as an injectable, long-term contraceptive. The reason given for disapproval as a contraceptive in the United States was based in part on research that indicated that it caused benign as well as malignant mammary tumors in dogs. Since then, long-term controlled clinical studies in other countries have shown a risk of breast cancer comparable to oral contraceptives and no increased risk for ovarian, liver, or cervical cancer. Based on these data, on December 10, 1990, the Food and Drug Administration approved an implantable contraceptive for marketing in the United States. The approval was for the Norplant System, which consists of six flexible, closed, tubular capsules, each containing the progestin levonorgestrel (FDA Medical Bulletin 1991). On October 29, 1992, the FDA approved medroxyprogesterone acetate as Depo Provera Contraceptive Injection. The dose recommended by the FDA is 150 mg administered every three months by deep, intramuscular injection in the gluteal or deltoid muscle (FDA Medical Bulletin, 1993).

Chapter 15

Estrogen and Hormone Treatment: Benefits

INTRODUCTION

Clearly, it is during perimenopause when hormone treatment is most sought after by women and recommended and prescribed to treat changes, sometimes referred to as symptoms. Hormones are also recommended to prevent osteoporosis and heart disease. The effects that hormones have on preventing heart disease and osteoporosis and increasing breast cancer risk are presently being studied via national studies, described later in this chapter. Unfortunately, the results of these studies will not benefit women of the baby boomer generation who are just now entering perimenopause, and questioning whether or not to be hormone users. The best-documented benefit to date from taking hormones is osteoporosis prevention, or stopping the progression of the disease once it is detected. This disease, typically called the "bone robber disease," affects both women and men. However, two factors combine to make osteoporosis more a women's disease. First, women live longer than men; so even though both are at risk of developing the disease, it is more prevalent in women simply because they live longer. Second, women generally have a smaller bone structure than men. Therefore, they have less bone to lose, and will feel the effects of bone loss sooner than men. For women then, both gender and age interact to increase the risk of developing this disease earlier than men. Gender and age also interact to increase the risk of developing heart disease in women, albeit at a later age than for men. I have devoted Chapter 18 to osteoporosis. Hormones and heart disease are discussed in this chapter.

SYMPTOM RELIEF

There is no doubt that hormone treatment, primarily with estrogen, benefits women in the form of symptom relief from hot flashes and atrophic vaginitis in particular. The dose of estrogen that is usually prescribed for women is that equivalent to the most widely-prescribed estrogen, estrone, in the form of Premarin. The dose of 0.625 milligrams once a day seems to be sufficient to reduce or eliminate symptoms. Even though there are documented risks to health from taking hormones, there is no doubt from the perspective of women that taking estrogen hormone spells *relief* of hot flash, vaginitis, and even some urinary problems. The words of The Tremin Trust women say it all. For example, a 49-year-old perimenopausal participant wrote about the relief she obtained:

> *When menopausal symptoms first appeared in 1990, I could have filled this page. Now that I've started estrogen, I feel 100 percent better and it's hard to remember how miserable I was. I also started menopause earlier than my peers—they're now catching up, and it's nice to be able to share the misery.*

A postmenopausal woman, age 54, writes about hot flashes and dry skin relief:

> *My hormonal therapy started in June 1990. I had hot flashes, wakefulness at night, dry skin. The initial two months on hormone therapy experience was prolonged bleeding, clotting. My doctor advised a gynecology follow-up and stopped the hormones. A GYN exam with Pap smear and biopsy in January of 1991 were all negative for pathology. So my gynecologist resumed therapy with estrogen and progesterone, and I have had no further problems.*

Regarding symptom relief, a 50-year-old perimenopausal woman said the following:

> *The hormones really helped my hot flashes—made me more confident and comfortable in public in the daytime and meant virtually uninterrupted sleep at night so I didn't always wake in the morning tired.*

A postmenopausal woman on hormone replacement therapy described the symptoms and misery she experienced, and the ambivalence she felt about the risk of breast cancer. In the final analysis, she decided that the relief she obtained with hormones is worth it:

> *Frankly, I had been looking forward to menopause for years. My periods had always been heavy with many cramps. Also, I sometimes had an "unreal" feeling a day or two before my period started—also severe migraine-type headaches that sometimes kept me home and in bed for a half to one-and-a-half days each period. Imagine my surprise as I moved into menopause to have such difficulties in something I was expecting to rather enjoy. Symptoms that started gradually at about age 45 were: heavy bleeding with clots large enough for me to feel them moving down, inability to stay asleep at night, heavy night sweats (although almost no daytime hot flashes), mood swings, usually extreme sadness that lasted from only ten minutes to several hours, and a general feeling of light-headedness and faintness that sometimes made me hesitant to leave the house or drive a car. For several years I was on an estrogen/progesterone schedule that gave me regular periods at about 29-day intervals. Then, last fall, some of the symptoms began returning, although not in a severe way. These symptoms were mood swings, night sweats and "unreal" feelings. My current* continuous *hormone schedule has eliminated all these symptoms except the occasional headache, and even these headaches are usually manageable. I am concerned about the long-range effects of estrogen and breast cancer, but my daily life on hormone therapy has so improved, I feel that at this time I have no choice but to continue it.*

Here is another woman's experience:

> *Have been on ERT for 14 months. Am quite irregular with my periods, generally they are 4-5 days—#2 light—but they never were very heavy. I skipped one month altogether. My hot flashes, night sweats, and sleeping have all improved. Though married, [I have] no intercourse; husband has diabetes and a heart condition, [thus] little interest. Went on estrogen after*

*discussing it with my doctor, and am not sure I will continue.
Will discuss it with my doctor next winter; perhaps things will
have stabilized by then.*

HEART DISEASE

Not since the 1960s, when healthy women were advised to take
hormones to protect against pregnancy, and Wilson's "estrogen
forever, feminine forever" philosophy for menopausal women,
have we seen such a push for women to take hormones to prevent
disease. Heart disease in older women has been proclaimed an
epidemic in the United States. Estrogen treatment of women at high
risk for developing the disease is recommended.

It is important to set the record straight at the outset regarding
women and heart disease. Yes, heart disease is an equal opportunity
disease–like osteoporosis, both men and women may develop
it–but women are more apt to develop it 10 to 15 years later than
men. Yes, women appear to be protected from heart disease during
menstrual/reproductive years, whereas men are at risk during this
same age range. The reason given that menstruating women are
protected is that they have estrogen hormone. The same estrogen
that protects women, however, was shown to worsen heart disease
in men. Years ago, when men were given estrogens to treat prostate
and breast cancer, they had heart attacks. Some died.

Estrogen treatment to prevent heart disease supports the menopause-as-disease ideology discussed in Chapter 6. How estrogen
functions to protect women is unknown. Schaefer and Levy (1985)
hypothesize that it increases the production of high-density lipoprotein (HDL) and an associated apolipoprotein, A-I, which is a major
protein associated with HDL, the so-called "good" cholesterol.
LaRosa (1992) thinks estrogen may act by enhancing the activity of
the low-density lipoprotein receptor. At menopause, then, the relative protection against heart disease present during menstrual years
declines. The decline is based upon changes in the lipid profile that
were identified as risk factors, based on research done on men. Yes,
it is a fact that at menopause a woman's lipid profile changes.
Again, however, rather than conceptualizing the changes as normal
metabolic events, they have been diagnosed as *hyperlipidemia*, a

documented risk factor for heart disease in men. Hyperlipidemia means that cholesterol levels, specifically total blood cholesterol and low-density lipoprotein-cholesterol, are high, requiring some form of intervention. The criteria used to identify those at risk were derived from research done on *men* who developed heart disease. Men whose total blood cholesterol approximated or exceeded 240 mg/dl (milligrams per deciliter) or higher, and whose LDL-C (low density lipoprotein-cholesterol) exceeded 160 mg/dl, were designated as high risk for heart attack. Hyperlipidemia leads to atherosclerosis, which is an accumulation of lipids in the coronary arteries. Fuster and colleagues (1992) note that high concentrations of blood lipids can themselves be injurious agents, or contribute to plaque formation following a vascular injury.

THE CHOLESTEROL STORY

I am grateful to Thomas J. Moore, who in 1989 wrote "The Cholesterol Myth," an article published in *The Atlantic Monthly*, and the book *Heart Failure*. In these publications, Moore argued against the evidence that lowering cholesterol levels lengthens life. Nonetheless, much research has gone forward based on the assumption that heart disease can be prevented if atherosclerotic (lipid-laden) plaques do not form in the coronary arteries. Not being able to examine coronary arteries directly to evaluate whether plaques are forming required having a valid metabolic indicator to diagnose hyperlipidemia. Enter cholesterol!

The Framingham, Massachusetts study, begun in 1948, is the most frequently cited research to demonstrate that high blood cholesterol levels are linked with heart disease in men. These results, reported in the 1960s, also documented that extensive heart disease existed among individuals with low or average cholesterol levels, but these results were less publicized. In the individuals studied, the researchers reported a considerable range of serum cholesterol levels, as well as inability to manipulate cholesterol levels through diet. The significance of the Framingham study findings for U.S. citizens (the study is ongoing today) was that it launched a national attack on heart disease. And, since it was 40- and 50-year-old men who were dying of heart attacks, U.S. dollars to fund this national attack went to study heart disease in men.

Two large-scale studies were carried out over a period of more than ten years. The first was the Multiple Risk Factor Intervention Trial (MR. FIT), which cost $115 million. The overall objective of the MR. FIT study was to evaluate the effect of a behavior modification program (diet, exercise, smoking) on a group of unfit men. It involved 28 medical centers across the nation (I can still remember the signs identifying the laboratory at the University of Minnesota), and employed more than 250 researchers. It took the MR. FIT researchers almost four years to find, screen, and recruit the experimental sample of men who were diagnosed at very high risk for heart attack. As Moore observed, these men were not exactly ready to run the Boston Marathon–they smoked, ate a high-fat diet, had high blood pressure, most were obese, etc. In other words, there was plenty of risk to modify.

The men were randomly divided into two groups, an experimental intervention group, and a control group who would receive "usual care" from their own physicians. It was hypothesized that men in the intervention group (who received the behavior modification) would make substantial changes in their lives, and as a result, would experience fewer deaths from heart attacks than men in the control group. The results of the study were terribly disappointing. No significant difference between the two groups in the overall number of deaths was found.

A second study, the Coronary Primary Prevention Trial, began about the same time as MR. FIT, and focused on lowering cholesterol through drug intervention. The study hypothesis was that lowering the blood level of low-density-lipoprotein-cholesterol ("bad" cholesterol) using the drug cholestryamine, over the long term, would decrease the incidence of heart disease. This study cost $142 million; it took three years to locate 3,810 men for the trial, which required examining and screening 480,000 middle-aged men, whose cholesterol levels averaged 290mg/dl. When data were examined in year seven, researchers found that cholesterol levels in the treatment group were only 6.7 percent lower than those measured in the placebo (control) group. At the end of the study those receiving the drug showed an average decrease of 13.4 percent and they had fewer heart attacks. Dr. Robert

Levy called it a milestone study. Nonetheless, Moore (1989) disagreed. He argued that both of these studies failed, citing as the reason that high cholesterol levels are a condition frequently *associated* with heart disease, but not the *cause* of it.

Nonetheless, efforts to identify and treat people with high cholesterol levels, including both adults and children, gained momentum. In 1991, the *Report of the Expert Panel on Blood Cholesterol Levels in Children and Adolescents* was published by the U.S. Department of Health and Human Services. The report, endorsed by more than 40 organizations, recommended screening children and adolescents for high cholesterol, and to begin treatment if the LDL-C was over 130 mg/dl (U.S. Department of Health and Human Services, 1991).

A 1992 editorial in *Circulation*, written by Hulley, Walsh, and Newman, challenged the national policy of widespread cholesterol education and treatment, recommending a change. Based upon analyses of cohort and clinical trials, the authors reached three conclusions. First, an association between *low* cholesterol and non-cardiovascular deaths in *men* and *women* was found. In other words, individuals who had total cholesterol levels less than 160 mg/dl were found to be more at risk of dying of other diseases, not heart disease. Second, no association was found between *high* levels of blood LDL-C and cardiovascular deaths in *women*. Low levels of high-density lipoprotein-cholesterol (HDL-C) were identified as a stronger risk factor for women than high levels of LDL-C (which has been identified as a definite risk factor for men). High LDL-C levels appeared to increase risk for recurrence of coronary heart disease in women who already had the disease. The third point made by the authors was that interventions utilized in primary prevention trials were ineffective, i.e., the death rates of participants in these studies from noncoronary heart disease increased rather than decreased. Only secondary prevention trials, that is, intervention research on individuals who were at high risk because they already had heart disease, were found to have a beneficial effect on death rates. Based on these findings, the authors requested clinicians to "pull back" on aggressive treatment of high cholesterol in primary prevention settings. They recommended treatment only when convincing evidence was present that the effects of a particular treatment were beneficial in reducing high blood cholesterol. They concluded that aggressive treatment to reduce cholesterol levels in healthy individuals should be reevaluated.

Has this advice been taken seriously?

Since the 1980s, increasing numbers of healthy menopausal women have been encouraged to take prescription estrogens to prevent heart disease. The change in a woman's lipid profile at menopause, declared as unfavorable by many, was said to increase the risk of developing heart disease. The era of treatment with estrogen hormone began, based on observations that women estrogen users had lower LDL-C levels and higher HDL-C levels than nonestrogen users. A sample of some study findings follows.

ESTROGEN AND HEART DISEASE

In the absence of basic research to indicate the exact mechanism by which estrogen transforms the lipid profile from unfavorable to favorable, there are several points to keep in mind. First, the issue of whether estrogen could prevent heart attacks, according to Barrett-Connor (1987), in either pre- or postmenopausal women was not even a topic for medical debate until the 1980s. Research on use of oral contraceptives (OCs) suggested that the most serious risks to women were those related to the cardiovascular system. Heart attacks and strokes were known to occur more often in women who used OCs than in women who did not. A study on men documented high levels of estrogen (estradiol) in heart attack victims. In the 1970s, two studies by Jick and co-workers (1978a,b) reported an increased risk of heart disease in menopausal women estrogen users. Then, in the 1980s two studies, one by Ross and co-workers (1981), the other by Bush and co-workers (1983), reported a decreased risk of developing heart disease in women estrogen users. Research on estrogens and heart disease in women proliferated.

The second point to keep in mind regarding hormone use and prevention of heart disease is that research on the topic is confusing and controversial, and most studies have been evaluated as being inherently flawed. For example, in 1985, Stampfer and co-workers reported data from the now highly-publicized Nurses' Health Study, that estrogen use reduced the risk of developing severe coronary disease. Another study, the same year, based on data from the Framingham Longitudinal Study, concluded that no cardiovascular benefit from estrogen use was found. In other words, mortality from all causes, including cardiovascular disease, did not differ between women who took estrogen and those who did not. One finding from this study, and one that is not generally cited, was the increase in vascular disease in estrogen users.

In 1987, another report based on the Nurses' Health Study, authored by Graham Colditz and colleagues, concluded that women who experienced menopause naturally and never used estrogen did not have an increased risk of developing heart disease when compared with premenopausal women. Women who were identified as being at risk were those who had both ovaries removed and had never taken estrogen.

Using changes in lipoprotein levels as an indirect indicator of risk for developing heart disease in estrogen users, in 1989 Matthews and colleagues reported an increase in LDL-C and a decrease in HDL-C in women who did not receive hormone treatment. The study participants were 69 naturally menopausal women (no period for 12 or more months), and 32 women who had stopped menstruating for about six months and who were on hormone replacement. Unfortunately, the differential effects of estrogen from estrogen and progesterone replacement (HRT) were not taken into account. The women on hormones were taking a variety of hormones, confounding analysis. The 69 naturally menopausal women were declared menopausal based on FSH levels of more than 30 international units (IUs) per liter. Yet, only 24 of the 32 women hormone users had FSH levels measured. Of the 24, only 19 were menopausal based on FSH data.

In 1991, another report from the Nurses' Health Study authored by Stampfer and co-workers concluded that nurses who were estrogen users had a 50 percent reduction in the incidence of coronary artery disease. When study data were reexamined, which meant including nurses who had been excluded from analysis because of cancer, preexisting heart disease, obesity, diabetes, etc., the risk reduction for total mortality (not just deaths from heart disease) was evaluated as insignificant. In other words, the study findings, rather than supporting that estrogen users have a lower incidence of heart disease, suggest instead that women who elect to take hormones are probably healthier than women who do not, and as such, would neither develop nor die of heart disease—with or without estrogen.

In 1991 Prior severely criticized the findings of the Nurses' Health Study. According to her, the study is biased in design and methodology. The study design was neither blinded nor randomized, and only risks for healthy women were reported. Wilson and co-workers (1985) criticized the report for not including data on women with preexisting diseases, and whether these women stopped taking estrogen because of migraines, swelling, or high blood pressure (which would indicate that blood vessels were being affected). Having this information could mean that estrogens in some women increased, rather than decreased, the risk for heart attack and/or other vascular problems.

The findings from a study of healthy postmenopausal women estrogen users by Walsh and co-workers in 1991 reported favorable alterations in low- and high-density lipoprotein cholesterol levels. This study also found that the blood levels of plasma triglycerides in women who took 0.625 mg and 1.25 mg of Premarin increased 24 percent and 38 percent, respectively. The researchers concluded that the increase in triglycerides did not induce clinical hypertriglyceridemia (which means high levels of blood fatty acids). The researchers advised women with preexisting hypertriglyceridemia to use estrogens with caution.

The validity of using changes in blood levels of lipoprotein-cholesterol levels to support the use of estrogen hormone treatment to prevent heart disease in healthy women is not supported by clinical trials. Evidence to date is either epidemiological or indirect. Related to the Nurses' Health Study, eliminating women who were smokers, obese, consumed more than 28 ml of alcohol per day, diabetic, hypertensive, had abnormal blood lipids, etc., limits the findings of this study. In the 1991 study by Walsh and colleagues, a progestin, medroxyprogesterone acetate (MPA), was given to women who used a weak estrogen, estrone, ten days after completion of the study to remove any hyperplastic endometrium (to ensure that the women menstruated). Study findings therefore are limited to the effects of estrone only given by mouth, to healthy women who had uteruses. In the long run, study findings are academic since healthy postmenopausal women who have not had a hysterectomy must take an estrogen with a progestin to prevent uterine cancer.

That menopausal changes in blood cholesterol levels are considered "unfavorable" is an assumption based upon research done on men. Barrett-Connor (1989) says the argument to support estrogen use is based on another assumption, that estrogen exerts a favorable effect on cholesterol metabolism. Proponents of estrogen therapy, for example LaRosa (1992), argue that the exclusion of women from most major studies on heart disease has led to the erroneous conclusion that cholesterol-altering therapy is either unnecessary or ineffective in women. Until data on women are available, proponents believe that the benefits of intervention (based on research done only in men) would occur in both sexes.

In summary, case control and cohort studies demonstrate a consistent bias in the selection of participants. A consensus of epidemiologic reports demonstrates that women who are given postmenopausal estrogen therapy reduce their risk of ischemic heart disease when compared with women who do not receive such therapy. However, epidemiologists are quick to agree that epidemiologic association does not establish cause and effect. Women who choose to take estrogens may have other characteristics that explain the lower risk of developing heart disease. The need for clinical trials was viewed as urgent. In a 1991 editorial in *The New England Journal of Medicine,* Goldman and Tostesen urged that a clinical trial of sufficient size be undertaken to document that the epidemiologic evidence of benefit of estrogen on heart disease is not just a function of bias or statistical legerdemain. They noted that the literature is replete with reports of randomized trials that failed to document benefits. In their opinion, there is no substitute for a randomized trial of estrogen replacement therapy. They advocated the use of control groups who would take placebos, even though there would be ethical contraindications and debate. The end points of interest they said would be those related to heart disease, osteoporosis, cancers of the breast and uterus, quality of life, and costs.

Somebody was listening here! Enter The Women's Health Initiative and the Heart and Estrogen Replacement Study.

The Women's Health Initiative (WHI)

The Women's Health Initiative, funded by the U.S. National Institutes of Health in 1992, will enroll between 55,000 and 60,000 women who will be randomly assigned to one of three treatment groups. The goal of the study is, for the most part, as outlined by Goldman and Tosteson (1991) is to evaluate through clinical trials the effects of fat, hormones, calcium, and vitamin D supplementation. The studies are designed to answer the following questions: What is the effect of a low-fat dietary pattern on the prevention of breast and colon cancer and coronary heart disease? What is the effect of hormonal replacement therapy on prevention of coronary heart disease, osteoporosis, and/or increased risk of breast cancer? What is the effect of calcium and vitamin D supplementation on prevention of osteoporosis and colon cancer? It will require about four years for protocol development and nine years of follow-up before these research questions can be answered. A total of 14 years and the investment of over 600 million dollars will be made. It is hoped by all that the outcome at the end of the 14 years will prove to have been a productive use of taxpayer money.

The Heart and Estrogen-Progestin Replacement Study (HERS)

The HERS began in 1993. It is a secondary prevention clinical trial, which means it is designed to evaluate whether women with documented heart disease who receive estrogen and a progestin combined will have fewer heart attacks than women not taking hormone treatment. The plan is to enroll 2,340 postmenopausal women with documented coronary heart disease who have not undergone hysterectomy.

When the WHI and HERS are completed, data will be available to support whether women who take estrogen can or cannot prevent heart disease and heart attack. The HERS is similar to the Coronary Prevention Trial conducted on men who had heart disease. The differences are gender and the drug—women and hormones versus men and cholestyramine.

While the results of these studies will provide much-needed information, there are also concerns, particularly in the WHI long-term hormone trial, wherein healthy women are recruited as experimental subjects. The research has barely started. Screening and recruitment of women has proved to be as onerous a task as it was for the MR. FIT and Coronary Prevention trials. And, nine years is a long time to be a participant in an intervention research protocol. Attrition over the long-term could affect study outcome, and risks to health are important factors to consider in any research. It is especially worrisome for the women who have been randomly assigned to the hormone treatment group, and do so knowing that they risk developing breast cancer.

The third point to keep in mind regarding estrogens and heart disease is that the mechanism of cholesterol uptake by liver cells and other cholesterol-utilizing cells was clearly delineated in the 1970s. Nowhere, and I repeat, *nowhere* in the basic research that was done, then or now, is there evidence in humans that estrogen directly facilitates cholesterol metabolism. From a cell-molecular perspective, the role estrogen plays in mediating lipid metabolism is still pretty hypothetical. In the WHI heart clinical trial, thousands of women will be placed on estrogen treatment to evaluate its effect on preventing heart disease. Heart disease is very complex; many factors can work independently or in combination with each other to change the lipid profile, some known (diabetes, obesity), some still unknown. These risk factors will not go away by taking an estrogen pill. In fact, some risks to health may increase, as observed in the cholesterol primary prevention trials and reported by Hulley, Walsh, and Newman in 1992. Schaefer and Levy (1985) suggest that estrogen use in women increases the production of HDL and apoprotein A-I in the liver and intestines. If this is so, this effect is probably indirect; that is, the effect is due to estrogen's ability to trick the receptor, and thus bind with a receptor that is not its primary target.

In addition to the clinical trials, studies are also needed at the cell level to verify how estrogen functions to alter lipid metabolism. If taking estrogen does increase the synthesis of HDL and apoprotein A-I in the liver, a favorable response, one wonders what other mechanisms are being initiated as well. Women with known preexisting metabolic diseases should not take hormone treatment. What about women who are healthy? Will taking estrogens over the long term alter gastrointestinal metabolism, increasing risk of developing a disease?

Postmenopausal Estrogen/Progesterone Intervention Trial

As discussed in Chapter 16, menopausal women with a uterus need to take a progestin with estrogen to protect against developing uterine cancer. At first, the hypothesized cardioprotective effect of estrogen was thought to be compromised in women who took an estrogen plus a progestin. There is some good news here. Data from the three-year Postmenopausal Estrogen Progesterone Intervention (PEPI) trial on 900 women found that estrogens, with or without a progestin, lowered the bad cholesterol, LDL-C, and did not lower (lower than base-line) HDL-C, the good cholesterol (see Newman and Sullivan, 1996). The bad news from this study is that women with a uterus need to take two hormones, estrogen and a progestin. One-third of the women in the PEPI study who were on estrogen alone developed precancerous uterine lesions. Much more data on the long-term effects of progestin use related to developing disease in other tissues and organs is needed. The results of the PEPI study add to the knowledge base on select physiological changes that occur with hormone treatment of healthy women. They do not, however, prove anything about heart disease and hormone use.

The silly news associated with those who argue on behalf of estrogen and its cardioprotective effect is that the benefit of *not* developing heart disease (this being said while the WHI studies are just beginning) is worth the risk of developing breast cancer. The data used to justify this statement are the often-quoted statistics regarding deaths from heart disease in women: 250,000 a year versus 41,000 a year for breast cancer. Women hear from care providers that the fear of getting cancer from estrogens is irrational. Breast cancers grow more slowly, can be detected and treated. Yes, I suppose this is so. But why should healthy women risk developing one disease to prevent another based on statistical probability? At the 1995 Annual Meeting of the North American Menopause Society, Isaac Schiff declared that woman and man do not live by statistics alone. It is a fact, he said, that the death rate from breast cancer is lower than it is for heart disease. Breast cancer, however, from the perspective of women, is a more feared and dreaded disease. Plotkin, a breast cancer specialist, knows that the treatments associated with the disease are not only disfiguring, but painful and agonizing, and for some women the word cancer is a death sentence (1996). No woman needs to hear from a health professional that her fears are irrational and unfounded regarding the fear of breast cancer. Even at the conclusion of the WHI, we may not know whether the risk of breast cancer increases with estrogen use; some breast cancers take 20 years to manifest (for example, the increased incidence in DES mothers as reported by Greenberg and colleagues in 1984).

HYPERLIPIDEMIA

Hyperlipidemia is high blood cholesterol. It is one cause of atherosclerosis, being a form of arteriosclerosis in which localized accumulations of lipid-containing material are found within or beneath the intimal surfaces of blood vessels. In coronary-prone individuals, atherosclerosis is associated with high levels of cholesterol circulating in the blood. If cholesterol is deposited in an artery, forming a plaque, this is especially dangerous if the plaque is in the artery of the heart or brain. A plaque that continues to grow can fill the entire lumen (the diameter of the artery), shutting off blood supply to the area surrounding the blockage. Or, the plaque can rupture, which happens more readily in the heart than other tissues due to normal bending and twisting of the coronary artery during the cardiac cycle, normal pressure changes during the cycle, or changes in resistance to blood flow, or coronary artery spasm. Rupture can also occur while undergoing diagnostic cardiac catheterization through catheter manipulation. With rupture, the cap on the plaque separates, exposing the core to blood constituents. A thrombus (clot) forms, and may cause total blockage of the coronary artery, resulting in a heart attack.

Theories of Atherosclerosis of the Coronary Arteries

Statistics indicate that every year approximately 500,000 U.S. women will have a heart attack. The cause: atherosclerosis. There are two major theories regarding plaque formation via atherosclerosis. The first is that plaques form in response to frequently recurring injuries to arterial walls, which can be due to high blood pressure, carbon monoxide from smoking, and high blood lipids. Whatever the agent, once the wall has been injured, substances reach the middle, or smooth muscle layer. This means that now LDL-C can supply cholesterol to the developing plaques. At the same time, platelets (blood cells that promote blood clotting) adhere to the newly-exposed tissue, clump together, and release a growth factor that stimulates smooth muscle cell proliferation. These cells migrate to the inner layer where the initial injury occurred. A central question related to this theory is Why do smooth muscle cells proliferate when injured? The answer appears to be related to the presence of low-density lipoprotein-cholesterol (LDL-C).

The second theory proposes that plaques are benign tumors, each of which has formed as a progeny of a single cell that has lost control of its growth, referred to as the monoclonal hypothesis. According to this theory, monocytes (white blood cells) are drawn to a protein secreted by endothelial cells, which line blood and lymphatic vessels. The protein is called monocyte chemoattractant protein. In most animal studies, the endothelium is not injured as the arterial lesions begin to form. Once the monocytes are attracted to the protein, they move through gaps in the inner layer of the vessel, causing smooth muscle cells to move from the wall of the blood vessel into the inner layer where blood flows.

Recruitment and proliferation of smooth muscle cells is the basic lesion that leads to plaque formation, according to this theory. Abnormalities in lipid metabolism and deposition in the arterial wall are said to play a role. The hypothesis is that some abnormal lipoproteins may cause the endothelial cells to secrete a substance called monocyte chemoattractant protein. The two theories are now integrated into a more complex "response to injury" hypothesis.

The Lipid Profile

Based upon research on men, a good lipid profile is the following: a total serum cholesterol level of 200 milligrams per deciliter (mg/dl) or less; a high-density lipoprotein-cholesterol (HDL-C) level of 35 mg/dl and higher; a low-density lipoprotein-cholesterol (LDL-C) less than 130 mg/dl; very low-density lipoprotein-cholesterol (VLDL-C) less than 38 mg/dl; triglyceride level between 10 and 190 mg/dl; and a total cholesterol/HDL-C ratio less than 3:5. To calculate the cholesterol ratio, divide the value of total cholesterol by the value of the HDL-C; for example, if total cholesterol is 200 mg/dl and HDL-C is 50 mg/dl, the result of the division is a ratio of 4 HDL-C to the total cholesterol, which is a below-average risk for heart disease.

Good and Bad Cholesterol

I have heard my colleague Judy Lutter, President of Melpomone Institute, ask the following question as she presents seminars on health and fitness. Invariably, when she asks, "Who believes that high cholesterol/fat foods are bad?" almost every hand in the audience is raised. Common sense indicates that, in most instances, what is bad about cholesterol is the quantity ingested or what is made in the body despite the amount ingested. Physiologically, cholesterol is not bad. On the contrary, it is a very good and much-needed molecule in the body. It is the building block for all steroid hormones. It is the major constituent of all cell and intracellular membranes. It is, so to speak, the bricks that hold the membranes together, yet at the same time affording it functionality. If an individual were to restrict fat intake to almost zero, the body would compensate by manufacturing cholesterol in the cells in order to maintain the integrity of the cells. Many individuals probably maintain "good" physiological levels of both the good and bad (that is, if LDL-C *is* bad for women) in the body by exercising discipline and restraint with regard to the excessive fat consumed in the diet, and also by engaging in some form of physical activity on a regular basis. Still some individuals do nothing; they are inactive slugs and eat what they want, and cholesterol levels do not change to what would be considered unhealthy. Still other individuals, in fact, 1 in 500 individuals, have a genetic defect called familial hypercholesterolemia (FH), which affects lipid metabolism. It is now possible through laboratory analyses to detect and identify whether one has FH as well as other specific disorders of lipid metabolism. In medical jargon, according to Schaefer and Levy (1985), identifying these disorders is referred to as lipoprotein phenotyping. This means that in the future, lipid abnormalities will increasingly be classified according to unique molecular defects. Whether the WHI and HERS have included within the research protocols measurement of

factors that comprise the lipid profile to identify the lipid pheno-
types of study participants is not known.

Familial Hypercholesterolemia

Individuals with familial hypercholesterolemia (FH) have inherited one normal gene for cholesterol metabolism and one mutant
gene. They have elevated levels of blood cholesterol and may die
from premature ischemic heart disease in their fifties or sixties. The
condition is relatively common (1 in 500). It is not uncommon for
affected individuals to marry (called heterozygotes in medical jargon). Since they have each inherited one bad gene, one-quarter of
the offspring from such marriages will be unaffected, one-half het-
erozygote-affected (the 1 in 500), and one-fourth will be homozygous-affected, which means these individuals inherit two copies of
the mutant gene. Individuals who are *homozygous FH* are unable to
make a functional receptor critical to moving cholesterol inside
cells. In homozygous-affected individuals, the disease is precocious
in onset. Death from heart attack may occur in childhood, since
these individuals have six to ten times the concentration of LDL-C
in the blood.

Fortunately, homozygous FH is rare, only occurring in 1 in 1
million persons. The basic defect is the inability to make a fully
functional receptor protein in order to remove cholesterol from the
blood. Absolute inability and/or decreased ability to remove LDL-C
leads to hyperlipidemia, which increases the risk of heart attack at
an early age.

What does information on FH have to do with a discussion of
estrogen and heart disease? Plenty! It was the basis for a Nobel
Prize award for Michael Brown and Joseph Goldstein in 1985, who,
beginning in 1972, set as a research goal to understand this human
genetic disease as one that represented a failure of end-product
repression of cholesterol synthesis.

MECHANISM OF REGULATING CHOLESTEROL

Experimentally, Brown and Goldstein hypothesized that the availability of FH-homozygous individuals (those with two mutant genes

for the receptor defect) would allow study of the effects of these genes without confounding effects from an FH-heterozygote individual who had one normal gene. When they began their research, there was agreement in the scientific community that all important events related to cholesterol metabolism occurred in the liver or intestine. To do their research, the researchers realized that they could not subject humans to multiple manipulations and liver biopsies in order to carry out their experiments. What they proposed to do was to take skin samples from individuals with homozygous FH, assuming that the mutant phenotype would be present in skin fibroblasts. It was.

During the course of many experiments, Brown and Goldstein discovered the following. The low-density lipoprotein-cholesterol receptor is a glycoprotein. High concentrations of the receptor are found in the liver and certain nonhepatic (other than liver) cells, such as in the adrenal gland, the testes and ovaries, and the brain. The receptor is formed in an intracellular structure called the endoplasmic reticulum, and then shuttled around in the cell until it reaches the cell membrane. One end is anchored in the membrane, and a small portion extends into the inside of the cell. The remainder extends into the circulation. Think of it as a lock protruding from the membrane, waiting for the right key to fit in the lock. The right key happens to be the low-density lipoprotein-cholesterol molecule. This molecule is formed via a series of metabolic degradations in which very low-density lipoprotein-cholesterol (VLDL-C), which contains three apoproteins on its surface (apoproteins C, E, and B-100), is enzymatically stripped of apoprotein C to form intermediate-density lipoprotein-cholesterol (IDL-C). This molecule has a high affinity for the LDL-C receptor, and much cholesterol is taken up by the liver and other cells that have a high requirement for cholesterol. IDL-C is rapidly converted into LDL-C by removal of another protein molecule, apoprotein E. LDL-C is left with apoprotein B-100, for which the receptor has a low affinity. The liver LDL-C receptors recognize the B-100 component of LDL-C. Binding leads to cellular uptake and internalization of both the receptor and the low-density lipoprotein- cholesterol molecules.

The process of cellular internalization of the cholesterol molecule with its carrier protein and the receptor is another important story. After the LDL-C molecule binds with the LDL-receptor, it is referred to as a complex molecule. Once formed, the complex diffuses laterally in the plane of the cell membrane until it reaches an area called *coated pits*. Once in the pit, the complex is swallowed by the cell (the process called endocytosis). Inside the cell, the receptor is separated from the LDL-C and returned to the cell membrane *only* if the concentration of cholesterol in the cell is low. The purpose of returning the receptor is to facilitate the entry of more cholesterol into those cells that need cholesterol. If the cells have sufficient quantity of cholesterol (in other words, they are stuffed, lipid-rich), and if liver and other high-cholesterol user cells are unable to metabolize the cholesterol load, the feedback to the cell is to repress the gene that directs the synthesis of the LDL-receptor protein molecule. In this way, cells regulate the intercellular concentration of cholesterol. Cells that are stuffed with cholesterol do not take in what they do not need. Consequently, any excess cholesterol circulates in the blood, increasing the risk in coronary-prone individuals that some LDL-C may be deposited in coronary arteries, initiating or contributing to plaque formation.

Brown and Goldstein also discovered that in individuals with familial hypercholesterolemia, cells are unable to make a fully functional low-density lipoprotein-cholesterol receptor; the receptor can bind LDL-C and cluster in the coated pits, but the receptor and the molecule to which it is bound cannot be transported into the cell. The basic defect in the receptor protein is that it lacks the last 90 amino acids at a location which would be the terminus (end) of the normal receptor. The receptor is therefore shorter than it should be. It can embed but it cannot span the cell membrane as the normal receptor does. Even though the receptor can bind LDL-C, it cannot diffuse into the coated pits. It is now known that individuals with FH may have an overall deficiency of LDL-C receptor, or a decreased ability to bind LDL-C as well.

The implications of Brown and Goldstein's research for individuals who do not have FH, but who do have high levels of blood cholesterol, is that a high dietary intake of cholesterol and saturated fat can reduce the number of LDL-C receptors. Reducing the intake of lipids increases the concentration of LDL-receptors. Through diet, then, not drugs or hormones, non-FSH individuals should be able to maintain blood levels of cholesterol within normal (nonatherogenic) limits.

The role of the good cholesterol, HDL-C, in the regulation of cholesterol metabolism is still not well understood. HDL-C serves as an acceptor of lipids in various tissues, rendering these molecules nonatherogenic. Women, on average, have higher levels of HDL-C molecules (which has been declared *cardioprotective*, meaning it is good cholesterol) than men. Gender differences in the risk of developing heart disease and the specific role played by the various cholesterol molecules, apoproteins, and other factors associated with heart disease may be better understood at the completion of the HERS and the WHI clinical trials.

Until then, what is a woman to do?

ANN'S ADVICE

1. *Don't take estrogen without first undergoing a complete physical examination, including a baseline lipid profile, to identify whether you have a condition that precludes taking estrogen (diabetes, hypertension, obesity, liver disease, etc.).* Do not take estrogen based upon age as the sole criterion. Often, care providers will use midlife as the time to start women on estrogen therapy to prevent heart disease and osteoporosis. Having a lipid baseline profile run prior to menopause will provide comparative data on total cholesterol, LDL-C, HDL-C, VLDL-C, and triglyceride levels, as well as identification of your lipid phenotype as you move to menopause and beyond.

2. *If your lipid profile is normal and if the HDL-C (good cholesterol) is not low (e.g., lower than 35 mg/dl), then just keep on doing whatever you are doing. If your lipid profile is abnormal (and remember, abnormal means it is being compared to what has been identified as abnormal for men), then ask your care provider to identify the specific lipoprotein disorder you have.* If, after discussion, estrogen is recommended, obtain a second opinion, preferably from a cardiologist. Gynecologists are more apt to prescribe estrogens since they are more convinced than others that the risk of heart disease increases postmenopausally. Estrogens are absolutely contraindicated in several lipoprotein disorders, for example, Types I, IV, and V hyperlipoproteinemia. If your physician states that lab data indicates a lipoprotein disorder, ask about other conditions that might be causing it. For example, hypercholesterolemia

can be caused by a diet high in saturated fat and cholesterol, as well as hypothyroidism, liver disease, kidney disease, etc.

3. *If you smoke, have high blood pressure, and have a lipoprotein disorder, it is especially important that something be done.* Diet is still the cornerstone of treatment for hyperlipidemia. Consult a dietician. Specific diets for individual types of hyperlipidemia are available. Follow Heart Association guidelines for a baseline diet, which suggest restricting dietary fat to less than 30 percent of total daily caloric intake, maintaining a low ratio of polyunsaturated fat to saturated fat, and restricting cholesterol to less than 300 mg/day. If you restrict cholesterol, but not fat, you will defeat the purpose of the diet. The fat will be broken down in the body via a process called beta oxidation, which effectively chops apart the long chain fatty acid molecules into 2-carbon fragments. These fragments are used by the body to make cholesterol.

A research study by McMurray and colleagues in 1991 on the Tarahumara Indians in Mexico revealed that they eat a largely vegetarian, low-fat diet. Their average plasma total cholesterol level is 121 mg/dl, LDL-C is 72 mg/dl, and HDL-C is 32 to 42, all in the low risk range for heart disease. In fact, coronary artery disease is virtually nonexistent in these individuals. When researchers changed the diet to a more typical "affluent" U.S. diet, mean blood cholesterol increased by 31 percent, primarily in the LDL-C fraction. The HDL-C increased, as did plasma triglycerides. The HDL-C increase was explained by the need to increase fat metabolism.

4. *If you have confirmed heart disease, and a high LDL-C, employ the therapeutic measures identified from the research on men that will lower LDL-C and raise HDL-C: diet, exercise, maybe even take drugs. It can't hurt!* Do what you need to do to get total cholesterol and LDL-C within normal limits, or at least move them out of the risk range. The key here is diet and exercise. Some studies suggest that a low-fat diet and exercise have less of an impact on decreasing LDL-C in women than men. Nonetheless, lower fat and cholesterol intake, exercise, and lose weight if you are overweight. Fuster and colleagues recommend steps to prevent progression of atherosclerosis in

coronary-prone individuals, and whatever it takes to enhance regression of the disease should be the single objective in the attempt to stabilize the atherosclerotic process. They believe that high HDL levels appear to exert a protective lipid-modifying effect. While it is not known exactly how HDL functions, the most favored hypothesis suggests that it promotes *reverse cholesterol transport;* that is, instead of depositing cholesterol in the arterial cells, HDL-C seems to prevent the deposition of cholesterol, remove it from arterial cells, or do both (possibly mediated via lipoprotein A). Here again, even though the effects of diet and exercise are not as pronounced on increasing HDL-C levels in women as they are in men, *do it,* as levels will increase, albeit modestly.

5. *Consider taking antioxidant vitamins.* Recent research suggests a possible benefit, particularly with vitamins C, E, and beta carotene. The Women's Health Study at Brigham and Women's Hospital in Boston is assessing the possible benefits of these vitamins on the prevention of heart disease and cardiovascular disorders. The doses of vitamins they will be administering are as follows: 500 mg vitamin C daily, plus a 50 mg beta carotene every other day, alternating with 600 IUs of vitamin E. *Do not* start vitamin therapy without consulting a care provider, and do not take megadoses of them. Too much of a vitamin can be as toxic as taking an overdose of a drug. Vitamins are cofactors in cell reactions. Too much can cause reactions in certain cells, while depriving other cells of needed cofactors. In general, antioxidants work to stabilize the cellular membranes by neutralizing free radicals. Enhancement of this process, therefore, could prevent arterial cell injury and plaque formation.

Recently, flavonoids have been identified as *cardioprotective.* Individuals with typically high fat intake and high flavonoid intake have a low death rate from heart disease. To get flavonoids in your diet, eat plenty of fresh fruits and vegetables, drink tea, and, if you do not drink wine or other alcoholic drinks, do not start drinking them in order to increase the intake of the nutrient. Related to heart disease, flavonoids probably act as an antioxidant of LDL-C, which prevents deposition of cholesterol in arteries. The highest levels of flavonoids are found in onions, kale, green beans, broccoli, endive, celery, cranberries, and citrus fruits (peel and pulp). Medium levels are found in wine, tea, lettuce, tomatoes and tomato juice, red peppers, strawberries, apples, grapes, and grape juice.

6. *Remember, estrogen is not a miracle drug.* Heart disease is a complex disease. It does not develop overnight. Taking estrogen, vitamins, or flavonoids, without modifying other risk factors, could serve only to increase risks to health in other organ systems. If you are healthy and you decide to take estrogen primarily to prevent heart disease, do so realizing that it will be nine to ten years before the WHI primary prevention trial generates reliable and valid data to say it works or it does not work. If you have a diagnosis of coronary artery disease, consider estrogen treatment as a therapeutic modality, one of many options that can be utilized.

7. *Keep in mind that just because a research report says there is a link between two phenomena, in this case, a favorable change in lipid profile with estrogen use, this does not mean cause and effect.* Correlations simply tell us that two variables are associated statistically. For example, high cholesterol levels in men are a condition frequently associated with heart disease, but not necessarily the cause of it. However, if more than one well-designed study reaches a similar conclusion, then there is a possibility that a finding is valid. The key here, however, is study design. There are rules researchers need to follow when doing research. Too often, design assumptions are violated, and methods used to do a study are biased.

8. *Weigh the kind of risk you want to take if a substantial benefit is associated with a treatment.* The risk of breast cancer is hypothesized to increase the longer one remains on hormone therapy. If quality of life is affected by menopause symptoms or heart disease, then it is time to consider hormone treatment along with other nonhormonal options.

Chapter 16

Estrogen and Hormone Treatment: Cancer Risks

INTRODUCTION

There is no pill for every ill, or to coin another old saying, there is no free lunch! For every touted benefit of any drug or hormone, there is always some side effect. For some compounds, rather severe side effects occur. For example, tamoxifen chemotherapy used to treat breast cancer results in menopausal symptoms and increases the risk of developing uterine cancer. Some treatment side effects are labeled as nuisances. However, what is described in pharmaceutical company patient inserts as an annoying side effect may be a major problem for consumers. For example, breast tenderness, headaches, and bloating are associated with estrogen use. Other "unwanted" effects of medicinals that require a prescription can be quite lethal, as in the estrogen uterine cancer connection established in the 1970s, the risk of eye problems and uterine cancer with tamoxifen use, and the risk of breast cancer in peri- and postmenopausal women who take hormones, etc. Women are very concerned about these risks in the risk-to-benefit equation presented to them related to hormone treatment, especially if the risk associated with taking these substances is cancer–no matter what the benefit.

UTERINE CANCER

The best-documented risk associated with estrogen taken in tablet form for women who have a uterus is cancer of the uterus. When

estrogen alone was found to cause endometrial cancer in menopausal women, a progestogen was added to the estrogen. Women
are now reassured that the risk of uterine cancer has been all but
eliminated by adding a progestogen. Also, some clinicians, well-
knowing what the impact of the word cancer has on women, minimize this particular risk by referring to cancer of the uterus as a
"good cancer." In other words, women are assured that should
uterine cancer develop from hormone use, it can be detected in an
early stage and treated. Treatment usually means hysterectomy.
Physicians claim that endometrial cancer is curable in most cases
(and it is), and that death rates from this disease are low (they are).
They also argue that cancer of the uterus cannot develop in women
who have undergone hysterectomy. It is easy for care providers to
state that uterine cancer can be cured, or better yet, prevented, by
removing a woman's uterus. But, is this what women really want to
do? A hysterectomy precludes the possibility of cancer developing.
But it does not prevent complications or side effects related to the
surgery, or those associated with estrogen use. (See Chapters 12 and
13). For women who keep their uterus and choose to take estrogen,
protecting their uterus from cancer with a progestin increases health
risks related to other body tissues and systems.

Women will tell you that no cancer is a good cancer, and no
woman wants to or needs to hear these words from her care provider. Nonetheless, the fact is that the risk of developing uterine
cancer is very high without a progestin to antagonize the proliferative effects of estrogen. As described in Chapter 3, during menstrual
cycle years, when endogenous progesterone is present, it stops
estrogen in its tracks; that is, it prevents estrogen from binding with
its receptor. When it does this, endometrial cells stop dividing and
stop proliferating. Without progesterone around to stop estrogen,
the cells continue to proliferate, to increase in number. Clinicians
refer to this process as *hyperplasia*, and until recently, hyperplasia
was thought to be the precursor to cancer, or neoplasia. Traditionally, endometrial hyperplasia was considered to represent a continuum of morphologic changes in uterine cells, the most severe being
atypical adenomatous hyperplasia, or carcinoma in situ. If
untreated, the hyperplasia was thought to carry a significant risk of
cancer. It was assumed that the less severe form of hyperplasia

preceded a more severe form. In fact, until recently, all forms of endometrial hyperplasia were considered precursors of invasive endometrial carcinoma. Recently, however, this traditional view has been revised. Gelfand, Ferenczy, and Bergeron suggest that it is women who have a preexisting precursor lesion, referred to now as *cellular atypia*, who are at high risk for developing uterine cancer. Today, it is cytologic atypia that is the only important diagnostic morphological feature that distinguishes endometrial lesions with invasive cancer potential from those that are noncarcinogenic.

For women who are hyperestrogenic (anovulatory or obese women, or women on estrogen replacement therapy), who have no source of progesterone production, or who do not take progesterone supplementation, estrogen has an essentially growth-promoting effect on uterine cells, *some of which have been cancer-initiated and some of which have not!* It is estrogen stimulation of the atypical, cancer-initiated cells that results in cancer, or, to use the medical term, *neoplasia*. Estrogen stimulation of noninitiated cells, on the other hand, leads to hyperplasia but with no, or at least minimal, risk of cancer. The risk of cancer developing in women diagnosed as *hyperestrogenic*, or diagnosed with cellular atypia, ranges between 11 percent and 35 percent. According to Gelfand, Ferenczy, and Bergeron, what is most interesting is that both cancer-initiated and non-cancer-initiated cells have been found in the same endometrium. So what is a woman to do if she has both kinds of cells? Take estrogen and add a progestogen!

Adding progestogens antagonizes estrogen's effect on cancer-initiated as well as non-cancer-initiated cells. Taking progestogens for 12 days each month causes the uterine endometrium to regress. Some women experience a bleed as they slough the endometrial cells. Others do not. The daily dose of commonly used progestogens needed to protect against endometrial abnormalities are as follows: norethindrone 0.7 nanograms; dl-norgestrel 150 micrograms; oral progesterone 300 milligrams; and medroxyprogesterone acetate (Depo Provera) 10 milligrams. A new product, Prempro, has recently received clearance from the FDA. Prempro is a combination of estrogen (premarin 0.625 mg), and a progestin (medroxyprogesterone acetate, 2.5 mg). This is the first product to combine estrogen and progestin in one tablet. The Wyeth-Ayerst ad claims that the continuous administration of the low dose progestin provides endometrial protection even though the total amount of progestin taken by a woman over four weeks of therapy is 70 mg (Menopause Management News Briefs, 1996). As indicated, there are few studies on the efficacy or safety of these various progestogens on body tissues, to include the breast and uterus. While progestogens do indeed antagonize estrogens at the level of the uterus, Schenken and Pauerstein (1989) believe more research is needed to identify the optimal compound, dose, and regimen for women in order to minimize negative consequences.

BREAST CANCER

Mechanisms induced by steroid hormones in the uterus are not the same as those which occur in human breast tissues. In other words, uterine and breast cells function differently. What neoplastic (cancer) or hyperplastic (uncontrolled growth) processes are initiated in breast tissue through exogenous estrogen alone or in combination hormone treatment is unknown. Reproductive hormones do play critical roles in normal breast development during menstrual and reproductive years. If these hormones are present in an altered form of the estrogen molecule (DES, ethynyl estradiol, medroxyprogesterone acetate) and/or in nonphysiological concentrations during the menstrual cycle or menopause, the probability of these substances either initiating tumor formation, or promoting a pre-existing breast cancer, exists. The mechanism of steroid hormone action is described in Chapter 14. The mechanism of action in cells that are target tissue for sex steroids is the same. The steroid, e.g., estrogen and/or progesterone, binds with a cell receptor inside the cell. The steroid and the receptor translocate through the nuclear membrane into the nucleus to bind with the DNA. Marc Lippman (1989), a breast cancer researcher, does not think that the mechanism of action of steroids with respect to breast cancer is mutagenic; in other words, no DNA damage has been found. This probably means that in the breast, the sex hormones function via the second mode of action described in Chapter 14–they stimulate the production of proteins. In the case of breast cancer, this can mean either synthesis of growth factors or factors that inhibit a suppressor substance that is normally present to prevent uncontrolled growth of cells.

In the June 1996 issue of *Atlantic Monthly*, David Plotkin, MD, a breast cancer specialist made clear that there are few things that frighten a woman more than discovering a lump in one of her breasts. With good reason Plotkin said:

> Breast cancer can transform a woman's breast into a vehicle of her death. Breast cancer is twice as likely to be diagnosed in American women today than 60 years ago. Once diagnosed, the treatment, beginning with surgery, is usually followed by radiation and chemotherapy, and is disfiguring, painful and, all too often unsuccessful. (p. 53)

The increase in diagnosis of breast cancer is growing by a rate of 4 percent a year, and of the women who have a diagnosis of breast cancer, 9,200 will be under the age of 40, which is nearly twice the number in 1970. Breast cancer is now the leading cause of death in American women age 40 to 55, and it causes more women to lose more years of productive life than any other disease.

A variety of factors, in addition to the sex hormones, have been identified as increasing a woman's risk of developing breast cancer; for example, ionizing radiation, sex (just being female), diet (fat particularly), obesity, socioeconomic status, and genetics. The $BRCA_1$ gene (BR = breast, CA = cancer) was the first major breast cancer gene to be isolated. As reported in *Science* in 1994, it is a large gene found on chromosome 17 and it codes for a protein that has a tumor suppressor function. Loss of this function may result in tumor development. Inherited loss of $BRCA_1$ function is said to place a woman at risk for increased susceptibility for both breast and ovarian cancer.

Some scientists believe there is a connection between a woman's endogenous estrogen production (made in a woman's body) and breast cancer. They cite the following reasons. First, women who have an early menarche and late menopause are at increased risk. Second, early menopause (induced by surgery) decreases the risk. Third, the increase in recurrence of breast cancer in obese postmenopausal women who have increased levels of estrone and estradiol and a decreased level of the hormone that binds these estrogens.

If a woman's own hormone production might increase the risk of breast cancer, does taking hormones at menopause also increase the risk? Lippman (1989) notes that all breast tissue is hormone dependent, and breast tissue is target tissue for the sex hormones. Breast cells require estrogen and progesterone for growth and development of the functional mammary gland. Women who take estrogen or a combination of estrogen and progesterone may not appreciate the risks involved. According to Plotkin, "Estrogen and progesterone, like aspirin, have such familiar sounding names that people often don't realize how powerful their effects are" (p. 58). Recall estrogen's effect on the uterus. It causes uterine cells to multiply exponentially unless and until progesterone is present to stop the process. A similar process occurs in the breast, where a multiplication of cells occurs (keeping in mind that the function of the uterus and the function of the breast are very different).

Many women today (with the exception of teens who become pregnant) delay childbearing until their late twenties or thirties, thus exposing their breasts to years of continued hormonal stimulation coincident with ovulatory menstrual cycles. These menstrual cycles are rarely interrupted by a full-term pregnancy. Under the influence of menstrual cycle hormones, the number of cells in some parts of the breast can increase by a factor of a 100 or more. This constant cellular multiplication may increase the likelihood of genetic accidents. Thus, Plotkin suggests that the menstrual cycle can be a precursor to breast cancer.

Jocelyn Peccei (1995), an anthropologist, has advanced a hypothesis about the necessity of menopause in terms of evolution and survival of the human species. The core of the hypothesis is based on the menstrual cycle and has relevance for breast cancer. Peccei suggests that our ancestral, hunter-gatherer, prehistory women were most likely either pregnant or lactating, not menstruating, and became menopausal at about age 45 in order to mother the last of the children born to ensure survival. Peccei speculates that menarche probably did not occur until the late teens instead of the average age of 12 today, and women probably menstruated fewer than 20 or 30 times during their reproductive lifetime. This situation is remarkably different than that which occurs with contemporary women residing in developed countries who, on average, may menstruate 300 to 400 times during reproductive life, a span of almost 40 years from age 12 to 51. Peccei's hypothesis is not so far-fetched. Beyene's study of Yucatan women documented an incredible number of pregnancies, 14 to 17 on average during reproductive life with menopause occurring around age 45 (1989). Women today, then, experience longer years of exposure of breast tissue to menstrual cycle hormones (gonadotrophic and ovarian), have either none or one or two years of exposure to hormones associated with the pregnancy cycle, experience a later age onset of first full-term pregnancy, and spend decreased or zero time nursing their babies.

THE BASICS OF BREAST DEVELOPMENT

No matter what text one reads on reproductive biology, the breast is described as a modified sweat gland. It was designed to provide milk for infants through a specialized system of glands and ducts. The ducts are analogous to small tubes that run to the nipple from milk-producing lobules that are attached to the ducts like a cluster of grapes. As most women already know, the breast changes in size and shape during each menstrual cycle (and with hormone replacement at menopause), and it changes in size and shape from menarche to postmenopause. For example, at birth a mother may observe that her baby's breasts, male or female, may secrete a liquid called *witch's milk*. This secretion is a result of sex hormones that were passed on to the baby from the mother via the placenta. As the hormone levels decline, the glands become inactive until puberty in females, and remain inactive throughout life in males. Males who have undergone a sex change can increase breast size through estrogen therapy. These males are also at risk of developing breast cancer.

Prepubertal breast development occurs around age 11. Breast appearance is such that both nipple and breast project from the chest. The mature adolescent breast develops about age 15. There is no nipple projection, and the breast and nipple have a smooth contour in a profile view.

During mature menstrual/reproductive years, the breasts change in size and shape monthly due to cyclic secretion of the sex hormones, progesterone and estrogen. How the breast changes differs from woman to woman. Some women experience pain, some tenderness to touch, others only a sense of fullness. It is thought that these changes are due to fluid accumulation, but no research has been conducted on this. All women over age 20 need to monitor/examine their breasts, and get to know the feel of their breast tissue. And they need to do this monthly at a time when their breasts are least tender, usually five to seven days after menstruation has started. Information on the correct way to perform breast self-examination is available from the American Cancer Society. Any health professional who specializes in women's health in a breast care center can demonstrate the most effective method of breast self-examination.

At menopause, the breast structure and appearance again change. Breast tissue no longer undergoes menstrual or pregnancy cyclic stimulation by sex steroids, and the changes normally associated with being a cycling or pregnant female disappear. The appearance of the breast at this time is characterized by nipple projection, and due to an increased amount of fat, breast tissue becomes rope-like and more dense than tissue associated with a menstruating woman's breast. Menopausal women should continue breast self-examination on a monthly basis, and it is a *must* for women over age 65. American Cancer Society statistics document that the breast cancer rate is the highest in this age group, increasing from 1 in 17 at age 65, to 1 in 8 women in their eighties. For more details related to the anatomy of breast development, refer to Sharon Golub's 1992 book *Periods*.

THE PHYSIOLOGY OF BREAST DEVELOPMENT

To understand the basics of breast development is to understand how the sex hormones promote growth and differentiation of breast tissue structures—the lactiferous ducts, alveoli, lobules and their terminal ends, and specialized muscle cells (myoepithelial cells). Normal development in any tissue is characterized by two distinct phases. One phase is *proliferation*—that which gives rise to the growth of tissue—and the other distinct process is called *differentiation*, which is the process by which tissue acquires the ability to express its unique function. In normal cells, growth and differentiation are extremely well coordinated and, for the most part, factors that promote tissue growth are often incompatible with those that promote differentiation. An extremely important point to remember is that with the onset of differentiation, proliferation stops and the tissue progresses to develop its genetically programmed function. For the breast, this function is secretion of milk. For the uterus, this function is transforming the uterus into a soft, nutrition-secretory organ, hospitable to implanting a fertilized egg. Dr. G. Shyamala (1992), a researcher at Lawrence Berkeley Laboratory in California, says that it is well documented in the field of cell biology and tumor biology that when these two processes, which are otherwise well coordinated, come apart or uncouple, it can lead to cancer. The estrogen/uterine cancer connection is a case in point. Women who took estrogen only, without progestin, promoted cellular proliferation which, unfortunately for some, resulted in cancer.

ANIMAL RESEARCH

Most of what is known about the normal processes of growth and differentiation in human breast tissue is derived from studies using experimental animals, e.g., mice and rats. The reason for this is obvious. It would be inhumane to subject women to multiple hormonal manipulations and breast biopsies at frequent intervals, as well as other kinds of surgical procedures. Shyamala, working with mice, characterized the changes that occur in the ducts and lobules of these animals pre- and postpuberty, and during pregnancy. At the onset of puberty, ducts that initially were rather primitive–like a tree with several branches and no leaves–branched out in many directions, and formation of bud-like (grape-like) structures occurred at the end of each branch. The presence of these bud-like structures, called end buds, is basically growth inhibiting. Even though there is space in the mammary fat pad for the ducts to grow, they stop growing.

During pregnancy, enormous growth was observed in breast structures of the mice, resulting in the ducts filling the entire mammary fat pad. Proliferation of epithelial cells during pregnancy produced lobulo-alveolar structures, which are the functional units in the breast that make milk postpartum. During lactation, the mammary tissue is almost totally composed of epithelial cells filled with milk to be secreted. Once the animal stops lactating, the epithelial cells self-destruct, a process called *apoptosis*, or programmed cell death. Shyamala observed also that the glands of animals that have finished lactating are similar to those of an animal that has never been pregnant. Through the process of apoptosis then, the epithelium that was formed during pregnancy is eliminated, and the cycle of growth and differentiation begins anew with the onset of another pregnancy.

The processes described, proliferation and differentiation of breast structures, are regulated by hormones, primarily estrogen and progesterone. Estrogen is the hormone that promotes epithelial growth whereas progesterone promotes glandular differentiation that results in the ability to produce unique milk components. Proliferation and differentiation are discontinuous events, occuring in discrete phases that are dictated by the physiological state of the animal, and that are regulated by hormones.

Even though many processes involved in normal breast development are known, very little is known about when breast cancer is initiated or promoted or what might cause it. A variety of environmental carcinogens, called EcoCancers by Janet Raloff (1993), have been suggested, such as pesticides that possess estrogenic properties (in other words, these substances can bind with the estrogen receptor). These include DDT, haptachlor, atrazine, as well as several polycyclic aromatic hydrocarbons, petroleum by-products, and polychlorinated biphenyls. Many of these pollutants are known to induce or promote mammary cancers in lab animal. Two findings unrelated to EcoCancers provided important leads for researchers: (1) epidemiological data that suggests an early full-term pregnancy before age 25 protects against breast cancer; and (2) a higher incidence of breast cancer in Japanese women between the ages of 10 and 19 was found following the atomic bombings of Nagasaki and Hiroshima.

Based on these findings, two researchers, Russo and Russo (1987), hypothesized that in the human female, the period between menarche and the first full-term pregnancy might be critical for initiation of breast cancer. The reason is that postmenarche is the time when mammary gland cells undergo a high rate of proliferation, making them susceptible to carcinogenic transformation. In experiments with rats, the Russos appeared to confirm their hypothesis. They first observed the morphological changes that occur in the gland of prepubertal rats. The first change, as described by Shyamala, was duct formation with branches forming off the ducts. By the second week of postnatal life, the ducts sprouted to form terminal end buds composed of three to six layers of epithelial cells. Then after three weeks, the end buds cleaved into three to five alveolar buds. The process of differentiation—from end buds to alveolar buds—was accentuated under the influence of the hormonal output of each estrous cycle. When the researchers introduced a carcinogen (an agent that is known to produce tumor formation) during the time the end buds were decreasing in number (due to transformation into alveolar buds), they observed the formation of a large number of intraductal structures. These *intraductal proliferations* became larger and formed microtumors. The researchers observed that not all of the end buds progressed to cancer; some differentiated. But the number of buds that differentiated was always lower than that observed in control animals who did not receive the carcinogen. When a carcinogen was administered after tissues had differentiated, from end buds to alveolar buds, no tumor formed. As the rats grew older, some end buds became smaller with age, atrophying into structures, which the researchers called terminal ducts. These terminal ducts in older animals were found to be very susceptible to neoplastic transformation when a carcinogen was administered.

When questioning why the end buds were most susceptible to carcinogenic transformation, the Russos hypothesized that it was probably related to the high proliferative rate of epithelial tissue since tumor development was inhibited in rats that had completed a full-term pregnancy and lactation prior to exposure of a carcinogen. The Russos' work with rats demonstrates that pregnancy protected the animals' mammary glands from chemically induced carcinogenesis. They concluded that pregnancy is the most physiologic and efficient means of protecting the breast from neoplastic transformation. They demonstrated this protection in later research by mimicking pregnancy in virgin rats through treatment with hormones.

IMPLICATIONS OF MICE AND RAT RESEARCH FOR WOMEN

First, the Russos hypothesized that the most vulnerable age range for women with respect to breast cancer is probably between ages 12 and 24, when the lactiferous ducts are undergoing a high degree of proliferation and low differentiation. Differentiation of mammary tissue as early as possible postmenarche would protect the breast from malignant transformation. This means that the earlier the first full-term pregnancy following menarche, the better, in order to promote epithelial differentiation, followed by lactation, and then apoptosis–a sort of biological house cleaning, if you will.

Second, mammary gland differentiation can be induced only during a well-defined period in the life span. Proliferation and differentiation are discontinuous events, occurring in discrete phases dictated by the physiological state of the animal, e.g., the reproductive years. This means that estrogen and progesterone are critically involved in the development of a woman's normal breast tissue, and these growth and development processes need to be regulated, not continuous, ongoing, and unregulated as occurs with hormone use. A woman who takes prescription estrogen or a combination of estrogen and progesterone, is, in effect, stimulating less receptive, older mammary gland tissue, tissue which may not have the suppressor agents, or inhibiting factors present, to ensure that tumor growth and spread will not occur.

Third, we learned from the tragic outcome of the atomic bombings of World War II, that the window of protection created by an early pregnancy can also be the window of susceptibility for tumor initiation. In other words, the earlier postpuberty end buds differentiate into alveolar buds/lobules, the better, as this minimizes the possibility of tumor formation by eliminating undifferentiated terminal ducts. In the absence of an early full-term pregnancy, the presence of proliferating, undifferentiated epithelial tissue during these formative years may increase the susceptibility to cancer *if a carcinogen is introduced*.

Fourth, breast lobular development is related to gynecological age and not chronological age. A full-term pregnancy in one's thirties or early forties is no assurance that breast tissue will differentiate sufficiently to afford protection against breast cancer. In fact, the reverse may be true–risk may increase with a late age onset of pregnancy since atrophied terminal ducts will be stimulated by the hormones of pregnancy.

HORMONES COULD CAUSE BREAST CANCER

Do ovarian hormones, whether endogenous or exogenous, in some way increase the risk of breast cancer? This is not only a sensible question to ask, but is very important. Unlike our prehistoric ancestors, many women are postponing first full-term pregnancies until their thirties, and sexually active teens are being placed on oral contraceptives in their early teens in order to prevent pregnancy. One of the most frequently asked questions concerning contraception is "At what age should a sexually active adolescent begin birth control?" The correct answer of course would be to wait until the young woman has experienced menarche and menstruations are regular. However, if a young woman is sexually active, the recommendation is to place her on oral contraceptives prior to menarche to prevent pregnancy–sort of a catch-22 on either end of a woman's menstrual/reproductive life. Women on oral contraceptives have in effect altered the normal processes of reproductive growth and differentiation, and shut down the regulatory mechanisms associated with the menstrual cycle. Oral contraceptives were designed to stop ovulation. If there is no ovulation, there is no endogenous estrogen or progesterone. Does this mean that these women are protected from breast cancer? Research indicates that women who do not have functioning ovaries do not develop breast cancer. If a young woman is taking oral contraceptive steroids and does not have endogenous hormones circulating, does breast development stop? If so, does the risk of breast cancer for this woman decrease? What happens physiologically when adolescents, at a later age, stop taking oral contraceptives, and become pregnant? Does the time clock for the window of protection begin ticking, as if reproductive maturation was on hold? Who knows?

STUDIES ON BREAST CANCER AND HORMONE USE

Numerous reports have been published based upon the Nurses' Health Study which was established in 1976, when 121,700 female registered nurses, ages 30 to 55, completed a survey. Many of these nurses have completed follow-up surveys every two years. From

1978 to 1992, the researchers, headed by Graham A. Colditz (1987, 1990), observed a significant elevation in the risk of breast cancer among the women using conjugated equine steroids alone (estrone). In June of 1995, researchers confirmed these findings in a report published in the *New England Journal of Medicine*, and also reported the finding of an increase in the risk of breast cancer in women taking combined hormone treatment, estrogen plus a progestin (Colditz et al., 1995). During 725,550 person-years of follow-up, 935 new cases of invasive breast cancer were diagnosed in women hormone users when compared with women who did not use hormones. The small number of women taking combined therapy previously precluded a detailed analysis of this risk. The relative risk of breast cancer was deemed highest among the oldest women, 65 to 69 years, which increased significantly among older women currently using hormones who had used them for more than five years. In sum, the increase in risk was most pronounced for women who were over age 55. The researchers concluded that these findings on U.S. women (the nurses) confirmed the findings of European researchers, those of Bergkvist and co-workers (1989), Ewertz (1988), and Hunt and co-workers (1987).

The findings of the study by Colditz and co-workers were directly opposite to those reported by Janet Stanford and her colleagues, which were also reported in June of 1995 in *The Journal of the American Medical Association*. This study was a population-based, case-control investigation. White women with breast cancer were identified through a cancer registry that covered 13 counties in northwestern Washington state. Of 660 women identified as eligible to participate in the study, 537 women ages 50 to 64, with confirmed breast cancer, were interviewed. These women were matched with 492 randomly selected women in King County who did not have breast cancer. The researchers found no overall association between breast cancer risk and the use of either estrogen alone or with a progestin. The researchers did acknowledge several limitations associated with the study. One limitation was the fact that the practice of prescribing a progestin with estrogen has only recently become widespread. Therefore, if, as has been reported previously (refer to the Greenberg study on incidence of breast cancer in DES mothers), it takes 10 to 20 years for breast cancer to surface, the findings of this study could not identify the effect on risk related to long-term use. Further studies will be required.

The researchers noted that recent studies conducted on premenopausal women indicate that breast mitotic activity (cell division) increases when endogenous progesterone levels are highest. This finding is consistent with the findings from animal studies wherein estrogen and progesterone work together to stimulate epithelial cell proliferation. Unfortunately, no data are available to support that the findings of how hormones work in breast tissue of premenopausal women are applicable to postmenopausal women. Hormonal stimulation of breast tissue in postmenopausal women is not regulated as it is during menstrual years. As Shyamala pointed out, when the processes, as they are known during reproductive years, come apart or uncouple, they can set the stage for carcinogenesis.

The reference citations to Colditz and Stanford studies are included in the bibliography, as are numerous other study citations. I invite you to read these studies and interpret the findings on your own. Also, read the Steinberg article published in 1991 in *The Journal of the American Medical Association*. The importance of this study is that it is a meta-analysis, which means that it was an analysis of the quality of research published on breast cancer and hormone use. When studies that were given high marks for design and method were examined (in other words, evaluated as high quality), an increase in breast cancer risk with hormone use was found. For those studies that were evaluated as low quality, no increase in breast cancer risk was found.

There will be no closure on this issue until the results of the Women's Health Initiative clinical trials on the risks and benefits of long-term hormone treatment are determined, which is some ten years down the road, in the twenty-first century. Concerns have been expressed about the clinical trials, that is, if positive effects (as are expected) are found related to hormone use and heart disease and osteoporosis, the trials will meet with an early ending. This will not be the case, however. The Data and Safety Monitoring Board, as reported by Prentice and colleagues, made clear that overall benefits versus risks will be the key for stopping the trial rather than any disease outcome. What this means is that the study will continue over the long-term in order to answer the breast cancer question.

IN THE MEANTIME–WHAT IS A WOMAN TO DO?

Dr. Isaac Schiff has some important insights on the issue. At the 1995 meeting of The North American Menopause Society, a special symposium was devoted to hormone therapy and breast cancer. Participants debated whether women who take estrogen or combined hormone therapy increase their risk of breast cancer. The debate, like the heart disease issue, was heated and controversial. No definitive answer to the question emerged. Dr. Schiff summarized the papers presented at the day-long conference, indicating that not one person in the room felt 100 percent confident that estrogens have no effect whatsoever on the incidence of breast cancer. He said that Dr. Trudy Bush suggested we may have reached the limits of the assay to determine whether or not estrogens cause breast cancer–epidemiologic studies are not going to provide the answer at this time. One warning flag that was raised, said Schiff, is the longer the duration of treatment, the greater the risk of developing breast cancer. Schiff concluded his presentation saying:

> ... if we coldly and insensitively went by statistics alone ... we might advise all of our patients to take hormones (for heart disease/osteoporosis), since more lives would be saved than would be lost to breast cancer. But, to coin a phrase, neither woman nor man lives by statistics alone and not every decision that is made is made simply to improve our chances of living longer. Living well and anxiety-free counts as well. Then again, the fear of cancer, especially breast cancer, remains an understandably potent dread to the possible victim–one that may lead her to a choice not supported by abstract statistical reasoning.

Many women have made and even more will make choices in the future not to take hormones at menopause for fear of breast cancer. The findings from basic laboratory research suggest that there is a process and a metabolic master plan that directs when hormonal stimulation of breast tissue is physiologically sound and when it is not. Knowing this, it is just plain silly for anyone to deny that taking hormones at menopause does not in some way alter breast cell metabolism, which might increase the risk of cancer.

Before making a decision to take hormones, it is important to discuss breast growth and development with a physician or a nurse practitioner. If these health professionals are not aware of the work done in cell biology, then recommendations made by them to use hormones are based solely upon data from case-control or epidemiological studies. The data emanating from these studies, according to Dr. Trudy Bush, are neither coherent nor reproducible.

OTHER RISKS

Other risks are associated with hormone use. These are described in detail in patient packet inserts. Gallbladder disease and high blood pressure are not unusual.

Gallbladder Disease

After about two years of estrogen use, a two- to threefold increase in the risk of surgically confirmed gallbladder disease in women receiving estrogens, versus women not on estrogens, has been reported.

High Blood Pressure

Blood pressure may increase with estrogen use. This is undoubtedly due to the water-retaining properties of estrogen, perhaps functioning at the cell level in much the same way as does aldosterone, the salt-retaining hormone in the body. Women with high blood pressure who decide to use estrogen hormone must have their pressure monitored frequently. And, of course, here is the first of many catch-22s that will emerge. A hormone is taken to treat symptoms or to obtain protection against developing heart disease or osteoporosis. A side effect from the treatment results in a disease, high blood pressure, which needs to be treated by another drug, which itself may cause other unwanted side effects, e.g., diuretic-induced loss of potassium, etc.

Adverse Reactions

In addition to these risks, other adverse reactions have been reported. These range from changes in the bleeding pattern, increase in uterine fibroids, changes in cervical secretions, painful and/or tender breasts, nausea, vomiting, migraine, increase in weight, loss of scalp hair, edema, changes in libido, etc. These changes are described also in patient package inserts that accompany hormone prescriptions. If one is not included with the hormone prescription, request it from the pharmacist, examine it carefully, and discuss any or all of the side effects with a health care provider.

Chapter 17

Ann's Advice on Estrogen or Hormone Treatment

1. *If symptoms are intolerable, or if there is a high risk of osteoporosis, or a diagnosis of osteoporosis, serious consideration should be given to hormone replacement.* Being able to live postmenopausal years with a high quality of life is desirable. If a decision to use hormones is made, a care provider, nurse, or physician must be consulted at least once a year. Twice is even better if insurance coverage is available. Tailoring hormone treatment to a woman's individual needs is complex. Side effects may occur that make the treatment seem worse than the symptoms.

2. *Research indicates that no specific mental disorder occurs during menopause, nor is there evidence that estrogens help in treating mental disorders.* In some women, however, the relief of a physical change of menopause, such as hot flash, may improve mood. Mood changes are quite normal during the menopausal transition. Mood changes are not a sign of mental illness. Depression is a bona fide mental illness. If a diagnosis of depression is made, drug therapy or psychotherapy is indicated.

3. *The research findings concerning sexuality changes at menopause are conflicting.* Some women report heightened sexual interest and arousal. Others report just the opposite. If changes have occurred, that is, a diminution of interest in sex, and sexuality is an important part of life, consult with a care provider; share this information with him or her. Hormone treatments help some women. The hormone may be applied locally (if interest in sex has diminished because of a painful vagina), or via patch or pill, which has a systemic effect. Also, androgen

replacement may help. Susan Rako (1996) has published information on androgen therapy and has a good discussion of side effects. Androgen therapy can increase the risk of heart disease by elevating blood lipids. If sexuality problems are serious, help is needed; consult a sexuality expert.

4. *There are serious risks associated with hormone use. Reread the sections on uterine and breast cancer to gain a full understanding of these risks.*

5. *If maintaining a youthful appearance is important, sorry, hormones and even wrinkle cream will not stop the process of aging.* Contrary to popular belief (created by Wilson's *Feminine Forever*), estrogens do not prevent age-related changes in skin, hair, and breasts. Sagging breasts are related more to loss of muscle and muscle tone than anything else. The skin, as an organ system, loses tone and elasticity with aging. Concerning hair, Claudia Bowe's excellent article in the April 1989 issue of *Lears* stated that each one of us has about 100,000 hairs on our bodies–head, arms, legs, trunk, pubic area, eyelids, eyebrows, and underarms. These hairs are lost throughout premenopausal life at a rate of about 100 or more a day. As they are lost, however, the process of replacing them has already begun. At menopause, as the concentration of estrogen decreases, the small amount of androgen that is always present in a woman's body now has an opportunity to interact with hair follicle receptors. Androgens normally inhibit hair growth. At least that is what research on bald men has shown. And so, as the hormonal picture changes at menopause, the hairs that fall out of the scalp may not grow back because growth is inhibited by androgens. In other areas, such as above the lip, for example, the "mustache" area, the opposite effect is observed. A typical male pattern of hair growth may occur here.

Estrogens may increase scalp hair growth and minimize the facial mustache and wild hairs that appear. A safe, inexpensive, and quick method of removing mustache hairs is to pluck them out with tweezers.

Hair loss can result from a variety of diseases, drugs (for example, for high blood pressure, antidepressants, cancer chemotherapies), and anemia, which may be more common than we think, because of episodic heavy bleeding perimenopausally. Drugs specifically for hair growth are on the market; one is Rogaine (Minoxidil), a widely advertised drug sold by Upjohn Company, which has been tested on men. Whether it will work on women remains to be seen. Hair loss and baldness are not restricted to men. Most of the time, when hair loss occurs, and is not related to illness or drugs, it is a result of our genetic composition.

6. *Take estrogens only with a prescription, and follow the instructions provided by a care provider.* Any woman taking hormones needs to remain under the care of a doctor or nurse who is familiar with her medical condition, who understands her general situation, and who discusses matters openly. Refer to Chapter 23 for tips on how to choose and interact with a care provider. Such care will help maximize the benefits of hormones, and minimize the risks associated with use, detecting dangerous side effects early, and discontinuing use as soon as possible. If vaginal estrogen is used daily and the prescribed dosage is exceeded, the concentration of estrogen circulating systemically can be increased. This can be risky if a woman has a condition for which estrogen is contraindicated, such as high blood pressure, gallbladder disease, frequent blood clots, or breast cancer that is estrogen-responsive. Hormones can aggravate or worsen a preexisting condition.

7. *Realize that estrogen use (with a progestin) interrupts the perimenopausal transition.* A woman who has been on hormones for several years and decides to stop can expect to experience some or all of the changes associated with menopause, no matter at what age the hormones are stopped!

8. *Being a woman does not increase the risk of developing Alzheimer's disease, contrary to the blitz in the popular media.* Seeing if you have a family history of the disease, like anything else, you may be at increased risk to develop this and other diseases. So far, scientists have yet to discover gender connection related to women, estrogen, and Alzheimer's disease. Women who continue to mentally challenge themselves seem to be protected against this disease. Connecting estrogen to Alz-

heimer's seems to be another instance of gender bias, i.e., using menopause to frighten and discriminate against women.

9. *Have the courage of your convictions.* To be or not to be a hormone user is a difficult decision to make. For now, only a small number of pre- and postmenopausal women who could benefit from hormone treatment choose to take the product–period! These women have decided that the benefits associated with hormone use outweigh the risks. Whether to be or not to be a hormone user is a very personal decision. When the decision is made, it does not need to be justified to anyone else. What is most important is that women who choose to use hormones remain under the care of a qualified health professional in order to assess both the risks and benefits associated with treatment.

10. *Abandon the terms "estrogen replacement therapy" or "hormone replacement therapy."* The terms imply that something is missing, causing a disease, and needs to be replaced. Women are not estrogen-deficient at menopause unless made that way through surgical castration or drugs and radiation. In any case, whether menopause is natural or induced, the correct terminology related to hormones should be consistent with that for any other drugs. To discuss estrogen use as "replacement therapy" softens the risk and heightens the benefits, while hiding the implication that menopause is a disease. Estrogen as treatment brings the menopause-as-disease ideology out of the closet, in the face of women and their care providers, where they can openly deal with the issues associated with treatments in general.

11. *Finally, remember, estrogen is not a miracle drug and menopause is not a disease.* Just because hormone levels drop at menopause–as we age–does not mean that this decrease will cause disease or that supplementing hormones reduces the risk of disease. On the contrary, supplementing hormones might result in disease, breast cancer for example. Both estrogen and progestogens are drugs which are administered in pharmacologic doses rather than physiological replacement.

Chapter 18

Osteoporosis

Osteoporosis is a disease. The Natural Osteoporosis Foundation's *Physician's Resource Manual on Osteoporosis* describes it as a condition in which bone tissue is reduced in amount. It is a demineralization and thinning of bone, increasing the likelihood of fracture. Two categories of osteoporosis have been identified, primary and secondary. Primary is the most common form of the condition and includes postmenopausal osteoporosis. Osteoporosis is not a disease in the usual sense of the term, as it is "silent" for many years after its onset; there may be no symptoms until a fracture occurs. Many victims of osteoporosis awake to the reality of a lifelong neglect of their bones when they suffer a fracture. Some bone loss occurs universally with aging, in both sexes, but the condition is more marked in females.

The process in individuals at-risk begins in the mid-thirties, and it occurs in both men and women. Osteoporosis has been defined as a multifactorial disorder. In women, early menopause, whether natural or induced, increases the risk of the disease, as do age, race, body shape, habits, and lifestyle.

PHYSIOLOGY OF BONE REMODELING

Many people think of bone as solid, inert, and/or inactive tissue that serves merely to provide structural support for the body. This view is far from the truth. Bone is an active metabolizing tissue; it is a depot for calcium, phosphorus, basic hydroxyl groups, and magnesium. During our lifetime, bone is in a dynamic state, constantly undergoing remodeling. Bone turnover, or remodeling, occurs in discrete packages called bone multicellular units, which are active on surfaces of both kinds of bone found in the body, cortical and trabecular.

In the resting state these bone surfaces are lined by flat, relatively inactive cells. However, when a remodeling signal is received, an area of bone is removed. The remodeling process involves two specialized bone cells, osteoclasts and osteoblasts. Osteoclasts remove tiny pieces of bone; a 0.1 millimeter piece of bone can be removed within a three week period. Once this has occurred, the osteoclasts are replaced by osteoblasts, another specialized cell which promotes the assimilation of calcium and other materials to lay down new bone. The osteoblasts essentially replace what the osteoclast has removed. The time from resorption (osteoclast removal of bone) to mineralization (osteoblast replacement of bone) is approximately three months. The balance between bone resorption and formation is known as the remodeling balance. If this balance is persistently negative, osteoporosis develops.

The process of bone remodeling (bone dissolution and bone repair) is regulated primarily by two hormones: calcitonin from the thyroid gland and parathyroid hormone (PTH), which is produced in the parathyroid gland. The primary function of these two hormones is to regulate and maintain blood calcium levels within very narrow limits, from 9 to 11.5 mg/deciliter. At this concentration, calcium does many things in the human body. It is very important in blood coagulation and in maintaining the acid-base balance of the body. It is involved in nerve conduction and muscle contraction, and it plays a major role in maintaining the permeability of all cell membranes. Regulation of blood calcium concentration *always* takes precedence over the maintenance of the structural integrity of bone. Thus, a lifetime of inadequate calcium intake and/or uptake by the intestine will be balanced by a depletion of bone mineral stores.

Restoration of a positive calcium balance via bone resorption does not seem to be either cost-effective or efficient. However, there is no other storage area for calcium in the body. The bones and teeth contain 99 percent of the calcium in the body. The other one percent is used for the various metabolic processes more than assimilation. If the resorptive process is allowed to continue in women who are at high risk for developing osteoporosis, the net result is a negative remodeling balance, and osteoporosis occurs, increasing the risk for fractures.

Bone density loss is a normal and natural condition of aging in both sexes. But, although it is natural, it can create hazards. Osteoporosis is the abnormal, unnaturally high acceleration of bone loss. For reasons unknown, bone loss in women which may lead to osteoporosis is said to be the most severe during the first five to six years after menopause. Prior to menopause, the sex hormones are thought to protect the bones, but how they do so is unknown. Scientists know that the effects of estrogens on bone are indirect, and probably related to the regulation and mediation of one or all of the mechanisms involved in maintaining calcium balance. I will discuss these mechanisms later.

PREVALENCE OF OSTEOPOROSIS

Fractures associated with postmenopausal and age-related osteoporosis are estimated to affect between 1.3 and 1.5 million Americans, most of whom are women. The rate of osteoporosis increases quite dramatically for women as they age, from a low of about 18 percent at ages 45 to 49, to 89 percent for ages 75 and higher. Winnifred Cutler (1988) describes osteoporosis as a worldwide medical problem confronting health care workers. This declaration emanated from reports of 247,000 hip fractures in 1985, mostly in white women. It was predicted from these data that eight percent of women who were then 35 years of age (in 1985) would experience a hip fracture in later life. In 1993 statistics reported in *The American Woman 1996-97*, the total female population of the United States was estimated at 134.7 million. Eight percent of these women over 30, or approximately 6 million, based on the 1985 estimates, would be at risk for hip fracture as they age. Based on these statistics, osteoporosis was described as *the* disease of American women. In 1987, Hall, Davis, and Baran recommended estrogen treatment for all menopausal women to prevent fractures and subsequent disability.

Epidemiological studies have documented the beneficial effect of estrogen with respect to a decreased risk of fractures in Caucasian women who are at risk for osteoporosis. Based on these studies, proponents of estrogen concluded that functional delay of menopause through administering estrogen would substantially decrease the risk of hip fractures. Even though other agents prevented bone loss leading to fractures, such as sodium fluoride, calcitonin, and a metabolite of vitamin D, the Food and Drug Administration approved the use of oral, short-acting estrogen (estrone) at a dosage of 0.625 mg. The dose of estrogen is to be taken for 25 to 26 days. However, as discussed previously, in order to protect a woman's uterus from cancer, a progestogen must be administered along with estrogen from days 12 to 15 through day 25. It is recommended that combination hormone treatment for women at risk be initiated as soon after the menopause as possible and continue for at least 5 to 15 years.

Most postmenopausal women, according to Yen (1986), do not need estrogen to prevent osteoporosis. Estrogen replacement may be unnecessary and even contraindicated for a significant number of postmenopausal women. The lack of valid and reliable predictive methods to identify who should receive some form of prophylactic therapy for osteoporosis poses a major dilemma. Yen argues that for those women who would benefit from estrogen, acceleration in bone loss would have occurred before definitive evidence of entry into the menopausal transition was observed. Robert Lindsay agrees. Identification of women at risk is a major problem. Lindsay says that risk factor assessment used in combination with bone mass measurement offers the closest approximation to the ideal (1989; 1993).

The linking of osteoporosis with menopause has given new meaning to the horrors of Wilson's living decay. This message has been translated into fear and concern and even some hysteria in women's magazines and popular books on the topic. Gail Sheehy, in her book *The Silent Passage*, also perpetuates the doom and gloom by citing questionable statistics, stating that one-third to one-half of all postmenopausal women and nearly half of all people over age 75 will be affected by this disease. While it is true that osteoporosis is a disease, it is also a multifactorial disorder. For women who have a family history of osteoporosis, heredity is a definite risk factor. But so are age, race, and body build. Sheehy provides some hope for the baby boomers, whom she describes as bouncing from work to gym in nitrogen-cushioned aerobic shoes, popping calcium, and snacking on veggies and yogurt. She contrasts these women with the elderly "frail" women who are now immobilized in nursing homes, implying that these women are stricken with osteoporosis because their formative years were calcium deficient and physically inactive. Perhaps there have been women born with silver spoons in their mouths, who spent their lives sitting idly in parlors, one cross-stitching while another lazed at a game of solitaire. Perhaps there have been a few. But most of our mothers, grandmothers, and great-grandmothers were hard-scrabble, hard-working, physically active women who grew up in the heyday of milk and cheese, when food was real and fast food was a wary chicken.

Sheehy has far too limited a perspective on the socio-historical dynamics and multifactorial aspects of both menopause and osteoporosis, which leads her into false conclusions. To Sheehy's credit, she forcefully notes that the politics concerning osteoporosis are scandalous, that most medical plans do not reimburse for osteoporosis screening, nor has a national screening program been established or endorsed for medical reimbursement to diagnose early changes consistent with osteoporosis, as there is for breast cancer (no doubt due to the fact that not all women are at risk for the disease). Given the serious consequences of osteoporosis for some women, experts recommend that women have their bone mineral density measured at menopause, and those with the lowest bone mineral density (BMD) be offered hormone treatments. Even though the Office of Technology Assessment (OTA), Congress of the United States, convened a task force in 1993 to study the policy implications related to women's health and estrogen treatment, no policy for either screening or hormones has been forthcoming. The OTA estimates that the societal expenditures for hip fractures in 1990 (not all osteoporosis-related) were $5 billion.

Whether or not women will develop osteoporosis depends on three main factors: (1) how much bone is present at maturity, (2) how fast bone is lost, and (3) longevity. These conditions are influenced by many circumstances, some of which are controllable, some not.

FACTORS THAT CANNOT BE CONTROLLED

Age at Menopause

The earlier the natural menopause, the greater the risk. If a woman has menopause induced, whether surgically, by radiation, or with drugs, estrogen levels fall precipitously. Early menopause places a woman at about a 50 percent risk of developing osteoporosis. So if a hysterectomy is recommended for any reason, get a second opinion, and utilize the resource material I have recommended. This is very important, as too often, healthy ovaries are removed with the uterus. When this happens, menopause is instantaneous, increasing the risk of developing osteoporosis.

Family History

Osteoporosis appears to run in families. If a woman's mother, grandmother, aunt, or sister has the condition, she can consider herself at high-risk through genetic inheritance alone.

Ethnic or Racial Differences, Bone Mass, and Skin Pigmentation

It is assumed that fewer black women than white women develop osteoporosis. However, this factor has not been supported by research. Furthermore, black women have been excluded from the prospective longitudinal studies that are most cited, such as the Framingham Longitudinal Study, the Nurses' Health Study, Leisure World (a California retirement community), and the Lipid Research Clinics. The few studies that document a relationship between the risk of developing osteoporosis and ethnicity indicate that women whose ancestors originated in Great Britain, Europe, China, or Japan are thought to be at higher risk for developing osteoporosis than women of African, Mediterranean, or Hispanic ancestry. But we do not know for sure. My own ethnicity is Slavic (European). My ancestors were hard-working, big-boned, farm people. I have no history of osteoporosis in my family. I have strong, big bones, eat a well-balanced diet, take no calcium supplements or estrogen replacement, have never fractured a bone, and have not lost height. I consider myself to be as sturdy as an old oak tree. Nevertheless, the possibility of developing osteoporosis is a frightening prospect for women. In addition to taking hormones, there are nonhormonal methods women can use to minimize the risk of developing osteoporosis and to cope with the fear.

BONING UP: FACTORS THAT CAN BE CONTROLLED

Nutrition and Diet

There is a lifelong need for good nutrition, whether we are discussing prevention of osteoporosis, heart disease, or breast cancer. At perimenopause, related to osteoporosis, this becomes even more critical because of age-related changes in the body's ability to absorb digested nutrients. According to Bruce Ettinger (1993), an osteoporosis researcher, from about age 60, the rate at which calcium is absorbed declines. Combined with this decline in absorption may be a decreased intake of calcium rich foods, such as fortified cereals, breads, juices, milk, cheeses, sardines, broccoli, kale, etc. Also, older women may synthesize less of the active vitamin D metabolite in the kidney, called 1,25 dihydroxy vitamin D (1,25-dihydroxyvitamin D_3) or $1,25(OH)_2D_3$.

To protect against osteoporosis, a daily calcium intake of between 800 and 1,000 milligrams (which is the amount found in a little more than a quart of milk) is required if it is less than five years since menopause. If more than five years have passed since menopause, then the daily calcium requirement per day is increased to between 1,000 (if on estrogen) and 1,500 milligrams per day (if not). An NIH Consensus Statement, *Optimal Calcium Intake* (1994) lists optimal calcium requirements across the life span. It also discusses the important cofactors for achieving optimal calcium intake (vitamin D), factors that decrease calcium availability, and risks associated with increased levels of calcium. Free copies of the booklet are available by calling a 24-hour voice mail at 1-800-NIH-OMAR. A plentiful intake of calcium during youth will help to "bone up" against the advent of osteoporosis in later years, but it is never too late to start boning up. Dairy products are the best source of calcium, as well as green leafy vegetables. However, according to Ettinger, some green leafy vegetables–spinach and Swiss chard, as well as cranberries, rhubarb, and, yes, even gooseberries–contain substances called oxalic acids, which leech the calcium from the body. When these substances are eaten they should be accompanied by rather liberal portions of calcium-rich foods, such as eggs, beans, and milk. Robert Heany at Creighton University in Nebraska suggests that by adding nonfat powdered milk to coffee; drinking calcium-fortified orange juice; and eating one serving of lowfat yogurt a day, a serving of a dark green, leafy vegetable, and a one-inch cube of cheese a day will add about 1,000 mg of calcium to the daily diet (Wymelenberg, 1994).

Differences in bone mass have been found in both men and women vegetarians when compared with red meat eaters. The average bone density of vegetarians in their seventies is more than that of meat eaters in their fifties. Reasons for these differences are only speculative, but it may be related to red meat being rich in phosphorous and vegetarian diets being low in acid. Consider decreasing the intake of red meat and increasing vegetable consumption. Consult a dietician, nurse practitioner, or physician in order to construct the best plan.

Calcium Supplementation

Do not take calcium tablets to increase calcium intake unless it is done under the supervision of a qualified health professional. There are many calcium preparations on the market and the amount of calcium in over-the-counter preparations varies in each product. The highest amount of calcium for the dollar is obtained through calcium carbonate preparations. The calcium in a carbonate preparation is 40 percent by weight. What this means is that calcium, as an inorganic ion, must always be bonded covalently (that is, it has two charges) to another inorganic ion. It cannot be found or prepared in isolation. In the case of calcium carbonate, calcium is bound to carbonate. The total gram molecular weight of one molecule of calcium carbonate is 100. Of this, 40 grams is calcium, or 40 percent of the total weight. This figure is useful for calculating how much calcium will be available for absorption. For example, if tablets in a bottle of calcium carbonate are labeled as 500 milligrams of calcium carbonate, then 40 percent of the 500 milligrams (200 mg), is the amount of calcium available for absorption. To ensure an intake of 1,000 milligrams of calcium a day, then, would require taking five of these 500 milligram tablets. Many calcium supplements now state directly on the bottle how much elemental calcium is contained in one tablet. Nonetheless, it is important to check with a pharmacist to determine whether the calcium supplement recommended by your health care professional is in fact providing the daily requirement. Dr. Bruce Ettinger did a cost analysis of the various calcium preparations. As mentioned, the dollar value obtained per calcium tablet is greatest with calcium carbonate. Oyster shell (generic), Tums-Ex and calcium rich Rolaids were identified as expensive calcium supplements, ranging from $40 to $55 per year to ensure an intake of 1,000 milligrams of calcium a day.

Dr. Ettinger also recommends the chewable form of calcium replacement because chewing enhances both the dispersion and bioavailability of the calcium. Another long-standing concern about calcium replacement via tablet form has been the safety of large doses, for example 1,500 milligrams a day, with respect to kidney stone formation. This problem has not been observed to occur with any great frequency in older women. However, to be on the safe side, it is recommended that these preparations be taken in chewable form and that an optimum state of hydration is maintained. In other words, drink *at least* six to seven glasses of water per day. Dr. Ettinger also recommends that the calcium tablets be taken at bedtime to maximize absorption. I do not believe this is based on any osteoporosis research. This finding is based on a study of hospitalized bedridden patients who lost both muscle and bone mass with prolonged bed rest.

I recommend Dr. Ettinger's article in the May 1993 issue of *Menopause Management*. Dr. Winnifred Cutler, in her 1988 book *Hysterectomy Before and After,* ranks calcium supplements in terms of their dissolution rate (p. 188). Giant Foods Natural was first in dissolution; Safeway calcium was last (number 52 out of 52 products tested).

Exercise

Regular exercise is important throughout life for development and maintenance of strong, healthy bones. Just as muscles atrophy and become weak through disuse, so do bones. Increasing the stress on your bones by carrying out exercises will have a positive influence on bone. Strong muscles and strong bones in youth are good preventative measures against osteoporosis, but, as with nutrition, it is never too late to start exercising.

Body Weight

Obese women generally do not develop osteoporosis. Two factors may explain why. First, the increase in body weight places more stress on the bones. The more stress, the more the bone is forced to maintain its strength, and therefore it does not deteriorate. Second, obese women (as discussed in the chapter on bleeding changes) make more estrogen in their bodies than thin women. Body fat is a synthesizer for estrogen. The catch-22 here is that obesity is a risk factor for developing heart disease, cancer of the uterus, stroke, diabetes, and perhaps breast cancer. Consequently, obesity is not a valuable prescription for avoiding osteoporosis.

Drug Use

Women who smoke tend to have an earlier menopause. This may be due to the fact that these women have less fatty tissue. But the real reason is unknown. In any event, a smoking woman may have fewer years in the premenopause than nonsmokers. So, there is less estrogen made within the body over a shorter period of time. Smoking is also a risk factor for developing heart disease; it is the major cause of lung cancer. Alcohol use, more than a couple of ounces a day, may impair calcium absorption.

Antacids are known to increase calcium excretion. For women with hypertension, a benefit associated with taking thiazide diuretics, in addition to treating hypertension, is that these diuretics significantly decrease the rate of bone mineral loss in both men and women because they reduce the amount of calcium lost in the urine. If the amount of calcium lost is decreased, there is less resorption of bone to provide calcium for important metabolic reactions, and therefore, fewer fractures.

It is best to consult with a pharmacist or other health care professional about the possible effect that any drug may have on calcium absorption and/or excretion. Drug-induced increase in calcium excretion can lead to a condition called *secondary osteoporosis*. Related to drugs and their effects on calcium metabolism, I recommend reading the book *Worst Pills, Best Pills*, by Dr. Sidney M. Wolfe and Rose Ellen Hope (1993), of the Public Citizen Health Research Group. This book should be required reading for all older adults. The cost is about $15.00 in paperback. The book may be ordered from Public Citizen, 2000 P Street, N.W. Suite 600, Washington, DC 20036.

HORMONE AND DRUG TREATMENTS

Hormones

Estrogen

Estrogen use after menopause results in a positive calcium balance. For women with clinically diagnosed osteoporosis, estrogen is a must to prevent further bone loss. Exactly how estrogen functions to maintain bone and prevent the breakdown of bone is not known entirely. Estrogen therapy may increase calcitonin levels to promote bone-building activity, and, thus, it may inhibit parathyroid hormone-mediated bone resorption (osteoclastic activity). Recall the mechanism of action of estrogen described in the hormone chapter. In order for estrogen to do its job in body cells, it must bind with specific receptors in the cell. After binding, it moves into the nucleus and binds with DNA. This binding initiates a series of events, one of which may be synthesis of proteins that can function as growth factors, hormones, enzymes, or even as receptors for other steroids or for estrogens. To date, no estrogen receptors per se have been found in bone. So, even though we know that estrogen stops the osteoporotic process, we do not know exactly how it works.

Estrogen may function as a vitamin D antagonist on the bone to prevent resorption. Or, it may function as an agonist in the intestine to promote calcium absorption. Or, it may promote the synthesis of calcitonin, inhibit parathyroid hormone at the level of the bone or at the site of synthesis, or function synergistically with Vitamin D to increase absorption of calcium, increase the sensitivity of the bones to calcitonin, increase the synthesis of vitamin D, etc. The bottom line here is that we do not know how estrogens stop bone resorption. No matter! For women who have a diagnosis of osteoporosis, that is, they have an amount of bone loss that places them at high risk for fracture, estrogen, unless contraindicated, is an option. Proponents of estrogen say that the benefit of stopping additional bone loss with hormone use outweighs most risks associated with it.

This recommendation should not be interpreted to mean that I unequivocally recommend that all women take estrogen to prevent osteoporosis. Such a recommendation is not morally, ethically, or professionally sound. Only about one-third of pre- and postmenopausal Caucasian women have been estimated as being at risk for developing osteoporosis. Why then should the other two-thirds risk compromising health by taking a hormone to prevent a disease that may never develop? Nordin and co-workers (1990) believe that the role of estrogen therapy in preventing osteoporosis and fracture may have been overstated. These researchers argue that it is not clear how much of the bone loss that occurs around menopause should be attributed to aging, and how much should be attributed to menopause. On the one hand, these researchers are quick to note that women do not lose bone as long as estrogen therapy is continued and in adequate dosage. But on the other hand, they caution that there is little data on older women who have a long history of hormone use. Furthermore, they note that if a woman starts estrogen therapy and then stops, the beneficial effect of past estrogen therapy appears to be obscured with time. That is, five years after a woman discontinues the treatment, there is little difference in bone density between treated and untreated women. The catch-22 of this story is that women are advised to take estrogen(s) at menopause and for about five to six years thereafter, the time when bone loss is observed to be the greatest. This therapeutic regimen was thought to afford women with fracture-preventing protection. Nordin and colleagues note that once therapy is stopped, bone loss is rapid. The estrogen protection that was obtained is lost.

Knowing that estrogen's osteoporotic protection is only good as long as the hormone is being used has prompted a new-age version of pharmaceutical company ads, which advocate a return to "estrogen forever" for women–to encourage women to continue taking estrogen until the end of life to either prevent osteoporosis in the first place, or to treat women who have a clinical diagnosis of osteoporosis in order to prevent further bone demineralization. This is a concept that is not likely to be acceptable to women or to many health care providers.

Should a woman choose to use estrogen, therapy must be implemented as soon as a diagnosis of osteoporosis is made, or before menopause if evaluated as high-risk to develop the disease based on lifestyle and/or family history. The Food and Drug Administration recommends the equivalent amount of estrogens found in 0.625 milligrams of conjugated estrogens, which is taken in a cyclic manner (three weeks on and one week off) for osteoporosis prevention. However, since each woman reacts differently to a standard dose of any drug or hormone, it is important that bone scans be done at a minimum of six-month intervals to be sure the dose of estrogen is therapeutic, i.e., that no additional bone has been lost on a particular dosage. Keep in mind that bone loss is most rapid five to six years after menopause. Therefore, it is important to begin taking the hormone as early as possible, that is, premenopausally. It is also important to keep in mind that when hormone therapy is stopped, bone loss accelerates and all of the gains made while on therapy may be eliminated. So, a commitment to estrogen replacement and the risks associated with hormone use (for women with a clinical diagnosis or at high risk of developing osteoporosis) may have to be a lifelong commitment. But a decision to use estrogen should not be a source of fear, guilt, or shame. *Osteoporosis is a disease and should be treated!* Even though risks are associated with estrogen use and combination hormone therapy, frequent consultation with a health care provider will ensure that everything possible is being done to identify early on any potentially lethal side effects.

Whether or not a woman needs to be an estrogen user related to osteoporosis depends on several factors. The main factors are having a family history of the disease, being Caucasian and having small bones and a small stature, being a smoker and/or a drinker of alcohol, and having a history of physical inactivity. My best advice to women considering estrogen therapy is to climb their family tree. Do some genealogical research. Discover what the chances might be for developing osteoporosis by asking mothers, grandmothers, and other family members about their pre- and postmenopausal health and bone condition, and that of the family's ancestry, if possible. As mentioned, I am fortunate that I inherited a strong and large bony frame. I was raised in the country, where walking to get anywhere was the norm. As a teenager I was very active, riding a bicycle, engaging in sports in high school, and continuing with walking, hiking, swimming, and biking as an adult. My diet as a youngster, and, in fact, for most of my life, has been full of calcium-rich dairy products and the right kind of green leafy vegetables that are not calcium leeching. Fractures of any kind by any female members in my family are rare. Unfortunately, my good genetic inheritance and nutritional intake is not a given for all women.

Progestogens

Synthetic progestogens, and perhaps endogenous progesterone, appear to have an anabolic effect on bone, which means they can stimulate bone formation. Does a decrease in the production of this hormone cause bone loss? In 1990, Prior, Vigna, and Schechter examined the effects of various levels of physical activity on bone mass in three groups of menstruating women, age range 21 to 42, who were experiencing regular menstrual cycles. One group of 21 women were training intensively for a marathon. Another group of 22 women ran regularly but less intensively than the marathon group. The third group of 23 women engaged in normal levels of activity. Prior and her researcher colleagues hypothesized that ovulating women runners would have accelerated bone loss if disturbances of ovulatory cycle length developed during training for a marathon, since maintenance of peak bone density throughout adulthood requires normal production of both estrogen and progesterone. After one year, measurements of spinal bone density made on the 66 women decreased, on average, 3.0 milligrams per centimeter per year (which calculated to about 20 percent bone loss). None of the women developed amenorrhea. Prior's group concluded that the decrease in bone density was due to asymptomatic disturbances of ovulation, especially anovulatory cycles. Recall in the chapter on menstruation that I emphasized that menstruation cannot be equated with ovulation. Related to Prior's study, none of the women were amenorrheic; this does not mean that they were ovulating.

This study has been criticized mainly on the basis of its methodology. However, whether or not it is progesterone that is the cause of bone loss in these healthy women, the findings of the study are important. Additional work is needed to find out how common bone loss may be with exercise. An interesting question to emerge from this study, which needs to be answered, is whether the bone loss that occurs in elite athletes or artistic performers (gymnasts, ice skaters, track and field runners/sprinters, ballet dancers, etc.) can be corrected when menstrual cycles return to normal.

Another question in need of answering related to osteoporosis is What is the effect of progestogen replacement on bone? Women who have a definitive diagnosis of osteoporosis and who have their uterus intact must replace estrogen along with progestin. To evaluate the effects of hormone replacement on bone loss, a group of Australian researchers headed by Richard Prince in 1991 compared the effects of an exercise regimen alone, exercise plus calcium, and exercise plus continuous replacement of estrogen and a progestogen. Over a two-year period, they studied 120 women. The study was randomized, double-blind, and placebo-controlled, which means that neither the researchers nor the women knew whether they were taking hormone, calcium, or a sugar pill combined with exercise. What they found was that exercise plus calcium supplementation (in the form of calcium lactate or gluconate) was effective in slowing or stopping bone loss. However, the exercise program alone was ineffective. The exercise plus hormone regimen reduced bone resorption, as well as increased bone density 5.4 percent in the forearm. The researchers concluded that the continuous estrogen and progestogen combination not only stopped bone loss, but it also increased bone density. Side effects associated with the hormone regimen, however, were cited as problems by the women, particularly vaginal bleeding and breast tenderness. Nonetheless, this study has important implications for women with osteoporosis. The researchers recommended that it may be appropriate to advise women with intermediate bone density to adopt the exercise calcium supplementation regimen and to reserve the estrogen or hormone replacement regimen for women with low bone density. This seems like good advice based on a sound research study.

Vitamin D (Calcitriol)

The function of vitamin D, which, incidentally, is both a vitamin (when supplied in the diet), and a hormone (which is the active form of vitamin D synthesized in the skin in the presence of ultraviolet light), is to increase the serum calcium concentration in the blood. It does this by (1) increasing absorption of calcium in the intestines (presumably by initiating the synthesis of a protein, a calcium transport molecule); (2) increasing resorption of bone mineral; and (3) probably by functioning at the level of the kidney to retain calcium. It has been known since the early 1970s that vitamin D functioned as a steroid hormone–binding with a receptor in the cell, etc.

Whether vitamin D deficiency is a major cause of osteoporosis is uncertain, since serum levels of this hormone have been found to be both low and normal among women with postmenopausal osteoporosis. The results of major clinical trials have generated conflicting results, and no studies have been large enough to evaluate the effect of vitamin D on the rate of new fracture incidence as well as safety of the drug for women. In 1989, Tilyard, Spears, and Thompson initiated a three-year randomized clinical trial to determine the rate of new vertebral fractures in women treated with calcitriol (vitamin D), as compared with women on calcium supplementation alone; 622 women, ages 50 to 79 enrolled in the study. None were taking estrogen. In February of 1992 they reported that of the 622 women who enrolled, 515 completed one year of treatment, 476 two years, and 432 completed all three years. The women who took calcitriol, 0.25 micrograms two times a day, had a significant reduction in the number of vertebral fractures experienced: 25 per 100 patient years, versus the women who took 5.2 grams of calcium gluconate supplementation every day. The fracture rate for the calcium group was 31.5 fractures per 100 patient years. The researchers noted that the protective effect of calcitriol was evident in women who had five or fewer fractures on entry into the study. They also felt that taking vitamin D for the three years was not associated with dangerous side effects.

Vitamin D supplementation should be done under the supervision of a health care provider. It is extremely important not to take more than the recommended daily allowance, 400 to 800 international units (IU) per day for men and 200 for women. Most multivitamins contain 400 IU vitamin D. For premenopausal women, 200 IUs is recommended. The dose for menopausal women in their fifties to sixties, and older women in their late sixties to seventies and beyond, may range from 400 to 800 IU/day. One egg yolk, for example, contains 265 IUs; one cup of vitamin D-fortified milk has 100 IUs. So vitamin D supplementation can be enhanced by eating foods that naturally contain it, or by drinking beverages (milk, orange juice) that are fortified with the vitamin. It is always safer to obtain required vitamins and inorganic ions the natural way, in food. Unlike water-soluble vitamins, the body cannot eliminate excess vitamin D. It is a sterol; it is lipid in nature, so the vitamin can accumulate to dangerous, even toxic levels, and can initiate a variety of undesirable side effects. For individuals with heart problems who take digoxin, a drug that regulates the heart rate, vitamin D enhances the side effects of this drug. For more information refer to *Worst Pills, Best Pills*, written by Sydney Wolfe and Rose Ellen Hope.

Calcitonin

In the normal process of regulation of bone and calcium metabolism, the hormone calcitonin functions to block bone resorption, or bone breakdown. Calcitonin functions primarily to regulate blood calcium levels by inhibiting bone resorption. The most potent naturally occurring calcitonin is isolated from salmon. The FDA has approved a nasal spray of calcitonin, "miacalcin," made by Sandoz Pharmaceutical Co. It needs to be taken once a day and with the recommended amounts of calcium and vitamin D. Miacalcin is recommended for women who have osteporosis and are five years beyond menopause.

Drugs

Fosamax (Alendronate Sodium)

Fosamax is a biphosphonate. Its function is to turn off the cells that break down bones. Research indicates that Fosamax reduced the incidence of new spinal fractures by up to 63 percent and built healthy new bone. The maker of Fosamax, Merck, has received clearance from the FDA to market Fosamax after five clinical trials which involved 1,827 women with diagnosed osteoporosis. Merck estimates that the retail price for a 10 mg tablet will vary between $1.65 and $1.80 a day ($600 to $660 annually). Merck has entered into a promotional agreement with Wyeth-Ayerst Laboratories to promote Fosamax in the United States. Merck is also promoting an educational campaign targeted at women to raise consciousness about osteoporosis–that there now is an alternative to hormones. According to the National Women's Health Network, Merck has also subsidized efforts by two companies that make bone density screening equipment. The Network is concerned about these activities. First, through the education blitz, Merck is inflating the need for bone screening. Low bone density is based upon measured levels of bone that are significantly different than those found in healthy, young adults, which results in all older women eventually being diagnosed as osteoporotic. The Network believes that bone density levels need to be compared with women of the same age. The second concern is that the educational campaign will inflate the need for screening, and all women will be encouraged to take the drug.

The long-term safety of Fosamax, like estrogen, has yet to be established. The most frequently cited side effects of Fosamax are abdominal and musculoskeletal pain. Fosamax must be taken in the morning with a glass of water, and a minimum of 30 minutes before any other liquids or solids are ingested. Other biphosphonates are being researched as well as substances that might build bone.

Slow-Release Sodium Fluoride

A team of investigators at the General Clinical Research Center at the University of Texas Southwestern Medical Center in Dallas, headed by Dr. Charles Y. C. Pak, has shown that sodium fluoride, a nonhormonal chemical, reduces the rate of new fractures by 83 percent in women with mild to moderate osteoporosis, and 70 percent for all treated patients. Spinal bone density also increased. Researchers did not observe any of the side effects previously associated with sodium fluoride (peptic ulcers). Their preparation is "slow release" and it is administered with calcium citrate. The cost of the dual drug therapy is estimated at almost $1 per day ($365 a year).

Screening for Osteoporosis: Bone Scans

The areas normally scanned are the vertebrae of the spine, the hips, and the long bones, such as the arm. These are the areas that are most prone to fracture. The earlier prior to menopause that the scans are done, the better. It is important that a premenopausal baseline bone scan be done (if possible) in order to compare with subsequent measurements.

Most large hospitals with outpatient clinics have equipment on-line to do bone scans. Almost all hospitals that have women's centers affiliated with them have scanning equipment available. Prices may vary among institutions. The measurements that can be performed are single- and dual-photon absorptionometry, which is a fancy way of indicating that bone mineral is measured using radioactivity. The principle underpinning this form of measurement is how much energy (that is, photons, which are particles of energy) is absorbed by bone minerals, primarily calcium. The cost of having bone density measured using the dual-photon method may exceed $150; usually, the cost of single-photon measurement is less than this.

Another form of measurement is a modification of the dual-photon method, the dual-energy X-ray absorptiometry. The scan time here is less, which results in less radiation. The cost of this test is estimated to range between $150 to 200. However, it is anticipated that the cost will be less than the dual-photon method because the scan time is faster.

Quantitative computed tomography is an extension of CAT-scan technology, and differs from the photon and X-ray absorptiometry in several important ways. First, the results obtained with this form of measurement reflect three-dimensional density, rather than the two-dimensional density obtained with the other forms of measurement. Second, the radiation source is higher. Third, the cost of the procedure, on average, may be more than $100, possibly as high as $400. (For more details on bone scans, see Melton, Wahner, and Delmas, 1994, p. 97. Also, the August/September 1996 issue of *A Friend Indeed* newsletter has an excellent update on osteoporosis.)

ANN'S ADVICE

1. *The very first thing a woman needs to do, is to "climb her family tree."* Identify whether or not anyone in the family had a diagnosis of osteoporosis or had bone problems.

2. *Women need to "measure up!" It is important to keep a height and weight record.* Height and weight measurements were made on all of us the day we were born. We have height and weight measurements made periodically, when we have a physical examination, in fitness clubs, in physical education classes in school, etc. It is important to continue to make periodic measurements to identify if

and when a change in height occurs. A method of height and weight record keeping is provided in Section IV, Keeping Records and Keeping in Touch.

3. *"Read up!" Be informed.* New information is reported almost daily on the effects of diet and exercise on calcium metabolism and how to maintain a healthy, strong body throughout life.

4. *Complete the following checklist to assess the risk of developing osteoporosis.* If the number of "yes" answers adds up to more than the "no" answers, it is time to "read up," and then begin to "bone-up."

__Yes __No	Do you have a small, thin frame, or are you Caucasian or Asian?
__Yes __No	Do you have a family history of osteoporosis?
__Yes __No	Are you a postmenopausal woman?
__Yes __No	Have you had an early or surgically induced menopause?
__Yes __No	Have you been taking excessive thyroid medication or high doses of cortisone-like drugs for asthma, arthritis, or cancer?
__Yes __No	Is your diet low in dairy products and other sources of calcium?
__Yes __No	Are you physically inactive?
__Yes __No	Do you smoke cigarettes or drink alcohol in excess?

Permission to use granted by the National Osteoporosis Foundation.

5. *Maintain at least 1,000 milligrams of calcium per day,* either by drinking four to five glasses of milk or eating foods high in calcium, especially dairy products, yogurt, sardines, collards, tuna, tofu, nuts, and sunflower seeds. Be careful to avoid calcium-leeching foods such as red meats. High-protein diets remove calcium from the body. Certain other foods and substances decrease calcium absorption, such as soft drinks, caffeine, chocolate, and foods high in fat. If you marinate some foods prior to cooking, do so in vinegar and use the marinade. Vinegar helps to remove calcium from the bone of meat.

6. *Take a calcium supplement only if you cannot take in the amount you need in food to offset losses.* The chewable form is

recommended and needs to be taken at bedtime on an empty stomach. Remember, if you buy over-the-counter calcium preparations, check with your pharmacist regarding how much elemental calcium is in the product. If your care provider recommends two 500 mg calcium carbonate tablets a day, question whether this is meant to provide less than 1,000 mg a day, which means the recommendation is based on total volume of calcium carbonate, rather than "elemental" calcium in the 500 mg product which would liberate only 200 mg (40 percent) of calcium for metabolic needs.

7. *Stress those bones.* Get involved in low impact weight-bearing exercises, such as walking or bicycling.

8. *Maintain adequate vitamin D intake of 400 International Units a day* and get out in the sun for at least 15 minutes a day to convert the inactive form of Vitamin D into the active form.

9. *Refer to Chapters 16 and 17 if you decide to use hormones for osteoporosis prevention or to treat it so that the disease does not progress.* Some of the risks associated with hormone use are documented. Others are still hypothetical. You need to decide what kind of risk you will take. After you have weighed the risks against the benefits, if you decide to take hormones or drugs, you do not need to justify your decision to anyone.

RESOURCES

The National Osteoporosis Foundation, Box MM, 1150 17th Street NW, Suite 500, Washington, DC 20036, will send a free packet of informational brochures that discuss everything from risk to treatment to how to live with osteoporosis.

The National Dairy Council (or your local dairy council if you have one in your city), 6300 N. River Road, Rosemont, IL 60018-4233, has pamphlets available on bone health, and information sheets on calcium, sodium, fat, and cholesterol.

The National Women's Health Network, 514 10th Street NW, Suite 400, Washington, DC 20004 has a packet of information available on osteoporosis, 160 pages. The cost is $8.00 for nonmembers.

SECTION IV.
KEEPING RECORDS
AND KEEPING IN TOUCH

Material in this section will show you how you can take charge, understand what is happening to you and what is to come, and figure out what to do. In this section I have included several methods of keeping records. One of the most important things you can do in coping with hot flashes, menopause, and other perimenopausal changes is to monitor what is happening with your body, and to keep records of these events. This will yield important information that is unique to you. Other books on menopause advise women to take charge of their lives to make informed decisions about their health care. This advice, while well intended, falls short of providing a *way* to take charge. Similarly, I am reminded of a popular commercial on television, wherein prominent actors and actresses promote an educational system that is guaranteed to improve students' grades in school. The program begins with the statement: "Where there is a will, there is an A," which is followed up with the speaker saying, "Don't just tell them [the children] to get better grades, give them the tools."

Here are some tools you can use to take charge, to be an informed consumer of health care:

- Tremin Trust Menstrual Calendar Card
- Menstrual and Ovulatory Calendar Card
- Mansfield/Voda/Jorgensen Bleeding Scale
- Basal Body Temperature Record
- Body Composition Measurement
- Hot Flash Diary

- Hot Flash Record Card
- Hot Flash Body Diagrams
- Breast Monitoring

And, because at some time in our life, each one of us will have to select a care provider, I have also included information on choosing a care provider.

The importance of collecting data cannot be overstated. Because you are unique, you need to collect data on *you*. You need to take your data with you when you consult with your health care provider. You and your data need to be taken seriously by your provider. If not, find someone who *will* take you seriously. Information gained from menstrual, body composition, ovulatory and hot flash records can help you anticipate and prepare for menopause and perimenopausal changes.

I cannot stress too strongly the need to keep records and to begin at any age. The importance of record keeping is validated in the voices of several long-time Tremin Trust participants. One woman wrote a long letter addressing how important a life of record keeping has been for her.

I must tell you how being a part of this research has affected me. My mother became a contributing member of MRH research while she was in college. When I reached menarche, I began contributing also. As much as I disliked the hassle, etc., when my period would start I kept careful notes for the research and enjoyed that so my period was more of a positive for me.

Each year I kept a copy of what I sent to the research project. I became more aware of my body and my menstrual cycle. After a couple of children were born, my cycle changed and for a year or so they were a few days closer together after one child and almost a week farther apart after another. I could usually count 28 days from the first day of my last period and my period would begin within that projected week. At 28 years of age I had delivered four babies and had one miscarriage. From that time my cycle has been 28 days and unless something would come up that caused anxiety or stress, I would ovulate as usual and my period was on time.

After my first child was born, I tried taking my temperature to find out when I was ovulating. Since I breast-fed all my children, I never wanted to take birth control pills. When I was breast feeding, my temperature was not changing much; then I got information about the Ovulation Method. Between the research data and the Ovulation Method, I could really keep a closer tab on my cycle. (I realize and have noted personally that the Ovulation Method works best if one has no drastic changes in emotions and no drastic changes in weight 365 days a year. My stress level has been high since I separated and divorced my first husband. It has been constant for various reasons so I just cope at this level and my periods generally are the same, but I know when my body is reacting to the stress.)

You asked for my thoughts and feelings. Thank you. As the years passed I became more pleased to be a contributor to this project. I am pleased to be a part of it and feel I've learned a lot, too. Each time you add questions to the Health Report Form, I am pleased as it adds to what you can compile in the research. I feel very lucky to be a part of this research and wish OB-GYN doctors and more than a few women could learn as much as this research allows.

I felt that I knew more about what was happening than my doctor when I was pregnant.

Other women responded to a question posed on a survey about the value of record keeping.

I know I talk to more people about menopause, especially asking them when they began (at what age?). I am 51 and think I must be beginning the process although my periods have not been too far off. But not the 26 days they always were. I have been especially interested in finding out who has taken and is taking hormones. Women with severe hot flashes seem to think it is worthwhile; others got along okay without. I am wary of side effects of estrogen. My female physician was almost on a campaign for it and recommended when the time comes to use it—but how does she know I would really need hormones or are they pushing it in medical school? (She is very young and I would be interested to know her decision when she has to make it.)

I'm pleased this research is being done, and proud to be a part of it. I began in 1965, so I'm truly a valid research member. Yes, I read and think about menopause much more openly than I would have years ago (thought it didn't seem real then!). I'm glad to find so many articles readily available on this still rather mysterious subject. I don't look forward to aging, while I'm not generally pessimistic in outlook, this midlife time takes a psychic-emotional toll. I don't buy that the second half of life is better than the first (if health has been okay). One of the certainties is that health won't be okay in this section of life—it has not been my experience in observing others that quality of life gets better with aging—sorry!

I feel it has made me more aware of my periods and things associated with it. I feel good to have been a part of the study all these years and hope it will help others in some way and maybe even me. I don't look at menopause as something to be feared, but a part of life. It is not difficult so far. I have heard others complain of it in the past, just as I have heard the same about raising teenagers; neither have been difficult.

By doing this study, I really pay more attention to the changes in my body, before, during, and after my period. I also am able to know pretty much to the day when I'll start so I am prepared and ready for it to come.

I think I'm better informed than most women (and all men) about menstrual/reproductive problems. The fact that I keep records helps predict the beginning and the next period. However, I experience a little anxiety when it arrives late.

I do think I've thought about it more and perhaps even talked more about it. My daughter just started her period so it is like we are in opposite ends—(can she get a card too?). I realize I really am happy to almost be over with this phase of my life.

I've gained through the years in really knowing my body better because of thorough record keeping. I'm scheduled for a hysterectomy in July, 1992. I have a good knowledge of my entire menstrual history because of the Tremin Trust. Because of the menopause questions I've thought about and identified my own changes or lack of them and I find it easier to work with my doctor and more comfortable to communicate very personal and private facts and feelings. Talking about the female reproductive system has always made me uncomfortable. It was a taboo when I was growing up and I never had pregnancy to help me normalize my feelings. The Tremin Trust survey has helped me so much.

Keeping the detailed calendar has helped me see patterns and made my heavy days more understandable. I've been far more aware of my menstrual changes and reasons why. Also assurances from your questions that I must be in fairly good shape as I have had very few symptoms described or listed as choice options.

Keeping track of my periods over the years has specifically made my life more predictable, and assured me that my menstrual health is normal, cyclical, dependably patterned. You have made me think more about menopause and ask questions of older relatives and read more. I feel better informed, less afraid.

Being from a medical family we have always talked about things like this freely. I'm probably the one who would ask more questions and talk about it more through the years though. My dad died when I was 18 and Mom died six years ago. My sister and I talk about menopause relatively often, just to compare notes. I hope I stop having periods this year so I don't have to do this questionnaire again. I feel very strongly though about not quitting with the research because my mom was one of the first people who started this program so she must have thought it very important. I will continue for her.

I think that keeping track of my periods and the flow patterns has made me more aware of my body. I think I've been influential in getting several female friends to go to a GYN when they were having problems. Being a widow and not having a consistent sexual or emotionally supportive partner has probably affected me more than any hormonal changes or PMS could.

I hadn't really thought about being close or into menopause age until participating in the study. I now recognize that weight gain, menstrual cycle changes, and irritability may be due to menopause or beginning menopause.

I'm happy to be part of research in this program. I've liked having the card for personal reference. My doctor likes the card as well, when I bring it to show how my periods have been.

Chapter 19

Calendar Cards
and the Bleeding Scale

I began my menstrual record keeping during my doctoral research. The accurate performance of hormone assays necessitated—in fact demanded—that I keep a record of my menstruations so that I knew when I was in the luteal phase of my cycle so I would not affect the hormone assays. When I took the necessary precautions, based on my records, my work proceeded smoothly. I continued to record my menstruation starts and stops so I would know when I was menopausal.

On October 7, 1981, I had my last menstrual bleed; actually, it was a spot. Following that day, I became a postmenopausal woman. But I would not be able to declare this until my record showed that one full calendar year had passed without a bleed. And you will not know when you become menopausal if you do not keep a record. Menopause is an event to remember, to claim as our own, to share with the next generation of women, daughters, and granddaughters who will have questions about the transition as well as the age of onset of menopause. Keeping menstrual records will keep us in touch, one with the other. I have included three methods of recording menstruations—the menstrual calendar card, the menstrual ovulation calendar card, and the Mansfield/Voda/Jorgensen bleeding scale.

THE MENSTRUAL CALENDAR CARD

The first is the menstrual calendar card, developed by Alan Treloar (see Figure 19.1). It is simple to use, and is being used today by

FIGURE 19.1. Menstrual Calendar Card (Front and Reverse Sides)

THE TREMIN TRUST

Circle first and last menstrual dates and join with a line.

Place dot above date for spot.

Place / thru date for non-menstrual bleed

Example: 9 10 11 12 13 14 15 16 17 18 19 20 21

Menstrual Calendar Card, Year

Please make notations here of:
1. Any flow period for which an accurate record was omitted from the calendar for any reason. This is VERY IMPORTANT
2. Any events which you think might have altered your normal menstrual pattern or which caused you to bleed between periods. This includes records of surgery (named), illnesses, medications, or any life event.
3. An explanation of any symbols you may have used on the other side of this card.

_____

_____

_____

_____

_____

_____

_____

_____

_____

_____

This is a research document of
The Tremin Trust
Rm. 501, College of Nursing
University of Utah
Salt Lake City, UT 84112

women participants in The Tremin Trust Research Program on Women's Health. To use this card:

1. Make several photocopies of the card.
2. Circle the first and last days of menstruation. Then, connect the circles with a straight line.

In the example provided, menstrual Day 1 was on January 1. This date is circled. The circles are joined by a straight line. This bleeding interval was of six days' duration. The back of the card can be used as a personal diary to record any unusual events associated with menstruation.

Be sure to mark your calendar for each menstrual bleed. It is easy to forget from one month to the next. This card is small and can easily fit inside a purse. In fact, some women in the research program carry it with them all of the time, and they take it with them when they travel.

Until you perceive the quality of your bleeds to change, the little menstrual calendar card would be the most efficient way to keep track of menstruations. However, once the bleeding pattern changes, you will want to begin collecting bleeding interval data using the bleeding scale described in the third method, and to share these data with your health care provider.

THE MENSTRUAL OVULATION CALENDAR CARD

The second method of collecting menstrual data allows you to systematically record your menstruations as well as your ovulations (see Figure 19.2). During the pre- and perimenopause, as I indicated in the chapter on menstruation, the frequency of ovulatory periods declines. Ovulation does occur, but sporadically. The variability in ovulation during the perimenopausal period no doubt explains why some women who are symptomatic for a period of time suddenly have a remission of symptoms. They have ovulated and their follicles are making estrogen and progesterone.

Keeping a record of your basal body temperature (which will be described in the next section) is important if for no other reason than that it is a way for you to collect valid data on your menstrual cycle:

FIGURE 19.2. Menstrual and Ovulation Calendar

Months											Days														Days								F	I	D
	1	2	3	4	5	6	7	8	9	10	11	12	13	14	15	16	17	18	19	20	21	22	23	24	25	26	27	28	29	30	31			
BBT																																		
	1	2	3	4	5	6	7	8	9	10	11	12	13	14	15	16	17	18	19	20	21	22	23	24	25	26	27	28	29	30	31			
BBT																																		
	1	2	3	4	5	6	7	8	9	10	11	12	13	14	15	16	17	18	19	20	21	22	23	24	25	26	27	28	29	30	31			
BBT																																		
	1	2	3	4	5	6	7	8	9	10	11	12	13	14	15	16	17	18	19	20	21	22	23	24	25	26	27	28	29	30	31			
BBT																																		
	1	2	3	4	5	6	7	8	9	10	11	12	13	14	15	16	17	18	19	20	21	22	23	24	25	26	27	28	29	30	31			
BBT																																		
	1	2	3	4	5	6	7	8	9	10	11	12	13	14	15	16	17	18	19	20	21	22	23	24	25	26	27	28	29	30	31			
BBT																																		
	1	2	3	4	5	6	7	8	9	10	11	12	13	14	15	16	17	18	19	20	21	22	23	24	25	26	27	28	29	30	31			
BBT																																		
	1	2	3	4	5	6	7	8	9	10	11	12	13	14	15	16	17	18	19	20	21	22	23	24	25	26	27	28	29	30	31			
BBT																																		
	1	2	3	4	5	6	7	8	9	10	11	12	13	14	15	16	17	18	19	20	21	22	23	24	25	26	27	28	29	30	31			
BBT																																		
	1	2	3	4	5	6	7	8	9	10	11	12	13	14	15	16	17	18	19	20	21	22	23	24	25	26	27	28	29	30	31			
BBT																																		
	1	2	3	4	5	6	7	8	9	10	11	12	13	14	15	16	17	18	19	20	21	22	23	24	25	26	27	28	29	30	31			
BBT																																		
	1	2	3	4	5	6	7	8	9	10	11	12	13	14	15	16	17	18	19	20	21	22	23	24	25	26	27	28	29	30	31			
BBT																																		
	1	2	3	4	5																													
BBT																																		

BBT = basal body temperature   F = flow   I = interval   D = diary

325

Am I ovulating or am I not? You do not need to go to a doctor to have the concentration of your sex hormones measured to find this out. These tests cost a lot of money, and they really don't tell you anything that you cannot figure out on your own. You will know how you are feeling and what symptoms you have. If you know that your periods have changed in quality and also in duration between bleeds, putting those data together with the information on whether or not you are ovulating will help explain why, as well as why you are or you are not, experiencing symptoms.

To use this menstrual ovulation calendar card, follow this procedure:

1. Make several photocopies of the card before you make any entries.
2. Print in the months on the left-hand side, starting with the month you will begin your record keeping.
3. When your period starts, either circle the number or mark an "X" through the day of the month. Do the same thing for every day of menstrual bleeding. Should you spot between periods, mark an S above the date the spotting occurs. The first menstrual day is the start of a new menstrual period.
4. Do the same thing at the onset of the next menstrual period. To calculate the number of days for a menstrual period, count from the day of onset of one menstrual bleed through to the day *before* the onset of the next bleed. As shown in the example calendar, the first period started on January 21, and lasted three days (21, 22, and 23). The onset of the next period was February 14. The menstrual interval, or days between menstrual bleeds, is calculated by counting the days from January 21 through February 13, which is 24 days. This information is recorded in the I column (I is for interval) on the right-hand side of the calendar.
5. To record the number of days of menstrual bleeding, count the number of days bleeding occurred, and record this information in the F (for flow) column. In the example calendar (Figure 19.3), three days of menstrual bleeding occurred during January.
6. To record whether a menstrual period was eventful (accompanied by cramps, back pain, excessive bloating, heavy bleeding,

FIGURE 19.3. Sample Menstrual and Ovulation Calendar

Months	1	2	3	4	5	6	7	8	9	10	11	12	13	14	15	16	17	18	19	20	21	22	23	24	25	26	27	28	29	30	31	F	I	D
January	1	2	3	4	5	6	7	8	9	10	11	12	13	14	15	16	17	18	19	20	21	22	23	24	25	26	27	28	29	30	31	3		24
BBT																																		
February	1	2	3	4	5	6	7	8	9	10	11	12	13	14	15	16	17	18	19	20	21	22	23	24	25	26	27	28	29	30	31	4		26
BBT																																		
March	1	2	3	4	5	6	7	8	9	10	11	12	13	14	15	16	17	18	19	20	21	22	23	24	25	26	27	28	29	30	31	5		24
BBT																																		
April	1	2	3	4	5	6	7	8	9	10	11	12	13	14	15	16	17	18	19	20	21	22	23	24	25	26	27	28	29	30	31	4		27
BBT																																		
May	1	2	3	4	5	6	7	8	9	10	11	12	13	14	15	16	17	18	19	20	21	22	23	24	25	26	27	28	29	30	31	3		25
BBT																																		
June	1	2	3	4	5	6	7	8	9	10	11	12	13	14	15	16	17	18	19	20	21	22	23	24	25	26	27	28	29	30	31	3		39
BBT																																		
July	1	2	3	4	5	6	7	8	9	10	11	12	13	14	15	16	17	18	19	20	21	22	23	24	25	26	27	28	29	30	31			
BBT																																		
	1	2	3	4	5	6	7	8	9	10	11	12	13	14	15	16	17	18	19	20	21	22	23	24	25	26	27	28	29	30	31			
BBT																																		
	1	2	3	4	5	6	7	8	9	10	11	12	13	14	15	16	17	18	19	20	21	22	23	24	25	26	27	28	29	30	31			
BBT																																		
	1	2	3	4	5	6	7	8	9	10	11	12	13	14	15	16	17	18	19	20	21	22	23	24	25	26	27	28	29	30	31			
BBT																																		
	1	2	3	4	5	6	7	8	9	10	11	12	13	14	15	16	17	18	19	20	21	22	23	24	25	26	27	28	29	30	31			
BBT																																		
	1	2	3	4	5	6	7	8	9	10	11	12	13	14	15	16	17	18	19	20	21	22	23	24	25	26	27	28	29	30	31			
BBT																																		
	1	2	3	4	5	6	7	8	9	10	11	12	13	14	15	16	17	18	19	20	21	22	23	24	25	26	27	28	29	30	31			
BBT																																		

BBT = basal body temperature   F = flow   I = Interval   D = diary

327

clots, etc.), put a check mark in the D (for diary) column, and use the diary page to record in your own words the changes you perceived in your body or in the quantity or quality of your menstrual flow.

MANSFIELD/VODA/JORGENSEN BLEEDING SCALE

At menopause, it is not unusual for the bleeding pattern to change along with changes in the duration of the menstrual and bleeding intervals. It is important to record the quality of the bleeding, since, as mentioned in Chapter 12, it is the perceived change in the quality of bleeding that is a major reason women seek out health care providers during the perimenopause. As such, bleeding data is important data to collect since it is on the basis of self-report of changes in the quality of bleeding that a care provider may suggest hormone or surgical treatment.

Dr. Phyllis Mansfield created a six-point rating scale to estimate the volume of blood lost. This tool is being used in our Midlife Women's Health Study to identify how the pattern of bleeding changes during perimenopause. The tool is called the Mansfield/Voda/Jorgensen Bleeding Scale. It is shown in Figures 19.4 and 19.5.

To use the MVJBS, use the following procedure:

1. Select a single digit code number from Figure 19.4 that best describes how light or heavy your menstrual flow is that day.
2. Write that number as clearly as you can on the menstrual calendar card above each day you are bleeding or spotting.
3. Write that number as precisely as you can in the space above the calendar date.

In the example provided, January 1 is circled as the first menstrual day. A "1" is placed above this date to indicate that the quality of the bleeding does not or would not require protection. On January 2, a rating of "4" indicates that the bleeding was moderate, that a change of regular absorbency tampon or pad was required every three to four hours. On January 3 and 4, the rating of "3" indicates light bleeding. And on January 5 and 6, a rating of "2" indicates that bleeding was very light, that the least absorbent type of product was required once or twice a day. A circle on January 6 indicates menstruation stopped.

Be sure to mark your calendar *every single day that you are menstruating*. It is very easy to forget from one day to the next, so to avoid problems remembering what happened to you yesterday, take a moment each day of your period and mark your calendar. At nighttime, before bed, is probably the best time to do this, when you know what your bleeding has been like all day. *Keep your calendar next to your bedside to make it convenient to mark before bedtime. Don't forget to take it along with you when you travel!*

FIGURE 19.4. Mansfield/Voda/Jorgensen Bleeding Scale

1= *Spotting.* You experience a drop or two of blood on your underwear, not requiring sanitary protection (although you may personally prefer to use a pantyliner).

2= *Very light bleeding.* You need to change the least absorbent type of tampon or pad once or twice a day to feel protected.

3= *Light bleeding.* You need to change a low or regular absorbency tampon or pad two or three times a day to feel protected.

4= *Moderate bleeding.* You need to change a regular absorbency tampon or pad every three or four hours to feel protected.

5= *Heavy bleeding.* You need to change a high absorbency tampon or pad every three or four hours to feel protected.

6= *Very heavy bleeding (gushing).* Sanitary protection hardly works at all. You need to change the highest absorbency tampon every hour or two to feel protected.

FIGURE 19.5. Menstrual Bleeding Calendar Card

Calendar year   only

JANUARY
1 2 3 4 5 6 7 8 9 10 11 12 13 14 15 16 17 18 19 20 21 22 23 24 25 26 27 28

FEBRUARY
29 30 31 1 2 3 4 5 6 7 8 9 10 11 12 13 14 15 16 17 18 19 20 21 22 23 24 25

MARCH
26 27 28 1 2 3 4 5 6 7 8 9 10 11 12 13 14 15 16 17 18 19 20 21 22 23 24 25

APRIL
26 27 28 29 30 31 1 2 3 4 5 6 7 8 9 10 11 12 13 14 15 16 17 18 19 20 21 22

MAY
23 24 25 26 27 28 29 30 1 2 3 4 5 6 7 8 9 10 11 12 13 14 15 16 17 18 19 20

JUNE
21 22 23 24 25 26 27 28 29 30 31 1 2 3 4 5 6 7 8 9 10 11 12 13 14 15 16 17

JULY
18 19 20 21 22 23 24 25 26 27 28 29 30 1 2 3 4 5 6 7 8 9 10 11 12 13 14 15

AUGUST
16 17 18 19 20 21 22 23 24 25 26 27 28 29 30 31 1 2 3 4 5 6 7 8 9 10 11 12

SEPTEMBER
13 14 15 16 17 18 19 20 21 22 23 24 25 26 27 28 29 30 31 1 2 3 4 5 6 7 8 9

OCTOBER
10 11 12 13 14 15 16 17 18 19 20 21 22 23 24 25 26 27 28 29 30 1 2 3 4 5 6 7

NOVEMBER
8 9 10 11 12 13 14 15 16 17 18 19 20 21 22 23 24 25 26 27 28 29 30 31 1 2 3 4

DEC-EMBER
5 6 7 8 9 10 11 12 13 14 15 16 17 18 19 20 21 22 23 24 25 26 27 28 29 30 1 2
3 4 5 6 7 8 9 10 11 12 13 14 15 16 17 18 19 20 21 22 23 24 25 26 27 28 29 30 31

Chapter 20

Basal Body Temperature and Ovulation Monitoring

A woman who has ovulated will find that her temperature rises each cycle after ovulation. Measurement of body temperature, using the method of basal body temperature measurement (BBT) is a simple, inexpensive, and reliable means of detecting ovulation. During the past 10 to 15 years there has been a virtual explosion of newly developed techniques marketed to detect ovulation. Commercial products on the market are useful for women who want to absolutely pinpoint the LH surge so that they can either avoid pregnancy (by avoiding intercourse or using protection), or try to become pregnant. These ovulation predictors are not entirely accurate, and they are expensive.

You will know whether ovulation has occurred if body temperature increases. In technical terms, the change in body temperature that occurs after ovulation, when it is plotted on graph paper, is referred to as a *biphasic curve*. This means that body temperature increases after ovulation and stays elevated until a day or two before menstration while at basal conditions (not moving, etc.). Why the temperature increases after ovulation is not absolutely understood. However, it is thought that it is an effect of progesterone. Any time there is an increase in metabolic activity, such as what occurs in the uterus related to prepregnancy preparations, theoretically, heat is generated as a by-product.

If you measure your temperature at basal conditions and you do not find an increase in temperature, you cannot absolutely infer that ovulation has *not* occurred. A flat kind of BBT curve is referred to as a monophasic curve; in other words, there is little or no change in temperature. A biphasic curve, however, is indicative of ovulation.

Measurement of BBT for women who have had a hysterectomy, but with ovaries retained, is a way to self-monitor for menopausal status.

Hysterectomized women have no outward indicator (change in bleeding) to tell them that the change process has started. The simple BBT method to detect that ovulation has occurred is as follows.

1. Take your temperature each and every morning either orally or rectally, whichever you prefer, but you must choose a site and use the same site every morning.
2. Use a regular fever-detecting thermometer. Special basal body thermometers are available, but you do not need one, and they are expensive.
3. Prior to taking your temperature, do not get out of bed to urinate, do not smoke, and do not engage in any physical activity. To do so disturbs basal conditions necessary for an accurate measurement.
4. Before taking your temperature, shake the thermometer down to 96° Fahrenheit or 35° Centigrade. If you shake it down before you go to bed at night and place it on your bedside table, you will not have to shake it down in the morning. Place the thermometer under the left side of the tongue as far back in the mouth as possible. Close your mouth and leave the thermometer in place for a minimum of three minutes. The longer you leave it in place, the more reliable the reading will be.
5. Record your temperature daily on the Menstrual Calendar (Figures 19.1 and 19.2) in the BBT column under the numbers.
6. Note the temperature change. If you have ovulated, your temperature will increase about 0.4 to 0.8° Fahrenheit *after* you have ovulated. The temperature will stay up until a day or two prior to your next menstrual period. On the sample Menstrual Calendar, note the progressive increase in BBT after February 1, which was sustained until two days prior to menstruation.
7. Family planners recommend recording BBT on a sheet of graph paper. This provides a visual method of determining whether or not cycles are ovulatory, since the sustained rise in temperature has been plotted on the graph. If you want to supplement this method of record keeping with your menstrual/ovulatory calendar, all you need do is buy some graph paper and a loose-leaf binder. Plot BBT on the graph paper per the sample BBT Graph (Figure 20.1) on page 333.

FIGURE 20.1. Sample Basal Body Temperature Graph

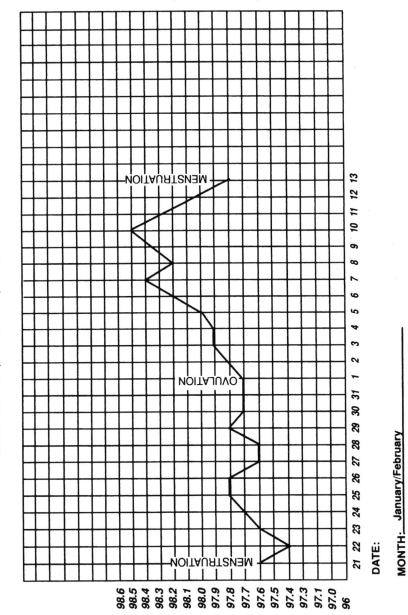

SAMPLE BASAL BODY TEMPERATURE CHART
Degree Fahrenheit

DATE:

MONTH: January/February

Chapter 21

Body Composition Monitoring: The Shape of Things to Come

Except for being a fat baby at birth (more than 8 pounds), I have always been on the lean or thin side. So, contrary to the old wives' tale, being a fat baby did not mean that I would be a fat woman. Whether this was due to my genes, or the fact that I have always eaten a fairly well-balanced diet, avoiding preservatives and emphasizing natural substances, fresh fruits, and vegetables, or that combined with the fact that I have generally been a physically active person, I do not know. I have monitored my weight on a yearly basis and know that I have changed over the years from a young adult weight of about 140 pounds, to 155 to 159 pounds in 1981, the year of my menopause. I do not know whether menopause had anything to do with weight gain, but I do know that in addition to weight gain, I experienced a redistribution of body fat. My body was changing, and areas which never had any fat, such as my abdomen, suddenly developed a "menopausal belly." After three months of reducing food intake, eating a well-balanced diet, plus increasing in physical exercise during the summer months, I returned to an earlier weight of about 141 to 142 pounds, and maintained this weight until the summer of 1983. I then took a new job, full of new stresses. I was experiencing hot flashes, and my physical activity had decreased, largely due to the fact that I wasn't riding a bicycle to work any longer. I slowly but surely put on about 10 pounds, which put me up to 152. But while I put on the weight, particularly when I increased to about 148 and above, I noticed a reduction in the frequency and intensity of my hot flashes.

This was great in terms of restful sleep, productivity during the day, and just plain comfort. As I started to exercise and firmed up without losing a lot of weight (3 pounds), returning to 149 pounds, I realized that my hot flashes had returned almost to the intensity that they had been prior to the increase in weight. I am not saying that the return of my hot flashes is a direct result of the change in body fat, but the association of an increase in hot flash intensity and frequency with the change in my body fat is supportive enough to suggest a real role for estrogen metabolism in fatty tissue. This indicates the need for more research to answer basic questions about changes in body composition, and the percent of body fat needed as we move into midlife, experience menopause, and progress into our later years.

Since the initial measurement of body composition was made and recorded for most people at birth, there is no easier or better way than to continue to do it on a yearly basis on one's birthday.

DIRECTIONS FOR MEASURING BODY COMPOSITION: HEIGHT AND WEIGHT RECORD

The equipment for measuring bone mass is not available to the average care provider. It is available at menopause clinics and women's health centers in large cities. Measurement of bone mass is very expensive. The methods of measurement are described in Chapter 18. You can supplement measurement data by studying your family tree, and by keeping records of regular height measurements.

The early bone changes related to osteoporosis occur in the upper body. They are called crush fractures, and they cause a shortening of the spinal column. Consequently, changes in height may possibly reflect bone demineralization. You will need assistance to measure your height accurately. *Accuracy* cannot be stressed too greatly. The decrease in height may be no more than a centimeter.

1. Paste a tape measure on a wall (much as you might have done to measure growth in children) and leave it there permanently.
2. Stand in bare feet, back against the wall, heels together and touching the tape. Permanently mark the position of your feet so that you can stand in the same spot each time you measure. Look at Figure 21.1 for a picture of the suggested way to do it.

3. As indicated in Figure 21.1, stand erect and have someone else place a flat object on your head. A small carpenter's level may be best in order to assure accuracy, but, until you get one, a ruler, book, board, etc., will have to do. Keep the object level and place it against the tape. The point where the underside of the object contacts the tape will measure your total height. Mark the tape.
4. Record the measurement on your Menstrual Calendar Card. You can also monitor your height another way. If you make a measurement from the head to the pubic bone, and from the heel to the pubic bone, the two measurements should be the same. The procedure is found in Figure 21.2. If height from head to pubic bone is less than that from pubic bone to heels, osteoporosis may be the cause. However, it is almost impossible to get repeatedly accurate measurements of the upper body, so do not panic if these measurements are not equal. People differ greatly in anatomical structure, and even though we would like to think that we are "perfectly proportioned," we are not. Some people are long-legged. Others have long torsos. The important point to remember is to start keeping records of your height and weight, hopefully before menopause. Then if you do measure a loss in height, especially upper body height, and you are at high risk for osteoporosis, there is cause to suspect osteoporosis. In this event, see a care provider and ask for a thorough evaluation of your bones. Request a bone densitometry examination, which will ascertain the density of your bones.

Recording weight can provide important information in coping with the hot flash. As I discussed, with weight gain you may notice a decrease in hot flash frequency and intensity. Conversely, the thinner you become, hot flashes may become more frequent and intense. You will want to record height and weight in the margins of your Menstrual Calendar Card.

If you want to be able to estimate what percent of your weight is fat and what percent is muscle mass, you can do so by having a care provider perform two simple body composition measurements: midarm circumference, and triceps skin-fold thickness.

FIGURE 21.2. Measurement of Upper Body Height

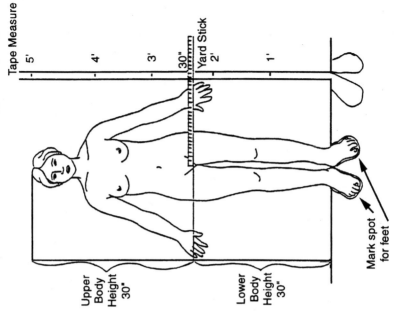

Tape Measure

5'
4'
3'
30"
Yard Stick
2'
1'

Upper Body Height 30"

Lower Body Height 30"

Mark spot for feet

FIGURE 21.1. How to Measure Height

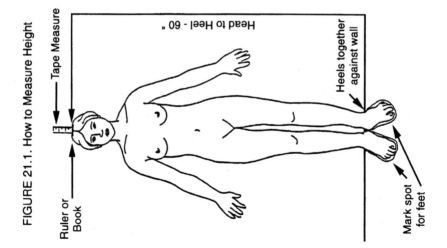

Tape Measure

Ruler or Book

Head to Heel - 60"

Heels together against wall

Mark spot for feet

Ross Laboratories (a division of Abbott Laboratories, Columbus, OH) produces a Nutritional Assessment Kit, which is distributed free to health care professionals. The kit contains materials and instructions on how to perform the measurements to estimate body fat. For nonprofessionals it is best to have the triceps measured by your care provider, since it is not possible to do alone, and the skin-fold caliper is expensive.

As with the other measurements, if you measure your triceps, keep a record and mark the value on your Menstrual Calendar Card each time you measure. Then eyeball your hot flash frequency from year to year and see if it changes if your percent of fat changes.

Chapter 22

Hot Flash Monitoring

HOT FLASH RECORD/DIARY

Because one of the first signs for many women that menopause is approaching is the hot flash, understanding your own hot flash experience is of great importance. In the beginning the hot flash may be merely a feeling of warmth, or it may be a one-time episode. Usually, the closer a woman gets to her last menstrual bleed, the more intense and frequent hot flashes become. Because certain foods, the time of day, and specific events can trigger a hot flash, keeping a record of your hot flashes may possibly help you alleviate or lessen them without the use of drugs. The record will provide you with a systematic examination of when, how frequently, and under what circumstances your hot flashes occur. It is possible, then, that avoiding what triggers your hot flash will help you to avoid the flashes themselves. See Figure 22.1 for an example of the hot flash record card. Keep the record for two consecutive weeks at least once a year. Any less time will not assure you of an accurate hot flash pattern. Follow these steps to use the hot flash record card:

1. Make several extra photocopies of the card before you make any entries.
2. Fill in the day and date on the left-hand side. When you have a hot flash, make a mark on the card that corresponds to the appropriate hour you had the flash. Look at the sample hot flash card (Figure 22.2). As an example, if a hot flash occurred at 6:20 a.m., put a mark in the space under the 6-7 a.m. section. In order to note the intensity (mild, moderate, severe) of the hot flash, we suggest you use three colored pens for marking

the flashes, such as green, blue, and red. Remember, your hot flash experience is unique to you.

3. In the box below the hot flash marks, record the event that preceded the hot flash. For example, if the hot flash is related to drinking hot coffee, record coffee. In order to have enough room on the record card, it will be necessary for you to develop a simple coding system that is workable for you. In the sample card, the following code is used:

C = coffee
A = activity (letting out the dogs, making coffee, etc.)
E = eating
W = working
S = sleeping
H = heat (from heat vent)
R = stress
T = television
B = alcoholic beverages
D = diary

The D code indicates that you have made a diary entry, explaining in more detail the circumstances of a particular hot flash. For example, it is important to indicate the subject matter on television that may have been the specific trigger, or it may simply have been the time of day that is the trigger, or the temperature of the room.

4. In the F column on the right-hand side of the card, keep a daily count of your hot flash frequency. Count the number of hot flashes for the day and enter the number in the appropriate box under F. At the end of two weeks, you will know your hot flash frequency per day and the total number you had over a two-week period. Our research indicates that most women have their highest frequency from 6 to 8 a.m. This does not mean that something is wrong with you if you have a different experience.

5. Note from your diary the events that seem to precede hot flashes, and develop ways of coping that may be different for you than those outlined earlier.

6. Keep the hot flash record once a year for as long as you experience the flashes. Do your record keeping at as close to the same time of year as possible. If you started recording January 21, 1983, do your next record in January for two weeks. Over the years, after menopause, you should note a decrease in both frequency and intensity.

HOT FLASH BODY DIAGRAMS

Since stress modification can help prevent many hot flashes, identifying your specific hot flash origin(s) is the first step in coping with the hot flash.

1. Photocopy several sets of the body diagrams (Figure 22.3). Some women have more than one hot flash origin and spread, and you will want to ensure that you have one or two extra diagrams.
2. On the origin portion of the diagrams, indicate the part of the body where your hot flash starts, i.e., where you first perceive the heat. Refer to the sample hot flash body diagram (Figure 22.4).
3. Name the area, that is, head, cheek, earlobe, neck, chest, belly, back, etc. Write it down on the page.
4. Draw an arrow pointing to where it starts. This will help you to localize the origin more specifically. Use as many of the diagrams as necessary.
5. Shade-in the specific area. If you named the head as the hot flash origin, shade in only the area affected. Some women experience hot flash origin only on the top of their heads; some women on the back of the neck.
6. On the spread diagrams, name the body area of the spread, and then draw an arrow to indicate the parts of the body involved. Then shade-in the area. Circle the intensity of the hot flash, i.e., mild (M), moderate (MO), severe (S).
7. Repeat the process at least three times. Some women have different origins and spreads for differing hot flash intensities.
8. Repeat the body diagram record keeping on a yearly basis.

FIGURE 22.1. Hot Flash Record Card

Day/Date	a.m. hours												p.m. hours												F
	12-1	1-2	2-3	3-4	4-5	5-6	6-7	7-8	8-9	9-10	10-11	11-12	12-1	1-2	2-3	3-4	4-5	5-6	6-7	7-8	8-9	9-10	10-11	11-12	
Hot Flash																									
Trigger																									
Hot Flash																									
Trigger																									
Hot Flash																									
Trigger																									
Hot Flash																									
Trigger																									
Hot Flash																									
Trigger																									
Hot Flash																									
Trigger																									

F = frequency

FIGURE 22.2. Sample Hot Flash Record Card

Day/Date	a.m. hours												p.m. hours												F
	12-1	1-2	2-3	3-4	4-5	5-6	6-7	7-8	8-9	9-10	10-11	11-12	12-1	1-2	2-3	3-4	4-5	5-6	6-7	7-8	8-9	9-10	10-11	11-12	
Dec. 20, 1996 Hot Flash	/		/		/		///	///		/			/	/	?				B	/	E				15
Trigger	S		S	S	S	A/E	A	W/C					E	C	?				B/E	/	/		T		
Dec. 21, 1996 Hot Flash			/	/		/	//	//		/	/			//	/				/	/		/			13
Trigger			S	S		A/E	A/H		C			W/C	?						B		T				
Dec. 22, 1996 Hot Flash				/	/		/	/					C	C	/			B	/	/		T			9
Trigger				S	S	A	A		C																
Hot Flash																									
Trigger																									
Hot Flash																									
Trigger																									
Hot Flash																									
Trigger																									
Hot Flash																									
Trigger																									

F = frequency

345

FIGURE 22.3. Hot Flash Body Diagrams

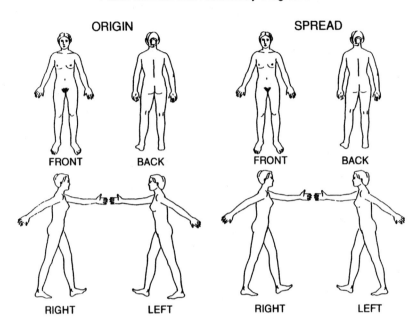

FIGURE 22.4. Sample Hot Flash Body Diagrams

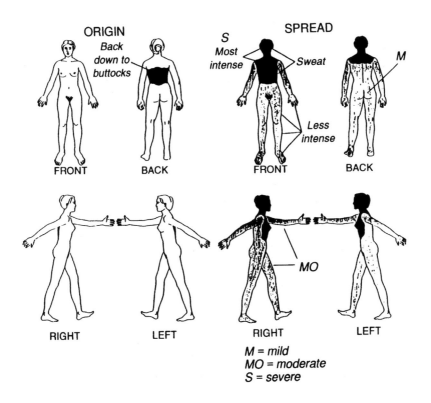

M = mild
MO = moderate
S = severe

Chapter 23

Choosing a Care Provider

At one time or another, each of us will need to consult a care provider. If hot flashes become unbearable, if periods become too painful, if moody episodes become too frequent, if bleeding becomes too frequent or too heavy and fatigue sets in, if joint pain becomes unbearable, if vaginal burning and itching interfere with sexual intercourse or cause painful urination, if urinary incontinence becomes more frequent despite exercising, if changes in sexual function create a problem, or if any other "ifs" become too great for you to care for yourself and you feel you need help, then it is time to consult a care provider. To delay doing so could worsen the problem.

HOW DO YOU FIND A CARE PROVIDER?

Choosing a care provider involves taking into consideration your personal value system, the acuity of the situation for which you need care (how bad is it?), where you live, and how much money you have to spend. In the past, women have sought out gynecologists for menstrual and menopausal concerns simply because there was no one else to turn to. Women have options now, and can choose whether they want to consult with a gynecologist (which until recently have mostly been male), or a certified family nurse practitioner (usually female). If they realize that their problem requires the resources of a specialized care provider, such as a psychotherapist, a sex counselor, marriage counselor, or any of a large variety of care practitioners, these options are also available.

In the final analysis, you are the one who must choose a provider. You can do so by picking a name out of a phone book, consulting with family and friends, or calling the local medical and nursing associations for a list of names. The National Women's Health Network has published a list of women's resource centers throughout the country in their *Resource Guide 7*. This list can be extremely useful in helping you contact those who can assist you in locating a care provider to meet your needs. For information on how to obtain it, write to them at 514 10th St. Suite 400 NW, Washington, DC 20005. The North American Menopause Society also has a list of professional practitioners in a variety of geographical areas who have agreed to be listed in a resource directory. Write to them at P.O. Box 94527, Cleveland OH 44101-4527.

RESOURCES FOR REFERENCES

1. Family and friends
2. Phone book
3. Associations such as the American Medical Association, State Medical Association, American Nurses Association, State Nurses Association, YWCA, Women's Resource Centers, etc.
4. Telephone interviews to ascertain costs and attitude toward women and health care

INTERVIEWING

During the initial consultation, and at any other time, feel free to interview your health care provider. You have certain rights and privileges as a patient. If those rights are not respected, you may want to choose someone different. Things to consider in such an interview include the following:

1. It is not unusual for sexism (attitudes male care providers have about women) to be in operation. Your provider may call you by your first name, but can you do the same with him? Does your provider call you "honey," "sweetie," "sugar," or some

other "pet" title, or tell you that you are a "good woman?" These may be indications of sexist prejudices.

2. You have the right to ask questions, including questions about the provider's attitudes regarding hormone use, hysterectomy, mastectomy, and why she or he advocates a particular approach to treatment. There are some providers who advocate the same treatment plan for all women. You need to know why they think the way they do. For example, many gynecologists remove ovaries routinely when doing a hysterectomy. You need to ask why. Others routinely place women on hormone replacement to prevent osteoporosis. Ask for the data used to make the diagnosis of osteoporosis, or that you are at high risk for osteoporosis.

3. It is okay to ask the provider about his or her experience and background, particularly if surgery is recommended.

4. It is okay and highly recommended to get a second opinion.

5. You have the right to refuse any treatment. In fact, it is best if you can take time to think over the options (if any were presented).

6. It is okay to call your provider if you think you are having a reaction to a drug or hormone replacement or treatment of any kind. Hormones can cause bleeding, headaches, leg pain, breast tenderness, bloating, etc. Some of the new drugs for osteoporosis can make you sick unless directions are followed precisely. Do not continue with treatment if you think you are having a reaction.

EVALUATING A PROVIDER

After initial consultation, evaluate the care provider by asking yourself the following questions:

1. Was I taken seriously? Were my concerns validated or invalidated?

2. Could I ask questions and get honest, straightforward answers?

3. Did I feel comfortable during the examination? Did I feel respected?

4. Was the care provider rushed? How much time did I spend with her or him for the money spent?
5. Was I satisfied with the treatment plan provided or suggested, i.e., drugs, surgery, therapy? Was I given options and time to think?
6. Was I treated like a child, an object, a uterus or a breast disassociated from a human body? A human being?
7. Was I advised to come in regularly or to call if problems should arise?
8. Was I encouraged to be self-assertive, and were my self-awareness questions and knowledge and perceptions of myself respected?
9. Did the care provider intimidate me by flaunting her or his degrees and professional status?
10. Was she or he receptive to using the information I have generated from my self-monitoring and record keeping?
11. Did the care provider understand what I was talking about?
12. Did I understand what the care provider was talking about?

There is no guarantee that a highly recommended professional will be more satisfactory than one chosen from a phone book, since both you and the care provider may very well operate out of differing value systems, and what may have worked for others may not work for you. The best approach is to make a choice using whatever data you can gather, and then evaluate the care provider and the care you received upon an initial consultation.

Two models of care have been described by Mari Ladi Londono: the patriarchal or traditional model, and a humanistic style of working with clients. I am indebted to Londono and the editors of *Women's Health Journal* (March 1991) for granting permission to include a slightly adapted version of the models here. The information provides a framework for evaluating the care provider you select.

PATRIARCHAL VERSUS HUMANISTIC MODELS OF CARE
Patriarchal Model

CARE PROVIDER'S ROLE	CLIENT'S ROLE
Is responsible for the health of the client.	Knows that it is the professional who cures, and therefore makes no effort of her own.
Decides what to do, how, when, and in what way, without discussing it with the client.	Does what she is told, so as not to disappoint the clinician or make her/him angry.
Care provider's time is more important. Care provider can't wait, although the care provider can make others wait, because he/she is very busy.	Goes to the care provider's office prepared to spend the entire afternoon there. Doesn't consider alternatives, since it's always been that way. Takes it for granted that the care provider is very busy.
Must be "objective." Doesn't show emotions for fear of getting involved.	Perceives the care provider to be on a higher level, a perception that inhibits her from adopting a critical attitude.
Doesn't take his/her own moods or personal problems into account. Deals with own concerns by masking them.	Expects infallibility. The professional must never make mistakes. Her health depends on this.
Forgets about straightforward communication. Uses esoteric terminology, which he/she judges as necessary for status.	Unfamiliar terms make things sound more serious. Looks for explanations from friends, which adds to her confusion.
Care provider feels that he/she has authority, that he/she is the responsible one. Scolds, gets angry or bothered when he/she sees someone who is very ill, because it means they didn't take care of themselves. Gets very angry if someone forgets to take medicine, etc. (Imagine if an architect or other professional got mad at clients requesting changes or more explanations!)	Submission is an effect of the patriarchal system. As a consequence, the client tends not to talk about symptoms, errors in taking medicines, etc.
Care provider thinks the client is simple-minded, and won't understand explanations. Doesn't bother to prove otherwise.	She feels ignorant, and even feels guilty for not understanding.

Patriarchal Model (continued)

CARE PROVIDER'S ROLE	CLIENT'S ROLE
Without realizing it, he/she can be coercive and use threats.	Increased dependence on the care provider, who represents an authority figure.
Views as tiresome the client who insists on seeking help for ailments considered unimportant.	Feels that the professional knows best. Lacks explanations or information about her complaints.
Follows what is new, doesn't criticize or question new "advances."	Lacks access to scientific information, research or experiences. Is taught to believe that she won't be able to understand.
Especially in the hospital, pays more attention to the norms than woman's individual biological response. If she doesn't eat because she feels that she can't or doesn't want to, she/he tries to convince her, or scolds her to be a "good patient."	Doesn't resist. Accepts what she is told by health personnel. Obeys even when she has doubts or doesn't agree. Gives in to health professional even if she knows a certain drug could harm her.
Feels uncomfortable and bothered by the "patient" who asks for explanations and information about risks, etc. Perceives them as creating problems.	Is afraid to be a bother, afraid of being mistreated for bothering, afraid of being ridiculed or seen as "stupid." Waits and probably asks friends.
Gets confused and sometimes offers moralistic treatment ("you should/you shouldn't"), reflecting his/her own values.	Feels that the professional should know, since she/he is always right. Doesn't ask questions or dissent.
Feels herself/himself to be the authority.	Is a patient.

Humanistic Model

CARE PROVIDER'S ROLE	CLIENT'S ROLE
Complete acceptance of the client.	Is tranquil, confident, and secure.
Respects client as an equal, with the right and the need to be informed. If the client doesn't know what's happening, she can't fight it, collaborate, or take responsibility for her health.	If the client doesn't understand, or can't decide on her own, she can't take responsibility for herself. Needs knowledge about her state in order to act appropriately.
Explains side effects, and the advantages and/or risks of treatments and surgery.	Takes responsibility for her body, which is to say, for herself.
Discourages dependence and encourages self-determination.	Grows and feels validated as a person because of the treatment she receives.
Investigates, observes, learns what is necessary to know about the client, her values, history, and environments, in order to understand her ailments.	Expresses herself in depth, without holding back information that could be important. Is not afraid to be herself, nor worried about how she might be judged.
Does not impose own opinions about hormones, birth control, or whether or not to use new medications.	Decides after being informed and assumes the corresponding risks.
Is flexible, uncomplicated, "a person just like me," understanding.	Has the right to change opinions, to make mistakes.
Allows herself/himself to feel affection and admiration (as opposed to seduction, which is an abuse of the position and the woman's psychologically fragile state).	Doesn't become infatuated with any health professional. Is clear about the professional's intentions and attends appointments enthusiastically.
Listens and pays attention to the client's fears, intuition, and feelings.	Knows she is understood, and is thus able to acknowledge her own worth and feel secure.
Modifies and/or puts aside traditional roles. Behaves spontaneously, without rigid masks.	Has the confidence to act with authenticity. Grows in the relationship. Will not be able to seek medical attention.
Feels like a professional who has been consulted because of the career his/her life has allowed him/her to pursue.	Looks for the help that she values and feels is necessary.
Feels like a person—not an authority figure.	Feels like a person who is consulting, not like a "patient."

Bibliography

Preface

Beyene, Y. (1989). *From Menarche to Menopause.* Albany, NY: State University of New York Press.

Davis, D. (1983). *Blood and Nerves: An Ethnographic Focus on Menopause.* St. Johns, Newfoundland: Memorial University of Newfoundland and Institute of Social and Economic Research.

Davis, D. (1986). The Meaning of Menopause in a Newfoundland Fishing Village. *Culture, Medicine, and Psychiatry,* 10:73-94.

duToit, B.M. (1990). *Aging and Menopause Among Indian South African Women.* Albany, NY: State University of New York Press.

Flint, M. (1975). The Menopause: Reward or Punishment? *Psychosomatics* 16: 161-163.

Kaufert, P. (1992). Public Policy and Ethics. Unpublished paper presented at the 1992 Meeting of the North American Menopause Society on September 18, 1992. Cleveland, Ohio.

Lock, M. (1993). *Encounters with Aging.* Berkeley: University of California Press.

Wright, A.L. (1982). Variation in Navajo Menopause: Toward an Explanation. In *Changing Perspectives on Menopause,* A.M. Voda, M. Dinnerstein, and S. O'Donnell (eds.). Austin, TX: University of Texas Press, pp. 84-89.

Introduction and Purpose

Averette, H.E., and H.N. Nguyen. (1994). The Role of Prophylactic Oophorectomy in Cancer Prevention. *Gynecologic Oncology,* 55:S38-S41.

Beyene, Y. (1989). *From Menarche to Menopause.* Albany, NY: State University of New York Press.

Diczfalusy, E. (1993). Contraceptive Prevalence, Reproductive Health, and Our Common Future. The C. Donald Christian Memorial Lecture. *Obstetrical and Gynecological Survey,* 48:321-332.

duToit, B.M. (1990). *Aging and Menopause Among Indian South African Women.* Albany, NY: State University of New York Press.

Graves, E.J. (1989). Summary: National Hospital Discharge Survey. Advance Data from Vital and Health Statistics. *Report No. 199.* Hyattsville, MD: National Center for Health Statistics.

Kaufert, P. (1992). Public Policy and Ethics. Unpublished paper presented at the 1992 Meeting of the North American Menopause Society on September 18, 1992. Cleveland, Ohio.

Lock, M. (1993). *Encounters with Aging.* Berkeley: University of California Press.

Plotkin, D. (1996). Good News and Bad News About Breast Cancer. *The Atlantic Monthly,* 277:53.

Pokras, R., and V.G. Hufnagel. (1987). Hysterectomies in the United States 1965-1984. *Department of Health and Human Services Publication No. DHS* 88-1753. Hyattsville, MD: National Center for Health Statistics.

Rodin, J., and J.R. Ickovics. (1990). Women's Health, Review, and Research Agenda as We Approach the 21st Century. *American Psychologist* 45:1018-1034.

Rosser, S.V. (1989). Revisioning Clinical Research: Gender and the Ethics of Experimental Design. *Hypatia,* 4:125-139.

Smith, D.C., R. Prentice, D.J. Thompson, and W.R. Herrmann. (1975). Association of Exogenous Estrogen and Endometrial Carcinoma Among Users of Conjugated Estrogens. *The New England Journal of Medicine,* 293:1164-1167.

Wright, A.L. (1982). Variation in Navajo Menopause: Toward an Explanation. In *Changing Perspectives on Menopause,* A.M. Voda, M. Dinnerstein, and S. O'Donnell (eds.). Austin, TX: University of Texas Press, pp. 84-99.

Ziel, H.K., and W.D. Finkle. (1975). Increased Risk of Endometrial Carcinoma Among Users of Conjugated Estrogens. *The New England Journal of Medicine,* 293:1168-1170.

Section I. Preparing for the Journey

Beyene Y. (1989). *From Menarche to Menopause.* Albany, NY: State University of New York Press.

Diczfalusy, E. (1993). Contraceptive Prevalence, Reproductive Health, and Our Common Future. The C. Donald Christian Memorial Lecture. *Obstetrical and Gynecological Survey,* 48:321-332.

Chapter 1

Abraham, G.E. (1974). Radioimmunoassay of Steroids in Biological Materials. *ACTA Endocrinological,* 183:7-42.

Guyton, A.C. (1986). *Textbook of Medical Physiology,* 7th Edition. Philadelphia: W.B. Saunders Co.

Hafez, E.S.E. (1980). *Human Reproduction: Conception and Contraception.* Hagerstown, MD: Harper and Row.

Martin, D.W. Jr., P.A. Mayes, V.W. Rodwell, and D.K. Granner. (1985). *Harper's Review of Biochemistry.* Los Altos, CA: Lange Medical Publications.

Mead, M. (1997). What Women Bring to Research. Unpublished paper in *Conference on the Participation of Women in Scientific Research.* Washington, DC: October 19, 1977.

O'Malley, B.W., and W.T. Schrader. (1976). The Receptors of Steroid Hormones. *Scientific American*, 234:32-43.

Pauli-Haddon, G. (1993). *Uniting Sex, Self and Spirit*. Scotland, CT: Plus Publications.

Segal, S. (1974). The Physiology of Reproduction. *Scientific American*, 231: 53-62.

Vigoda, R. (1993). "There's Passion in the Potion, says a Phila. Scientist." *The Philadelphia Inquirer*, p. G3, 9/26/93.

Voda, A.M. (1980). Pattern of Progesterone and Aldosterone in Ovulatory Women During the Menstrual Cycle. In *The Menstrual Cycle Volume 1: A Synthesis of Interdisciplinary Research*, A.J. Dan, E.A. Grahan, and C.P. Beecher (eds.). New York: Springer Publishing Co., pp. 223-236.

Voda, A.M. (1981). Climacteric Hot Flash. *Maturitas*, 1:1-21.

Voda, A.M., and M.P. Randall. (1982). Nausea and Vomiting of Pregnancy: "Morning Sickness." In *Concept Clarification in Nursing*, C.M. Norris (ed.). Rockville, MD: Aspen Publication, pp. 133-165.

Voda, A.M., N.S. Christy, and J. M. Morgan. (1991). Body Composition Changes in Menopausal Women. *Women and Therapy*, 11:71-96.

Chapter 2

Atwood, M. (1985). *The Handmaid's Tale*. Toronto: McClelland and Stewart.

Beauchamp, T.L., and L. Walters. (1978). *Contemporary Issues in Bioethics*. Belmont, CA: Dickensen Publishing Co.

Beer, A., and R.E. Billingham. (1976). *The Immunology of Mammalian Reproduction*. New York: Prentice Hall.

Beral, V. (1976). Cardiovascular Disease Mortality Trends and Oral Contraceptive Use in Young Women. *Lancet*, 2:1047-1052.

Beral, V. (1977). Mortality Among Oral Contraceptive Users. *Lancet*, 2:727-731.

Bleir, R. (1984). *Science and Gender: A Critique of Biology and Its Theories on Women*. New York: Pergamon Press.

Cooke, J. (1988). The Early Embryo and the Formation of Body Pattern. *American Scientist*, 76:35-41.

Corea, G. (1985). *The Mother Machine*. New York: Harper and Row.

Delaney, J.M., J. Lupton, and E. Toth. (1988). *The Curse: A Cultural History of Menstruation*. Urbana: University of Illinois Press.

Greenberg, E.R., A.B. Barnes, L. Resseguie, J.A. Barrett, S. Burnside, L.L. Lanza, R.K. Neff, M. Stevens, R.H. Young, and T. Cotton. (1984). Breast Cancer in Mothers Given Diethylstilbesterol in Pregnancy. *The New England Journal of Medicine*, 311:1393-1398.

Greep, R.O., M.A. Koblinsky, and F.S. Jaffe. (1976). *Reproduction and Human Welfare: A Challenge to Research*. Cambridge, MA: MIT Press.

Grimes, D.A. (1994). *The Contraception Report*. 4 NJ: Emrone, Inc.

Hatcher, R.A., F. Stewart, J. Trussel, D. Kowal, F. Guest, G.K. Stewart, and W. Cates. (1990). *Contraceptive Technology, 1990-1992*. New York: Irvington Press.

Hellman, I.M. (1975). Fertility Control at a Crossroad. *American Journal of Obstetrics and Gynecology,* 124:331-337.

Nash, M. (1992). Is Sex Really Necessary? In "Sizing Up the Sexes," Christine Gorman (ed.). *Time,* 139:47.

Pauli-Haddon, G. (1993). *Uniting Sex, Self, and Spirit.* Scotland, CT: Plus Publications.

Rodger, J.C., and B.L. Drake. (1987). The Enigma of the Fetal Graft. *American Scientist,* 75:51-57.

Wassarman, P.M. (1987). The Biology and Chemistry of Fertilization. *Science,* 235:553-560.

Chapter 3

Buckler, H.M., and D.C. Anderson. (1994). The Perimenopausal State and Incipient Ovarian Failure. In *Treatment of the Postmenopausal Woman: Basic and Clinical Aspects,* R. Lobo (ed.). New York: Raven Press, Ltd., pp. 11-23.

Grahn, J. (1993). *Blood, Bread, and Roses: How Menstruation Created the World.* Boston: Beacon Press.

Guyton, A.C. (1986). *Textbook of Medical Physiology.* Philadelphia: W.B. Saunders Co.

Hafez, E.S.E. (1980). *Human Reproduction.* Hagerstown, MD: Harper and Row, Publishers.

Hartman, C.G. (1962). *Science and the Safe Period.* Baltimore: Williams and Wilkins.

Henderson, B.E., R.K. Ross, R.A. Lobo, M.C. Pike, and T.M. Mack. (1988). Re-Evaluating the Role of Progestogen Therapy After the Menopause. *Fertility and Sterility,* 49:9S-15S.

Jackson, J.A., and H.M. Salisbury. (1921). *Outwitting Our Nerves.* New York: The Century Co.

Jones, H.W., A.C. Wentz, and L.S. Burnett. (1988). *Novak's Textbook of Gynecology.* Baltimore: Williams and Wilkins.

Profet, M. (1993). Menstruation as a Defense Against Pathogens Transported by Sperm. *The Quarterly Review of Biology,* 68:335-381.

Root, J.L. (1992). Women's Perceptions of the Experience of Menstruation. PhD dissertation, unpublished, Salt Lake City: University of Utah.

Segal, S.J. (1974). The Physiology of Human Reproduction. *Scientific American.* 23:53-62.

Shaw, S.T. Jr., and C.P. Roche. (1985). The Endometrial Cycle: Aspects of Hemostasis. In *Mechanisms of Menstrual Bleeding,* D. Baird and E. Michie (eds.). New York: Serona Symposium Publications.

Sherman, B.M. and S.G. Korenman. (1975). Hormonal Characteristics of the Human Menstrual Cycle Throughout Reproductive Life. *Journal of Clinical Investigation,* 55:699-706.

Treloar, A.E. (1974). Menarche, Menopause, and Intervening Fecundity. *Human Biology*, 46:89-107.

Vollman, R.F. (1977). *The Menstrual Cycle*. Philadelphia: W.B. Saunders Co.

Chapter 4

Associated Press (1992). Surgeons Say No, So Rape Suspect Won't Be Castrated. *Salt Lake Tribune*. March 17, 1992.

Czerwinski, B. (1991). Feminine Hygiene Considerations for the Space Environment. In *Menstruation, Health and Illness*, D. Taylor and N. F. Woods (eds.). Washington, DC: Hemisphere Publishing Company, pp. 65-71.

Frisch, R.E. (1981). Delayed Menarche and Amenorrhea of College Athletes in Relation to Age of Onset of Training. *Journal of the American Medical Association*, 246:1559-1563.

Frisch, R.E., and J.W. McArthur. (1974). Menstrual Cycles: Fatness as a Determinant of Minimum Weight for Height Necessary for Their Maintenance or Onset. *Science*, 185:949-951.

Golub, S. (1992). *Periods: From Menarche to Menopause*. Newbury Park, CA: Sage Publications.

McCullough, C. (1977). *The Thorn Birds*. New York: Harper and Row.

Neus, E. (1993). "Birth-Control Pill Breeds Controversy." *The Salt Lake Tribune*, A-16.

Rochon-Ford, A. (1986). Hormones: Getting Out of Hand. In *Adverse Effects in Women and the Pharmaceutical Industry*, K. McDonnell (ed.), The Hague, The Netherlands: International Organization of Consumers Unions, pp. 27-40.

Root, J.L. (1992). *Women's Perceptions of the Experience of Menstruation*. Unpublished dissertation. Department of Health Education, Salt Lake City: University of Utah.

Tanner, J.M. (1973). Growing Up. *Scientific American*, 229:34-43.

Tanner, J.M. (1978). *Foetus into Man*. Cambridge, MA: Harvard University Press.

Treloar, A.E., R.E. Boynton, B.G. Behn, and B.W. Brown. (1967). Variation of the Human Menstrual Cycle Throughout Reproductive Life. *International Journal of Fertility*, 12:77-126.

Vollman, R.F. (1977). *The Menstrual Cycle*. Philadelphia: W.B. Saunders Co.

Chapter 5

American Psychiatric Association. (1987). *Diagnostic and Statistical Manual of Mental Disorders*, 3rd Edition, Revised. Washington, DC: Author.

Asso, D. (1983). *The Real Menstrual Cycle*. Chichester, England: John Wiley & Sons.

Chuong, C.J., L.R. Pearsall-Otey, and B.L. Rosenfeld. (1994). Revising Treatments for Premenstrual Syndrome. *Contemporary OB/GYN*, 39:66-76.

Connors, D.D. (1985). Women's "Sickness": A Case of Secondary Gains or Primary Loss. *Advances in Nursing Science*, 7:1-17.

Corea, G. (1985). *The Mother Machine*. New York: Harper and Row.

Dalton, K. (1983). *Once a Month*. Claremont, CA: Hunter House.

Dan, A.J., E.A. Graham, and C.P. Beecher. (1981). *The Menstrual Cycle, Volume I: A Synthesis of Interdisciplinary Research*. New York: Springer Publishing Co.

de Beauvoir, S. (1949). *The Second Sex*. New York: Knopf Publishing Co.

DeCrow, K. (1990). Personal Communication.

Delaney, J.M., J. Lupton, and E. Toth. (1988). *The Curse: A Cultural History of Menstruation*. Urbana, University of Illinois Press.

Fausto-Sterling, A. (1985). *Myths of Gender*. New York: Basic Books, Inc.

Frank, R.T. (1931). The Hormonal Causes of Premenstrual Syndrome. *Archives of Neurology and Psychiatry*, 26:1053-1105.

Freud, S. (1927). Some Psychological Consequences of the Anatomical Distinction Between the Sexes. *International Journal of Psychoanalysis*, 8:133-143.

Gannon, L.R. (1985). *Menstrual Disorders and Menopause: Biological, Psychological, and Cultural Research*. New York: Praeger Publishers.

Golub, S. (1985). *Lifting the Curse of Menstruation*. Binghamton, NY: The Haworth Press.

Grahn, J. (1993). *Blood, Bread, and Roses*. Boston: Beacon Press.

Hedrick, C.A. (1992). Menopause Has No Part in the Year of the Woman. *The Society of Menstrual Cycle Research Newsletter*, 9:3.

Keye, W.R. (1988). *The Premenstrual Syndrome*. Philadelphia: W. B. Saunders Co.

Komnenich, P., M. McSweeney, J.A. Noack, and N. Elder. (1982). *The Menstrual Cycle, Volume II: Research and Implications for Women's Health*. New York: Springer Publishing Co.

Lander L. (1988). *Images of Bleeding*. New York: Orlando Press.

Lange, L. (1983). Woman Is Not a Rational Animal: On Aristotle's "Biology of Reproduction." In *Discovering Reality*, S. Harding and M.B. Hintikka (eds.). Dordrecht, Holland: D. Reidel, pp. 1-15.

Lauersen, N.H., and E. Stukane. (1983). *PMS, Premenstrual Syndrome and You*. New York: Simon and Schuster, Inc.

Lever, J., and M.G. Brush. (1981). *Premenstrual Tension*. London: McGraw Hill.

MacDonald, N.H., and W. Good. (1972). The Effects of Parity on Plasma Sodium, Potassium, Chloride, and Osmolality Levels during Pregnancy. *Journal of Obstetrics and Gynecology British Commonwealth*, 79:441-449.

Mitchell, S.W. (1888). *Doctor and Patient*. Philadelphia: Lippincott Publishing Co.

Moos, R. (1968). The Development of a Menstrual Distress Questionnaire. *Pyschosomatic Medicine*, 30:853-867.

Olesen, V.L., and N. Fugate-Woods. (1986). *Culture, Society, and Menstruation*. New York: Hemisphere, Harper and Row.

Profet, M. (1993). Menstruation as a Defense Against Pathogens Transported by Sperm. *The Quarterly Review of Biology*, 68:335-381.

Robinson, W.J. (1917). *Woman: Her Sex and Love Life*. New York: Eugenics Publishing Co., Inc.

Root, J.L. (1992). Women's Perceptions of the Experience of Menstruation. Unpublished PhD dissertation. Salt Lake City: University of Utah.

Sommer, B. (1983). Personal Communication.

Stall, S. (1904). *What a Young Man Ought to Know.* London: The Vir Publishing Co.

Stall, S. (1907). *What a Young Husband Ought to Know.* London: The Vir Publishing Co.

Voda, A.M., and M.P. Randall. (1982). Nausea and Vomiting of Pregnancy: "Morning Sickness." *Concept Clarification in Nursing.* C.M. Norris (ed.) Rockville, MD: Aspen Publications, 133-166. ·

Zeveloff, S.I., and R. Conover. (1991). The Sociobiology of Menopause: Implications from Parental Investment and Concealment of Ovulation. In *Proceedings of the 8th Society for Menstrual Cycle Research,* A.M. Voda and R. Conover (eds.). Salt Lake City, UT: Society for Menstrual Cycle Research, pp. 353-371.

Section III. Menopause: The Closure of Menstrual Life

Robinson, W.J. (1917). *Woman: Her Sex and Love Life.* New York: Eugenics Publishing Co., Inc.

Chapter 6

Barrett-Connor, E. (1987). Postmenopausal Estrogen, Cancer, and Other Considerations. *Women and Health,* 32:179-195.

Bart, P. (1979). How to do Research on Women, by Women and for Women. In *Women's Health Research: An Exchange of Ideas.* M.C. Mackey (ed.). Women's Health Research Group. Chicago: University of Illinois, pp. 5-11.

Beyene, Y. (1989). *From Menarch to Menopause.* Albany: State University of New York.

Flint, M. (1975). The Menopause: Reward or Punishment? *Psychosomatics,* 16:161-163.

Gambrell, R.D. (1992). Abnormal Vaginal Bleeding: Routes of Investigation. *Menopause Management,* 1:28-31.

Goodman, M. (1991). Menopause Research 1979-1989. In *Proceedings of the 8th Conference Society for Menstrual Cycle Research,* A.M. Voda and R. Conover (eds.). Salt Lake City, UT: Society for Menstrual Cycle Research, pp. 141-160.

Hatcher, R.A., F. Stewart, J. Trussell, D. Kowal, F. Guest, G.K. Stewart, and W. Cates. (1990). *Contraceptive Technology* 1990-1992. New York: Irvington Publishers.

Koeske, R.K. (1980). Theoretical Perspectives on Menstrual Cycle Research: The Relevance of Attributional Approaches for the Perception and Explanation of Premenstrual Emotionality. In *The Menstrual Cycle Volume 1: A Synthesis of Interdisciplinary Research,* A. Dan, E.A. Graham, and C.P. Beecher (eds.). New York: Springer Publishing Co., pp. 8-25.

MacPherson, K.I. (1981). Menopause as Disease: The Social Construction of a Metaphor. *Advances in Nursing Science,* 3:95-113.

MacPherson, K.I. (1985). Osteoporosis and Menopause: A Feminist Analysis of the Social Construction of a Syndrome. *Advances in Nursing Science,* 7:11-21.

MacPherson, K.I. (1991). Hormone Replacement Therapy for Menopause: A Contrast Between Medical and Women's Health Movement Perspectives. In *Proceedings of the 8th Conference of the Society for Menstrual Cycle Research*, A.M. Voda and R. Conover (eds.). Salt Lake City, UT: Society for Menstrual Cycle Research, pp. 196-208.

Martin, E. (1987). *The Woman in the Body: A Cultural Analysis of Reproduction*. Boston: Beacon Press.

National Women's Health Network. (1995). *Taking Hormones and Women's Health: Choices, Risks, and Benefits*. Washington, DC: National Women's Health Network.

Parker, S.L., T. Tong, S. Bolden, and P.A. Wingo. (1996). Cancer Statistics, 1996. *Cancer*. 46:5-27.

Root, J.L. (1992). *Women's Perceptions of the Experience of Menstruation*. Unpublished PhD dissertation. Salt Lake City: University of Utah.

Schenken, R.S., and C.J. Pauerstein. (1989). Effects of Progestogens on the Endometrium. In *Menopause: Evaluation, Treatment, and Health Concerns*, C.B. Hammond, F. I. Haseltine, and I. Schiff (eds.). New York: Alan R. Liss, Inc., pp. 1-28.

Seaman, B., and G. Seaman. (1977). *Women and the Crisis in Sex Hormones*. New York: Rawson Associates, Inc.

Utian, W.H. (1990a). Cardiovascular Implications of Estrogen Replacement Therapy. *Obstetrics and Gynecology*, 75:18S-35S.

Utian, W.H. (1990b). The Menopause in Perspective. In *Multidisciplinary Perspectives on Menopause: Annals of the New York Academy of Sciences*, 592:1-7.

van Keep, P.A. (1984). Menopause in Review. Unpublished paper presented at the Fourth International Congress on Menopause, Orlando, FL.

Voda, A.M. (1994). Risks and Benefits Associated with Hormonal and Surgical Therapies for Healthy Midlife Women. *Western Journal of Nursing Research*, 16:507-523.

Wilbush, J. (1979). La Menespausie: The Birth of a Syndrome. *Maturitas*, 1:145-151.

Wilson, R. (1966). *Feminine Forever*. New York: M. Evans & Co.

Wilson, R., and T.A. Wilson. (1963). The Fate of the Nontreated Postmenopausal Woman: A Plea for the Maintenance of Adequate Estrogen from Puberty to the Grave. *Journal of the American Geriatric Society*, 11:327-362.

Chapter 7

Treloar, A.E. (1981) Menstrual Cyclicity and the Premenopause. *Maturitas* 3:249-264.

van Keep, P.A., R. Greenblatt, and R. Albeaux–Fernet. (1976). *Proceedings, 1976 International Congress on Menopause*. Lancaster England: MTP Press.

Woods, N.F. (1982). Menopausal Distress: A Model for Epidemiologic Investigation. In *Changing Perspectives on Menopause*, A.M. Voda, M. Dinnerstein, and S. O'Donnell (eds.). TX: University of Texas Press, pp. 220-238.

World Health Organization. (1981). *Research on Menopause*. Technical Report Series 670. Geneva Switzerland: World Health Organization.

World Health Organization (1996). *Scientific Group on Research on Menopause in the 1990s*. Technical Report Series 886. Geneva Switzerland. World Health Organization.

Chapter 8

Callahan, J. (1993). *Menopause: A Midlife Passage*. Bloomington: Indiana University Press.

Mansfield, P.K., and A.M. Voda. (1993). From Edith Bunker to the 6:00 News: How and What Midlife Women Learn About Menopause. *Women and Therapy*, 14:89-103.

Mansfield, P.K., and A.M. Voda. (1994). Hormone Use Among Middle-Aged Women: Results of a 3-Year Study. *Menopause*, 1:99-108.

Mansfield, P.K., and A.M. Voda. (1995). Predictors of Sexual Response Changes in Heterosexual Midlife Women. *Health Values*, 19:10-22.

Theisen, S.C., P.K. Mansfield, B.L. Seery, and A.M. Voda. (1995). Predictors of Midlife Women's Attitudes Toward Menopause. *Health Values*, 19:22-31.

Chapter 9

William Bridges and Associates. (1992). *Managing Organizational Transition*. Mill Valley, CA: William Bridges and Associates.

Chapter 10

Callahan, J. (1993). *Menopause: A Midlife Passage*. Bloomington: Indiana University Press.

Mansfield, P.K., and A.M. Voda. (1993). From Edith Bunker to the 6:00 News: How and What Midlife Women Learn About Menopause. *Women and Therapy*, 14:89-103.

Mansfield, P.K., and A.M. Voda. (1994). Hormone Use Among Middle-Aged Women: Results of a 3-Year Study. *Menopause*, 1:99-108.

Mansfield, P.K., and A.M. Voda. (1995). Predictors of Sexual Response Changes in Heterosexual Midlife Women. *Health Values*, 19:10-22.

Theisen, S.C., P.K. Mansfield, B.L. Seery, and A.M. Voda. (1995). Predictors of Midlife Women's Attitudes Toward Menopause. *Health Values*, 19:22-31.

Chapter 11

Feldman, B.M., A.M. Voda, and E. Gronseth. (1985). Prevalence of Hot Flash and Associated Variables in Perimenopausal Women. *Research in Nursing and Health,* 8:261-268.

Greenwood, S. (1996). *Menopause Naturally,* 4th edition. Volcano, CA: Volcano Press.

Kronenberg, F. (1990). Hot flashes: Epidemiology and Physiology. *Annals of the New York Academy of Sciences,* 592:52-86.

Kronenberg, F. (1994). Hot Flashes. In *Treatment of the Postmenopausal Woman: Basic and Clinical Aspects,* R. A. Lobo (ed.). New York: Raven Press, Ltd., pp. 97-117.

Molnar, G.W. (1975). Body Temperature During Menopausal Hot Flashes. *Journal of Physiology,* 38:499-503.

Voda, A.M. (1981). Climacteric Hot Flash. *Maturitas,* 1:1-21.

Voda, A.M., B.M. Feldman, and E. Gronseth. (1986). Description of the Hot Flash: Sensations, Meaning and Change in Frequency Across Time. In *The Climacteric in Perspective,* M. Notelovitz and P. van Keep (eds.). London: MTP Press, pp. 259-269.

Chapter 12

Coffey, N. (1993). An Introduction to Hysterectomy, the Operation and Its Lifelong Consequences. *HERS Newsletter,* V:2-4.

Cutler, W.B. (1988). *Hysterectomy Before and After.* New York: Harper & Row.

Fraser, I. (1991). Personal Communication.

Fraser, I.S., G. McCarron, R. Markham, and T. Resta (1985). Blood and Total Fluid Content of Menstrual Discharge. *Obstetrics and Gynecology,* 65:194-198.

Gambrell, R.D. (1992). Abnormal Vaginal Bleeding: Routes of Investigation. *Menopause Management.* 1:28-31.

Hufnagel, V., with S. Golant. (1988). *No More Hysterectomies.* New York: New America Library.

Kronenberg, F. (1990). Hot Flashes: Epidemiology and Physiology. In: *Multidisciplinary Perspectives on Menopause. Annals of the New York Academy of Sciences,* 592:52-86.

Mansfield, P.K., and C.M. Jorgensen. (1991). Menstrual Pattern Changes in Middle-Aged Women. In *Menstrual Health in Women's Lives,* A. Dan and L. Lewis (eds.). Champaign: University of Illinois Press, pp. 213-225.

Mishell, D.R. (1994). Abnormal Uterine Bleeding: Combined Treatment Approaches. *Menopause Management,* III:24-28.

Patterson, E.T., and E.S. Hale. (1985). Making Sure: Integrating Menstrual Care Practices into Activities of Daily Living. *Advances in Nursing Science,* 4:18-31.

Rankin, G.L.S., N. Veal, R.G. Huntsman, and J. Liddel. (1962). Measurement with Cr^{51} of Red Cell Loss in Menorrhagia. *Lancet,* 1:567-569.

Reynolds, T. (1995). Midlife Health: A Guide for the 40-Something Woman. *National Women's Health Resource Center,* 17:1-5.

Seltzer, V.L., F. Beryamen, and S. Deutsch. (1990). Perimenopausal Bleeding Patterns and Pathologic Findings. *Journal of the American Medical Women's Association,* 45:132-134.

Smith, S. (1991). Historical Perspectives on Menorrhagia. In *Antifibrinolytic Therapy in Dysfunctional Uterine Bleeding, Report on a Workshop.* Uppusala Sweden: Kabi Pharmacia Therapeutics. KV1106:2-3.

Snowden, R., and B. Christian. (1983). *Patterns and Perceptions of Menstruation.* New York: St. Martin's Press.

Townsend, D.E., R.M. Richart, R.A. Paskowitz, and R.E. Woolfork. (1990). Rollerball Coagulation of the Endometrium. *Obstetrics and Gynecology,* 76:310-313.

Voda, A.M., and P.K. Mansfield. (1991). Menstrual Bleeding Patterns in Premenopausal Women. In *Proceedings of the 9th Conference of the Society for Menstrual Cycle Research, Mind–Body Rhythmicity: A Menstrual Cycle Perspective,* Donald Golgert. Seattle, WA: Hamilton and Cross, pp. 1-11.

Vollman, R.F. (1977). *The Menstrual Cycle,* Philadelphia: W.B. Saunders Co.

World Health Organization. (1981). A Cross-Cultural Study of Menstruation: Implications for Contraceptive Development and Use. *Studies in Family Planning,* 12:3-15.

Chapter 13

Callahan, J. (1993). *Menopause: A Midlife Passage.* Indiana University Press.

Chapin, J.L., and S.A. Pereles. (1992). Women's Access to the Health Care System. In *The Women's Health Data Book: A Profile of Women's Health in the United States,* J.A. Horton (ed.). Washington, DC: The Jacobs Institute of Women's Health.

Garcia, R., and W.B. Cutler. (1992). *Menopause: A Guide for Women and the Men Who Love Them,* New York: Norton Publishing Co.

Gelfand, M., A. Ferenczy, and C. Bergeron. (1989) Endometrial Response to Estrogen-Androgen Stimulation. In *Menopause: Evaluation, Treatment, and Health Concerns,* C.B. Hammond, F.I. Haseltine, and I. Schiff, (eds.). New York: Alan R. Liss, pp. 1-28.

Grodin, M., P.K. Siiteri, and P.C. MacDonald. (1973). Source of Estrogen Production in the Postmenopausal Woman. *Journal of Clinical Endocrinology and Metabolism,* 36:207-214.

National Center for Health Statistics (1987). *Department of Health and Human Services Publication #88–1753.* U.S. Department of Health and Human Services, PHS, CDC. Washington, DC.

Parker, S., L.T. Tong, S. Bolden, and P.A. Wingo. (1996). Cancer Statistics, 1996. *CA - A Cancer Journal for Clinicians,* 46:5-27.

Pinn, V. (1993). Keynote Address on Women's Health. Society for Menstrual Cycle Research Conference, Boston MA. Unpublished.

Schenken, R.S. and C.J. Pauerstein. (1989). Effects of Progestogens on the Endometrium. In *Menopause: Evaluation, Treatment, and Health Concerns*, C. B. Hammond, F.l. Haseltine, and I. Schiff (eds.). New York: Alan R. Liss, pp. 1-28.

Siiteri, P.K. (1975) Estrogens in Postmenopause. *Frontiers of Hormone Research*, 3:40-44.

Utian, W.H. (1990). The Menopause in Perspective. In *Multidisciplinary Perspectives on Menopause. Annals of the New York Academy of Sciences*, 592:1-7.

Voda, A.M. (1992). Menopause: A Normal View. In Estrogen Replacement Therapy, K. Parker Jones (ed.), *Clinical Obstetrics and Gynecology*, 35:923-933.

Voda, A.M., and R. Conover. (1991). *Proceedings: 8th Conference Society for Menstrual Cycle Research*. Salt Lake City, UT: Society for Menstrual Cycle Research.

Voda, A.M., M. Dinnerstein, and S. O'Donnell. (1982). *Changing Perspectives on Menopause*. Austin: University of Texas Press.

Wilson, R. (1966). *Feminine Forever*. New York: M. Evans.

Wilson, R. and T.A. Wilson. (1963). The Fate of the Nontreated Postmenopausal Women: A Plea for the Maintenance of Adequate Estrogen from Puberty to the Grave. *Journal of the American Geriatric Society*, 11: 347-362.

Chapter 14

FDA Medical Bulletin. (1991). The Norplant System Approved as New Contraceptive Implant. *U.S. Food and Drug Administration*, 21: 6.

FDA Medical Bulletin. (1993). 3-Month Contraceptive Injection Approved. *U.S. Food and Drug Administration*, 23: 6.

O'Malley, B.W., and W.T. Schrader. (1976). The Receptors of Steroid Hormones. *Scientific American*, 234:32-43.

Voda, A.M. (1982). Alterations of the Menstrual Cycle: Hormonal and Mechanical. In *The Menstrual Cycle, Volume 2: Research and Implications for Women's Health*, P. Komnenich, M. McSweeney, J.A. Noack, and N. Elder (eds.). New York: Springer Publishing Co., pp. 145-163.

Voda, A.M. (1993). Journey to the Center of the Cell. In *Menopause, A Midlife Passage*, J.C. Callahan (ed.). Bloomington: Indiana University Press, pp. 160-193.

Chapter 15

Barrett-Connor, E. (1987). Postmenopausal Estrogen, Cancer and Other Considerations. *Women and Health*, 32:179-195.

Barrett-Connor, E. (1989). Postmenopausal Estrogen Replacement and Breast Cancer. *The New England Journal of Medicine*, 321:319-320.

Brown, M.S., and J. Goldstein. (1986). A Receptor Mediated Pathway for Cholesterol Homeostatis. *Science*, 232:34-37.

Bush, T.L., L.P. Fried, and E. Barrett-Connor. (1988). Cholesterol, Lipoproteins, and Coronary Heart Disease in Women. *Clinical Chemistry,* 34:B60-B70.

Bush, T.L., L.D. Cowan, E. Barrett-Connor, M.H. Criqui, J.M. Koron, R.B. Wallace, H.A. Tyroler, and B.M. Rifkind. (1983). Estrogen Use and All Cause Mortality: Preliminary Results from the Lipid Research Clinics Program Follow-Up Study. *Journal of the American Medical Association,* 249:903-906.

Colditz, G.A., W.C. Willett, M.J. Stampfer, B. Rosher, F.E. Speizer, and C.H. Hennekens. (1987). Menopause and the Risk of Coronary Heart Disease in Women. *The New England Journal of Medicine,* 316:1105-1110.

Collins, J. (1991). Monocyte-Attracting Protein May Initiate Atherosclerosis. Research Resources Reporter, National Center for Research Resources XV:1-3.

Connor, J.M., and M.A. Ferguson-Smith. (1984). *Essential Medical Genetics.* Oxford: Blackwell Scientific Publications.

Freeman, R. (1996). Hormones and Heart Disease. *Menopause Management,* 5:10.

Fuster, V., L. Badimon, J.J. Badimon, and J.H. Chesebro. (1992). The Pathogenesis of Coronary Artery Disease and the Acute Coronary Syndromes. *The New England Journal of Medicine,* 326:242-318.

Goldman, L., and A.N.A. Tosteson. (1991). Uncertainty About Postmenopausal Estrogen. *The New England Journal of Medicine,* 325:800-802.

Greenberg, E.R., A.B. Barnes, L. Resseguie, J.A. Barrett, S. Burnside, L.L. Lanza, R.K. Neff, M. Stevens, R.H. Young, and T. Colton (1984). Breast Cancer in Mothers Given Diethylstilbesterol in Pregnancy. *The New England Journal of Medicine,* 311:1393-1398.

Hazzard, W.R. (1989). Estrogen Replacement and Cardiovascular Disease: Serum Lipids and Blood Pressure Effects. *American Journal of Obstetrics and Gynecology,* 161:1847-1853.

Hazzard, W.R. (1989). Why Do Women Live Longer Than Men? *Postgraduate Medicine,* 85:271-283.

Hulley, S.B., J.M.B. Walsh, and T.B. Newman. (1992). Health Policy on Blood Cholesterol: Time to Change Directions. *Circulation,* 86:1028-1030.

Jacobs, D., H. Blackburn, H. Higgens, D. Reed, H. Iso, G. McMillan, J. Neaton, J. Nelson, J. Potter, B. Rifkind, J. Rossouw, R. Shekelle, and S. Yusuf. (1992). Report of the Conference on Low Blood Cholesterol: Mortality Associations. *Circulation,* 86:1046-1060.

Jick, H., B. Dinan, and K.J. Rothman. (1978). Noncontraceptive Estrogens and Nonfatal Myocardial Infarction. *Journal of the American Medical Association,* 239:1407-1408.

Jick, H., B. Dinan, R. Herman, and K.J. Rothman. (1978). Myocardial Infarction and Other Vascular Diseases in Young Women: Role of Estrogens and Other Factors. *Journal of the American Medical Association,* 240:2548-2552.

LaRosa, J.C. (1992). Lipids and Cardiovascular Disease: Do the Findings and Therapy Apply Equally to Men and Women? *The Jacob's Institute of Women's Health,* 2:102-104.

Lip, G.Y., G. Beevers, and J. Zarifis. (1995). Hormone Replacement Therapy and Cardiovascular Risk: The Cardiovascular Physician's Viewpoint. *Journal of Internal Medicine,* 238:389-399.

Lobo, R.A. (1990). Cardiovascular Implications of Estrogen Replacement Therapy. *Obstetrics and Gynecology,* 75:18S-35S.

Lobo, R.A. (1994). *Treatment of the Postmenopausal Woman: Basic and Clinical Aspects.* New York: Raven Press.

Matthews, K.A., E. Meilahn, L.H. Kuller, S.F. Kelsey, A.W. Caggiula, and R.R. Wing. (1989). Menopause and Risk Factors for Coronary Heart Disease. *The New England Journal of Medicine,* 321:641-646.

McCance, K. and S. Huether. (1995). *Pathophysiology.* St. Louis: Mosby Publishing Co.

McMurray, M.P., M.T. Arqueira, S. Connor, and W.E. Conner (1991). Changes in Lipid and Lipoprotein Levels and Body Weight in Tarahumara Indians After Consumption of an Affluent Diet. *The New England Journal of Medicine,* 355:1704-1708.

Moore, T. J. (1989) *Heart Failure.* New York: Random House.

Newman, K.P., and J.M. Sullivan. (1996). Coronary Heart Disease in Women: Epidemiology, Clinical Syndromes, and Management. *Menopause,* 3:51-59.

Notelovitz, M. (1989). An Opposing View. *The Journal of Family Practice,* 29:410-415.

Phillips, G.B., W.P. Castelli, R.D. Abbott, and P.M. McNamara (1983). Association of Hyperestrogenemia and Coronary Heart Disease in Men in the Framingham Cohort. *American Journal of Medicine,* 74:863-869.

Plotkin, D. (1996). Good News and Bad News About Breast Cancer. *Atlantic Monthly,* 277:53.

Posner, B.M., Cobb, J.L., A.J. Belanger, A. Cupples, B. D'Agostino, and J. Stokes. (1991). Dietary Lipid Predictors of Coronary Heart Disease in Men. *Archives of Internal Medicine,* 15:1181-1187.

Prentice, R.L., J.E. Rossouw, S.R. Johnson, L.S. Freeman, and A. McTiernan. (1996). The Role of Randomized Controlled Trials in Assessing the Benefits and Risks of Long-Term Hormone Replacement Therapy: Example of the Women's Health Initiative. *Menopause,* 3:71-76.

Prior, J. (1991). Postmenopausal Estrogen Therapy and Cardiovascular Disease (letter to the editor). *The New England Journal of Medicine,* 326:705-706.

Ross, R.K., A. Paganini-Hill, T.M. Mack, M. Arthur, and B.E. Henderson. (1981). Menopausal Oestrogen Therapy and Protection from Death and Ischaemic Heart Disease. *Lancet,* 1:858-860.

Schaefer, E.J., and R.I. Levy. (1985). Pathogenesis and Management of Lipoprotein Disorders. *The New England Journal of Medicine,* 312:1300-1310.

Stampfer, M.J., G.A. Colditz, W.C. Willett, J.E. Manson, B. Rosner, F.E. Speizer, and C.H. Hennekens. (1991). Postmenopausal Estrogen Therapy and Cardiovascular Disease. *The New England Journal of Medicine,* 325:756-762.

Stampfer, M.J., W.C. Willett, G.A. Colditz, B. Rosner, F.E. Speizer, and C.H. Hennekens. (1985). A Prospective Study of Postmenopausal Estrogen Therapy and Coronary Heart Disease. *The New England Journal of Medicine,* 313:1044-1049.

U.S. Department of Health and Human Services, PHS. (1991). *Report of the Expert Panel on Blood Cholesterol Levels in Children and Adolescents.* NIH Publication 91-2732. Washington, DC: NIH.

Vandenbrouke, J.P. (1991). Postmenopausal Oestrogen and Cardioprotection. *Lancet,* 337:833-834.

Walsh, B.W., I. Schiff, B. Rosner, L. Greenberg, V. Ravnikar, and F.M. Sacks. (1991). Effects of Postmenopausal Estrogen Replacement on the Concentrations and Metabolism of Plasma Lipoproteins. *The New England Journal of Medicine,* 325:1196-1204.

Wilson, P.W.F., R.J. Garrison, and W.P. Castelli. (1985). Postmenopausal Estrogen Use, Cigarette Smoking, and Cardiovascular Morbidity in Women Over 50. *The New England Journal of Medicine,* 313:1038-1043.

Wolfe, S.M. (1992). Estrogen, Breast Cancer, Heart Disease. *A Friend Indeed,* VII:1-3. (Canadian Newsletter).

Chapter 16

Berg, J.W. (1984). Clinical Implications of Risk Factors for Breast Cancer. *Cancer,* 53:589-591.

Bergkvist, L. H. Adami, I. Persson, R. Hoover, and C. Schairer. (1989). The risk of Breast Cancer After Estrogen and Estrogen-Progestin Replacement. *The New England Journal of Medicine,* 321:293-297.

Beyene, Y. (1989). *From Menarche to Menopause.* Albany: State University of New York Press.

Bush, T.L. (1995). Hormones and Breast Cancer. Paper presented at the 6th Annual Meeting of the North American Menopause Society, San Francisco, CA. September 20, 1995.

Bush, T.L., and K.J. Helzlsouer. (1993). Tamoxifen for the Primary Prevention of Breast Cancer: A Review and Critique of the Concept and Trial. *Epidemiologic Reviews,* 15:233-242.

Colditz, G.A., S.E. Hankinson, D.J. Hunter, W.C. Willett, J.E. Manson, M.J. Stampfer, C. Hennekens, B. Rosner, and F.E. Speizer. (1995). The Use of Estrogens and Progestins and the Risk of Breast Cancer in Postmenopausal Women. *The New England Journal of Medicine,* 332:1589-1593.

Colditz, G.A., M.J. Stampfer, W. C. Willett, C.H. Hennekens, B. Rosner, and F.E. Speizer. (1990). Prospective Study of Estrogen Replacement Therapy and Risk of Breast Cancer in Postmenopausal Women. *Journal of the American Medical Association,* 264:2648-2653.

Colditz, G.A., W.C. Willett, M. J. Stampfer, B. Rosner, F.E. Speizer, and C.H. Hennekens. (1987). Menopause and Risk of Coronary Heart Disease in Women. *The New England Journal of Medicine,* 316:1105-1110.

Ewertz, M. (1988). Influence of Non-Contraceptive Exogenous and Endogenous Sex Hormones on Breast Cancer Risk in Denmark. *International Journal of Cancer,* 42:832-838.

Gelfand, M., A. Ferenczy, and C. Bergeron. (1989). Endometrial Response to Estrogen-Androgen Stimulation. In *Menopause: Evaluation, Treatment, and Health Concerns,* C.B. Hammond, F.I. Haseltine, and I. Schiff (eds.). New York: Alan R. Liss, pp. 1-28.

Glass, A., and R.N. Hoover. (1990). Rising Incidence of Breast Cancer: Relationship of Stage and Receptor Status. *Journal of the National Cancer Institute,* 82:693-696.

Golub, S. (1992). *Periods.* Newbury Park, CA: Sage Publications.

Hunt, K., M. Vessey, K. McPherson, and M. Coleman. (1987). Long-Term Surveillance of Mortality and Cancer Incidence in Women Receiving Hormone Replacement Therapy. *British Journal of Obstetrics and Gynecology,* 94:620-635.

Kelsey, J.L., and P. Horn-Ross. (1993). Breast Cancer: Magnitude of the Problem and Descriptive Epidemiology. *Epidemiologic Reviews,* 15:7-16.

Key, T.J.A., and M. C. Pike. (1988). The Role of Oestrogens and Progestogens in the Epidemiology and Prevention of Breast Cancer. *European Journal of Clinical Oncology,* 24:29-43.

Lippman, M. (1989). Growth Regulation of Breast Cancer. In *Menopause: Evaluation, Treatment, and Health Concerns,* C.B. Hammond, F.P. Haseltine, and I. Schiff (eds.). New York: Alan R. Liss, Inc., pp. 111-119.

Mack, T., M. Pike, B. Henderson, R Pfeffer, V.R. Gerkins, M. Arthur, and S.E. Brown. (1976). Estrogens and Endometrial Cancer in a Retirement Community. *The New England Journal of Medicine,* 294:1262-1267.

Miki, Y. et al. (1994). A Strong Candidate for the Breast and Ovarian Susceptibility Gene BRCA$_1$. *Science,* 266:66-71.

Menopause Management News Briefs. (1996). One Table HRT Product to be Available. *Menopause Management,* 5:3.

Peccei, J. (1995). The Origin and Evolution of Menopause: The Altriciality-Lifespan Hypothesis. *Ethology and Sociobiology,* 16:425-449.

Pike, M.C., D.V. Spicer, L. Dahmoussh, and M.F. Press. (1993). Estrogens, Progestogens, Normal Breast Cell Proliferation, and Breast Cancer Risk. *Epidemiological Review,* 15:17-35.

Plotkin, D. (1996). Good News and Bad News About Breast Cancer. *Atlantic Monthly,* 277:53.

Prentice, R.L., J.E. Rossouw, S.R. Johnson, L.S. Freedman, and A. McTiernan. (1996). The Role of Randomized Controlled Trials in Assessing the Benefits and Risks of Long-Term Hormone Replacement Therapy: Example of the Women's Health Initiative. *Menopause,* 3:71-76.

Raloff, J. (1993). EcoCancers. *Science News,* 144:10-13.

Russo, I. H., M. Koszalka, and J. Russo. (1990). Effect of Human Chorionic Gonadotrophin on Mammary Gland Differentiation and Carcinogenesis. *Carcinogenesis,* 11:1849-1855.

Russo, I.H., M. Koszalka, and J. Russo. (1991). Comparative Study of the Influence of Pregnancy and Hormonal Treatment on Mammary Carcinogenesis. *British Journal of Cancer,* 64:481-484.

Russo, J., and I.H. Russo. (1987). Biological and Molecular Bases of Mammary Carcinogenesis. *Laboratory Investigation,* 57:112-137.

Russo, J., B.A. Gusterson, A. Rogers, I.H. Russo, S.R. Wellings, and M.J. van Zwieten. (1990). Comparative Study of Human and Rat Mammary Tumorigenesis. *Laboratory Investigation,* 62:244-278.

Schenken R.S., and C.J. Pauerstein. (1989). Effects of Progestogens on the Endometrium. In *Menopause: Evaluation, Treatment, and Health Concerns,* C.B. Hammond, F.I. Haseltine, and I. Schiff (eds.). New York: Alan R. Liss, pp. 29-40.

Schiff, I. (1996). Summing Up the Risk:Benefit Equation. *Menopause,* 3:61-64.

Shyamala, G. (1992). Hormonal Factors and Breast Cancer. Unpublished paper presented at President's Cancer Panel Special Commission on Breast Cancer. Bethesda, MD.

Smith, D.C., R. Prentice, D.J. Thompson, and W.L. Herrmann. (1975). Association of Exogenous Estrogen and Endometrial Carcinoma Among Users of Conjugated Estrogens. *The New England Journal of Medicine,* 293:1164-1167.

Stadel, B. and N. Weiss. (1975). Characteristics of Menopausal Women: A Survey of King and Pierce Counties in Washington, 1973-1974. *Journal of Epidemiology,* 102:215-218.

Stanford, J.L., N.S. Weiss, L.F. Voigt, J.R. Daling, L.A. Habel, and M.A. Rossing. (1995). Combined Estrogen and Progestin Hormone Replacement Therapy in Relation to Risk of Breast Cancer in Middle-Aged Women. *Journal of the American Medical Association,* 274:137-142.

Steinberg, K.K., S.B. Thacker, S.J. Smith, D.F. Stroup, M.W. Zack, W.D. Flanders, and R.L. Kerkelman. (1991). A Meta-Analysis of the Effect of Estrogen Replacement Therapy on the Risk of Breast Cancer. *Journal of the American Medical Association,* 265:1985-1990.

Thomas, E.B. (1984). Do Hormones Cause Breast Cancer? *Cancer,* 53:595-604.

Ziel, H.K., and W.D. Finkle. (1975). Increased Risk of Endometrial Carcinoma Among Users of Conjugated Estrogens. *The New England Journal of Medicine,* 293:1168-1170.

Chapter 17

Rako, S. (1996). *The Hormone of Desire: The Truth About Sexuality, Menopause, and Testosterone.* New York: Harmony Books.

Chapter 18

Costello, C., and B.K. Krimgold. (1996). *The American Woman 1996-97.* New York: W. W. Norton and Company.

Cutler, W. (1988). *Hysterectomy Before and After.* New York: Harper and Row.

Deal, C.L. (1993). Bone Pain in Mature Women: Differential Diagnosis. *Menopause Management,* 11:26.

Ettinger, B. (1993). Calcium Intake After Menopause: When, How, How Much? *Menopause Management,* 2:26.

Hall, B.K. (1988). The Embryonic Development of Bone. *American Scientist,* 76:174-185.

Hall, F.M., M.A. Davis, and D.T. Baran. (1987). Bone Mineral Screening for Osteoporosis. *The New England Journal of Medicine,* 316:212-214.

Kirkpatrick, M.K., and M. Edwards. (1985). Osteoporosis: A Self-Care Checklist for Women. *Journal of Occupational Health Nursing,* 33:500-503.

Lindsay, R. (1989). Osteoporosis: An Updated Approach to Prevention and Management. *Geriatrics,* 44:45-54.

Lindsay, R. (1993). Osteoporosis: How to Predict Who is at Risk. *Menopause Management,* 2:11.

Melton, L.J., H.N. Wahner, and P. Delmas. (1994). Bone Mineral Measurement and Biochemical Markers of Bone Cell Function. In *Comprehensive Management of Menopause,* J. Lorrain, L. Plouffe Jr, V. Ravnikar, L. Speroff, and N. Watts. (eds.). New York: Springer-Verlag, pp. 97-109.

Menopause Management. (1996). Osteoporosis Update. *Menopause Management,* 5:10.

Merck and Co., Inc. (1995). *Fact Sheet on Fosamax.* West Point, PA: Merck and Co., Inc.

NIH (1994). Optimal Calcium Intake, 1994. *NIH Consensus Statement,* 12:1-31.

Nordin, F.F., N. Christopher, A.G. Need, B.E. Chatterton, and M. Horowitz. (1990). The Relative Contributions of Age and Years Since Menopause to Postmenopausal Bone Loss. *Journal of Clinical Endocrinology and Metabolism,* 70:83-88.

O'Leary-Cobb, J. (1996). Update on Osteoporosis. *A Friend Indeed,* XIII:1-4.

Pak, C.Y.C., K. Sakhaee, V. Piziak, R.D. Peterson, N.A. Breslan, P. Boyd, J.R. Poindexter, J. Herzog, A. Heard-Sakhaee, S. Hayes, B. Adams-Huet, and J.S. Reisch. (1994). Randomized Control Trial of Slow Release Sodium Fluoride in the Management of Postmenopausal Osteoporosis. *Annals of Internal Medicine,* 120:625-632.

Peck, W.A., B.L. Riggs, and N.H. Bell. (1987). Physician's Resource Manual on Osteoporosis: A Decision-Making Guide. Washington, DC: National Osteoporosis Foundation.

Polan, M.L. (1994). Value of Early Screening for Osteoporosis. *Contemporary OB/GYN,* 39:63-67.

Prince, R.L., M. Smith, I.M. Dick, R.I. Price, P.G. Webb, N.K. Henderson, and M.M. Harris. (1991). Prevention of Postmenopausal Osteoporosis: A Comparative Study of Exercise, Calcium Supplementation, and Hormone-Replacement Therapy. *The New England Journal of Medicine,* 325:1189-1195.

Prior, J.C., Y. Vigna, M.T. Schechter, and A.E. Burgess. (1990). Spinal Bone Loss and Ovulatory Disturbances. *The New England Journal of Medicine,* 323:1221-1227.

Sheehy, G. (1992). *The Silent Passage*. New York: Random House.

Tilyard, M.W., G.F.S. Spears, J. Thomson, and S. Dovey. (1992). Treatment of Postmenopausal Osteoporosis with Calcitriol or Calcium. *The New England Journal of Medicine*, 326:357-362.

Tosteson, A.N.A., D.I. Rosenthal, J. Melton, and M.C. Weinstein. (1990). Cost-Effectiveness of Screening Perimenopausal White Women for Osteoporosis: Bone Densitometry and Hormone Replacement Therapy. *Annals of Internal Medicine*, 113:594-603.

U.S. Congress, Office of Technology Assessment. (1995). *Effectiveness and Costs of Osteoporosis Screening and Hormone Replacement Therapy, Volume I: Cost Effectiveness Analysis*. OTA-BP-H-160. Washington, DC: US Government Printing Office.

Wallach, S. (1993). Osteoporosis Treatment Regimens: Past, Present, Future. *Menopause Management*, 2:4.

Winick, M. (1992). Lifestyle and Osteoporosis Prevention: Part II - The Role of Nutrition. *Menopause Management*, 1:17.

Wolfe, S., and R.E. Hope. (1993). *Worst Pills, Best Pills*. Washington, DC: Public Citizen Health Research Group.

Wymelenberg, S. (1994). Alternatives to Estrogen. *Harvard Health Letter*, 19:6-8.

Yen, S.S.C. (1986). Estrogen Withdrawal Syndrome. *The New England Journal of Medicine*, 255:1014.

Zones, J.S. (1995). *Letter to Members: Osteoporosis*. National Women's Health Network. Washington, DC: National Women's Health Network.

Chapter 20

Moghissi, K.S. (1976). Accuracy of Basal Body Temperature for Ovulation Detection. *Fertility and Sterility*, 27:1415-1421.

Vermesh, M., D.A. Kletsky, V. Davajan, and R. Israel. (1987). Monitoring Technologies to Predict and Detect Ovulation. *Fertility and Sterility*, 47:259-264.

Chapter 23

Londono, M.L. (1991). A Humanistic Approach to Health Services for Women. *Women's Health Journal*, 3:4-9.

Index

Abbott Laboratories, 339
Abraham, Guy, 27
Aging. *See also* Menopause
  reaction to, 124
  vs. menopause, 133,138
Alcohol and osteoporosis, 302
Aldosterone, 105. *See also*
  Hormones
Alendronate sodium. *See* Fosamax
Alzheimer's Disease, 291
Amenorrhea, 67,68. *See also*
  Menstruation
  and long-term oral contraceptive
    use, 89
  and osteoporosis risk, 68
  and protection from breast cancer,
    276
American Cancer Society, 299,278
American College of Obstetrics
    and Gynecology, 121
American Gynecological Society, 48
American Heart Association, 268
American Journal of Nursing, 20
American Medical Association, 350
American Nurses Association, 350
American Psychiatric Association
    (APA), 101,110
American Woman, The, 1996-97, 295
Anatomy, 6. *See also* Biology,
  as destiny
Androgens
  and hair growth, 290
  and sexual response, 289-290
Andrology, 211
Androstenedione, role in
    postmenopausal estrogen
    synthesis, 226
Anemia, 217

Ann's advice. *See* Bleeding; breast
  cancer; heart disease; hot
  flash
Anorexia nervosa, 68
  as contraceptive, 68
Antioxidants. *See* Beta carotene,
  as antioxidant; vitamin C;
  vitamin E
Apoptosis, 279,282
Aristotle, 40,95
  theory of women as imperfect,
    109
Ashton, Carol, 159
Athena Institute for Women's
    Wellness Research, 28
Atwood, Margaret, 51

Baby boomers, 247
Barrett-Connor, E., 121,254,257
Bart, Pauline, 124
Basal body temperature. *See* Record
  keeping
Bellergal, 178,181
Bergkvist, L.H., 284
Berman, Edgar, 100
Beta carotene, as antioxidant, 269
Beyene, Yewoubdar, 12,124,277
Biological deficit model, 226
Biology, as destiny, 95,99,118
Biphosphonate. *See* Fosamax
Bleeding
  abnormal, 194,228
    evaluation of, 195
  Ann's advice on understanding,
    217
  antifibrinolytic agents
    and tranexamic acid, 214

Order Your Own Copy of
This Important Book for Your Personal Library!

MENOPAUSE, ME AND YOU
The Sound of Women Pausing

_____ in hardbound at $49.95 (ISBN: 1-56023-911-5)

_____ in softbound at $24.95 (ISBN: 1-56023-922-0)

COST OF BOOKS _____

OUTSIDE USA/CANADA/
MEXICO: ADD 20% _____

POSTAGE & HANDLING _____
(US: $3.00 for first book & $1.25
for each additional book)
Outside US: $4.75 for first book
& $1.75 for each additional book)

SUBTOTAL _____

IN CANADA: ADD 7% GST _____

STATE TAX _____
(NY, OH & MN residents, please
add appropriate local sales tax)

FINAL TOTAL _____
(If paying in Canadian funds,
convert using the current
exchange rate. UNESCO
coupons welcome.)

☐ **BILL ME LATER:** ($5 service charge will be added)
(Bill-me option is good on US/Canada/Mexico orders only;
not good to jobbers, wholesalers, or subscription agencies.)

☐ Check here if billing address is different from
shipping address and attach purchase order and
billing address information.

Signature _____

☐ **PAYMENT ENCLOSED: $** _____

☐ **PLEASE CHARGE TO MY CREDIT CARD.**

☐ Visa   ☐ MasterCard   ☐ AmEx   ☐ Discover
☐ Diners Club
Account # _____

Exp. Date _____

Signature _____

Prices in US dollars and subject to change without notice.

NAME _____

INSTITUTION _____

ADDRESS _____

CITY _____

STATE/ZIP _____

COUNTRY _____ COUNTY (NY residents only) _____

TEL _____ FAX _____

E-MAIL_____
May we use your e-mail address for confirmations and other types of information? ☐ Yes   ☐ No

Order From Your Local Bookstore or Directly From
The Haworth Press, Inc.
10 Alice Street, Binghamton, New York 13904-1580 • USA
TELEPHONE: 1-800-HAWORTH (1-800-429-6784) / Outside US/Canada: (607) 722-5857
FAX: 1-800-895-0582 / Outside US/Canada: (607) 772-6362
E-mail: getinfo@haworth.com
PLEASE PHOTOCOPY THIS FORM FOR YOUR PERSONAL USE.

BOF96

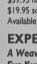